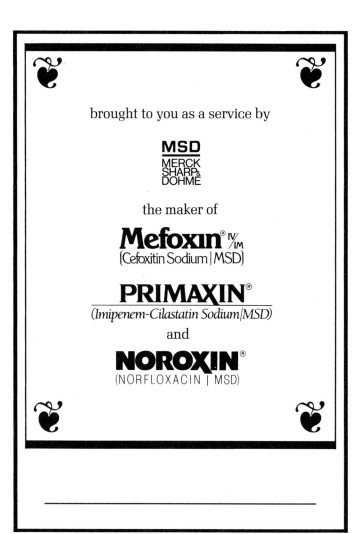

brought to you as a service by

MSD
MERCK
SHARP&
DOHME

the maker of

Mefoxin® ᴵⱽ/ᴵᴹ
(Cefoxitin Sodium | MSD)

PRIMAXIN®
(_Imipenem-Cilastatin Sodium/MSD_)
and
NOROXIN®
(NORFLOXACIN | MSD)

CONTEMPORARY ISSUES
in INFECTIOUS DISEASES
VOL. 6

SERIES EDITORS

Merle A. Sande, M.D.

Richard K. Root, M.D.

Volumes Already Published

Vol. 1 New Dimensions in Antimicrobial Therapy
Richard K. Root, M.D. and Merle A. Sande, M.D., Editors
Vol. 2 Endocarditis
Merle A. Sande, M.D., Donald Kaye, M.D.,
and Richard K. Root, M.D., Editors
Vol. 3 Bacterial Meningitis
Merle A. Sande, M.D., Arnold L. Smith, M.D.,
and Richard K. Root, M.D., Editors
Vol. 4 Septic Shock
Richard K. Root, M.D. and Merle A. Sande, M.D., Editors
Vol. 5 Respiratory Infections
Merle A. Sande, M.D., Leonard D. Hudson, M.D.,
and Richard K. Root, M.D., Editors

Forthcoming Volumes in the Series

Vol. 7 Parasitic Infections
Merle A. Sande, M.D., James H. Leech, M.D.,
and Richard K. Root, M.D., Editors

NEW SURGICAL and MEDICAL APPROACHES in INFECTIOUS DISEASES

Edited by

Richard K. Root, M.D.

Professor and Chairman
Department of Medicine
University of California, San Francisco
School of Medicine
San Francisco, California

Donald D. Trunkey, M.D., F.A.C.S.

Professor of Surgery and Chairman
Department of Surgery
Oregon Health Sciences University School of Medicine
Portland, Oregon

Merle A. Sande, M.D.

Professor and Vice Chairman
Department of Medicine
University of California, San Francisco
School of Medicine
Chief, Medical Service
San Francisco General Hospital
San Francisco, California

Churchill Livingstone
New York, Edinburgh, London, Melbourne   1987

Library of Congress Cataloging-in-Publication Data

New Surgical and Medical Approaches in Infectious Diseases.

(Contemporary issues in infectious diseases ; vol. 6)
Includes bibliographies and index.
1. Bacterial diseases—Treatment. 2. Surgical wound
infections—Treatment. I. Root, Richard K.
II. Trunkey, Donald D. III. Sande, Merle A., date–
IV. Series. [DNLM: 1. Bacterial Infections—therapy.
W1 CO769MQV v.6 / WC 200 I43]
RC112.I455   1987   616.9'2   87-11659
ISBN 0-443-08540-4

© **Churchill Livingstone Inc. 1987**

Distributed in the United Kingdom by Churchill Livingstone,
Robert Stevenson House, 1-3 Baxter's Place, Leith Walk, Edinburgh EH1
3AF, and by associated companies, branches, and representatives throughout
the world.

Accurate indications, adverse reactions, and dosage schedules for drugs are
provided in this book, but it is possible that they may change. The reader is
urged to review the package information data of the manufacturers of the
medications mentioned.

Acquisitions Editor: *Robert A. Hurley*
Series Development Editor: *Linda Panzarella*
Copy Editor: *Julia Muiño*
Production Designer: *Melanie Haber*
Production Supervisor: *Jocelyn Eckstein*

Printed in the United States of America

First published in 1987

Contributors

J. Davis Allan, Jr, M.D. Instructor in Medicine, Harvard Medical School, Boston, Massachusetts; Member, Infectious Disease Section, New England Deaconess Hospital, Boston, Massachusetts

Christopher C. Baker, M.D. Associate Professor of Surgery, Yale University School of Medicine, New Haven, Connecticut; Director, Trauma Center, Yale-New Haven Hospital, New Haven, Connecticut

James W. Brooks, Jr, M.D. Fellow, Division of Infectious Diseases, Department of Medicine, University of Alabama at Birmingham School of Medicine, Birmingham, Alabama

Richard E. Bryant, M.D. Professor of Medicine, Head, Division of Infectious Diseases, Oregon Health Sciences University School of Medicine, Portland, Oregon

George Cierny III, M.D. Associate Professor of Surgery, Department of Orthopaedic Surgery, Emory University School of Medicine, Atlanta, Georgia

J. William Costerton, Ph.D. AOSTRA Professor of Microbiology and Biology, University of Calgary Faculty of Science Calgary, Alberta, Canada; Adjunct Professor of Microbiology and Infectious Diseases, University of Calgary Faculty of Medicine, Calgary, Alberta, Canada

Ralph G. Dacey, Jr, M.D. Assistant Professor of Neurological Surgery, University of Washington School of Medicine, Seattle, Washington

E. Patchen Dellinger, M.D., F.A.C.S. Associate Professor of Surgery, University of Washington School of Medicine, Seattle, Washington; Harborview Medical Center, Seattle, Washington

William E. Dismukes, M.D. Professor and Vice Chairman, Department of Medicine, University of Alabama at Birmingham School of Medicine,

Birmingham, Alabama; Assistant Chief, Medical Service, Birmingham Veterans Administration Medical Center, Birmingham, Alabama

George M. Eliopoulos, M.D. Assistant Professor of Medicine, Harvard Medical School, Boston, Massachusetts; Member, Infectious Disease Section, New England Deaconess Hospital, Boston, Massachusetts

Finn Gottrup, M.D., Ph.D. Associate Professor of Anatomy, Assistant Professor of Surgery, University of Aarhus, Aarhus, Denmark

Betty Halliday, B.A. Research Specialist, Department of Surgery, University of California, San Francisco, School of Medicine, San Francisco, California

W. Scott Helton, M.D. Senior Fellow, Department of Surgery, University of Washington School of Medicine, Seattle, Washington

David C. Hohn, M.D. Associate Professor of Surgery, Department of Surgery, University of California, San Francisco, School of Medicine, San Francisco, California

Thomas K. Hunt, M.D. Professor and Vice Chairman, Department of Surgery, University of California, San Francisco, School of Medicine, San Francisco, California

R. Brooke Jeffrey, Jr, M.D. Associate Professor of Radiology, University of California, San Francisco, School of Medicine, San Francisco, California; Chief, Interventional Radiology, San Francisco General Hospital, San Francisco, California

Kent Jonsson, M.D., Ph.D. Assistant Professor of Surgery, Department of Surgery, Malmö General Hospital, University of Lund, Malmö, Sweden

David R. Knighton, M.D. Assistant Professor of Surgery, Department of Surgery, University of Minnesota Medical School—Minneapolis, Minneapolis, Minnesota

Daniel V. Landers, M.D. Clinical Instructor, Department of Obstetrics, Gynecology, and Reproductive Sciences, University of California, San Francisco, School of Medicine, San Francisco, California

Frank R. Lewis, Jr, M.D. Professor of Surgery, University of California, San Francisco, School of Medicine, San Francisco, California; Chief, Surgical Service, San Francisco General Hospital, San Francisco, California

Jon T. Mader, M.D. Associate Professor of Medicine, Division of Infectious Diseases, University of Texas Medical Branch, Galveston, Texas; Chief, Division of Marine Medicine, Marine Biomedical Institute, Galveston, Texas

Stephen J. Mathes, M.D. Professor of Surgery, Head, Division of Plastic, Reconstructive, and Hand Surgery, University of California, San Francisco, School of Medicine, San Francisco, California

Robert C. Moellering, Jr, M.D. Shields Warren-Mallinckrodt Professor of Clinical Research, Professor of Medicine, Harvard Medical School, Boston Massachusetts; Physician-in-Chief, New England Deaconess Hospital, Boston, Massachusetts

David C. Price, M.D. Professor of Radiology and Medicine, Department of Radiology, University of California, San Francisco, School of Medicine, San Francisco, California

Basil A. Pruitt, Jr, M.D. Commander and Director, United States Army Institute of Surgical Research, Fort Sam Houston, Texas

Mary P. Pugsley, M.D. Assistant Professor of Medical Microbiology, Assistant Professor of Medicine, Creighton University School of Medicine, Omaha, Nebraska

Martin I. Resnick, M.D. Professor and Chairman, Division of Urology, Department of Surgery, Case Western Reserve University School of Medicine, University Hospitals of Cleveland, Cleveland, Ohio

Sheldon D. Roberts, M.D. Resident in Urology, Case Western Reserve University School of Medicine, University Hospitals, Cleveland, Ohio

Richard K. Root, M.D. Professor and Chairman, Department of Medicine, University of California, San Francisco, School of Medicine, San Francisco, California

Robert H. Rubin, M.D. Associate Professor of Medicine, Harvard Medical School, Boston Massachusetts; Chief of Infectious Disease for Transplantation, Massachusetts General Hospital, Boston, Massachusetts

Merle A. Sande, M.D. Professor and Vice Chairman, Department of Medicine, University of California, San Francisco, School of Medicine; Chief, Medical Service, San Francisco General Hospital, San Francisco, California

Christine C. Sanders, Ph.D. Professor of Medical Microbiology, Department of Medical Microbiology, Creighton University School of Medicine, Omaha, Nebraska

W. Eugene Sanders, Jr, M.D. Professor and Chairman, Department of Medical Microbiology, Professor of Medicine, Creighton University School of Medicine, Omaha, Nebraska

Richard L. Sweet, M.D. Professor and Vice-Chairman, Department of Obstetrics, Gynecology, and Reproductive Sciences, University of California, San Francisco, School of Medicine, San Francisco, California; Chief, Obstetrics and Gynecology Service, San Francisco General Hospital, San Francisco, California

Donald D. Trunkey, M.D., F.A.C.S. Professor of Surgery and Chairman, Department of Surgery, Oregon Health Sciences University School of Medicine, Portland, Oregon

Lee Watkins, B.A. Administrative/Editorial Assistant, Department of Biology, University of Calgary, Calgary, Alberta, Canada

Preface

Infection is a serious risk in the surgical patient, yet surgery may be the treatment of choice in the control of infection in the nonsurgical patient. This volume presents surgeons and clinical specialists with the latest methods of infection diagnosis, treatment, and control, both medical and surgical. The choice of modality or sequence of modalities is discussed in view of specific clinical manifestations, and the background information on wound healing mechanisms, pathophysiologic events, and host defense alterations is presented as an aid to the team approach to treatment. The complexities of infection control in the intensive care unit are also presented, as is the use of radiology in both diagnosis and treatment.

Included in this volume are chapters dealing with specific conditions such as sepsis, endocarditis, abdominal abscesses, pelvic inflammatory disease, osteomyelitis, transplantation infections, and antimicrobial therapy.

Although variously termed throughout the volume as HTLV-III, LAV, and ARV, the AIDS-associated retrovirus is now officially designated as the human immunodeficiency virus (HIV) (International Committee on the Taxonomy of Viruses: Human immunodeficiency viruses. Science 232:697, 1986).

The authors presented their topics at a symposium held in San Francisco in 1985, and the chapters have been updated to reflect recent findings for inclusion in this volume. The San Francisco symposium was funded by Beecham Pharmaceuticals, and we are grateful for their contribution that helped make this publication possible.

Richard K. Root, M.D.
Donald D. Trunkey, M.D.
Merle A. Sande, M.D.

Contents

1 | Oxygen in the Prevention and Treatment of Infection*

Thomas K. Hunt   *Betty Halliday*
David R. Knighton   *Finn Gottrup*
David C. Price   *David C. Hohn*
Stephen J. Mathes   *Kent Jonsson*

In the prevention and treatment of infection physicians usually assume that granulocyte function is normal unless they have obvious evidence to the contrary. The purpose of this paper is to review evidence which shows this is not a fair assumption, that granulocyte function is often abnormal, and that with some forethought it can be enhanced. The net effect of enhancement can be clinically about as powerful as the effect of antibiotics.

The basic observation from which this assertion stems is that resistance to infection in tissue is proportional to blood supply. This is one of the axioms of surgery. A good surgeon would not seriously consider removing a minor skin lesion from the ischemic foot of a patient with severe peripheral arteriosclerosis, as he would expect the wound to become infected. The same surgeon, however, would not hesitate to remove the same lesion from the earlobe of the same patient. In the absence of evidence to the contrary no one would

* Portions of this paper appeared in Hunt TK, Heppenstall RB, Pines E, Rovee D (eds): Soft and Hard Tissue Repair. Biological and Clinical Aspects, Praeger Scientific, New York, 1984, p. 574. We thank the publisher and our fellow editors for permission to reprint them.

1

doubt the immune competence of the patient, but, while the earlobe wound would undoubtedly heal, one would expect a wound in this patient's foot to become infected no matter how careful the aseptic technique or how aggressive the antibiotic coverage. The only difference between the foot and the earlobe in this case is their blood flow. No one doubts that fact, but what property of blood flow confers immunity? The data now clearly indicate that at least a major portion of the difference resides in the degree to which oxygen is available to leukocytes.

Normally, leukocytes move and ingest bacteria as well on anaerobically as on aerobically derived energy. However, they depend on the availability of molecular oxygen for a major portion of their capacity to kill them.[1,2] Phagocytic killing is usually conceived of as having two major components. The first mechanism is degranulation, in which ingested bacteria are exposed within the phagosome to various antimicrobial compounds derived from leukocytic granules. These "packages" of enzymes are carried by leukocytes from bone marrow to the site of phagocytes, and the efficacy of this system is unrelated to the environment of the leukocyte. The second mechanism, called *oxidative killing*, depends upon molecular oxygen, which is captured by the leukocyte and converted to high-energy radicals such as superoxide, hydroxyl, peroxide, aldehydes, hypochlorite, hypoiodite, and others, all of which are toxic in varying degrees to bacteria. The rate of production of toxic radicals is directly proportional to oxygen tension.[3]

The oxidative pathway has some specificities. Organisms such as *Staphylococcus aureus, Escherichia coli, Proteus* spp, *Salmonella* spp, *Klebsiella* spp, etc., are killed at rates proportional to local oxygen tension, while the killing of other organisms, such as *Staphylococcus epidermidis, Bacillus subtilis*, and *Pneumococcus* spp, is not affected by oxygen tension.[2,3] Therefore these remarks do not apply to all infections. The organisms affected by the oxidative pathway, however, in general are those involved in abscesses and wound infections.

The first evidence of the oxidative killing mechanism came more than 50 years ago, when it was noted that shortly after white cells ingest bacteria their respiration (i.e., oxygen consumption) rises in a short burst to as much as 25 times basal rates. Eventually, this *respiratory burst* was related to a primary oxidase located in the white cell membrane and activated by phagocytosis; the substrate requirements are furnished largely by the hexose monophosphate shunt, which is also activated by phagocytosis.

The importance of the respiratory burst was established when absence or abnormality of the primary oxidase was found to be responsible for the genetic disease called *chronic granulomatous disease of childhood* (CGD). This enzyme converts molecular oxygen to superoxide, the first step in the respiratory burst. CGD is characterized by frequent bacterial infections due to organisms which normally are killed by the oxygen-dependent mechanism. Before antibiotics were available afflicted children almost always died within a few years. The appreciation that leukocytes from CGD victims failed to mount a respi-

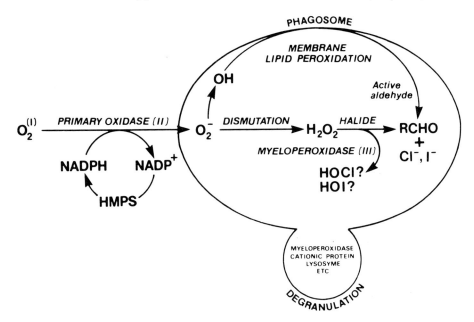

Fig. 1-1. Schema of the oxidative killing mechanism, showing how it relates to the nonoxidative pathway.

ratory burst led to the discovery that the burst coincides with a short period of bacterial killing. Eventually, it was found that oxygen radicals are produced by leukocytes and that they contribute to microbicidal mechanisms. Part of the sequence can be replicated in vitro by incubating (and killing) susceptible bacteria in the presence of halide ions, hydrogen peroxide, and myeloperoxidase.[1] A simplified schema of the present concept is given in Figure 1-1.

In chemical terms the absence of an enzyme is equivalent to the absence of the substrate on which that enzyme acts. The absence of the primary oxidase in leukocytes (as in CGD) is therefore equivalent to anoxia in normal cells. Therefore, in a normal granulocyte hypoxia should induce a disorder equivalent to some degree to CGD. A simple confirmation was made of this prediction by Hohn et al.,[4] who compared CGD cells with normal human cells while measuring bacterial killing at oxygen tensions ranging from zero to 150 mmHg, with *Staphylococcus* 502A as the test organism (Fig. 1-2). Normal leukocytes lost approximately half of their maximum killing capacity when oxygen tension was reduced to near zero. More important, their rate of killing became equivalent, as predicted, to that of cells from children with CGD. The major loss of killing capacity occurred when local PO_2 fell below about 30 mmHg. Oxygen tensions below this are commonly reached in injured animal and human tissues.[5,6]

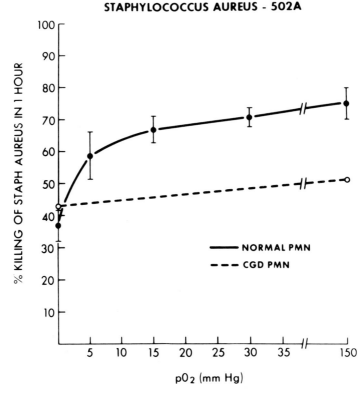

Fig. 1-2. Granulocytes and opsonized bacteria were mixed and rate of survival measured by culture count. The CGD cells, donated by children with chronic granulomatous disease, exhibited no respiratory burst. Anoxic leukocytes are equivalent to CGD leukocytes.

INITIAL EXPERIMENTS

The initial test of the surgical significance of these findings was simple. Bacteria was inoculated into cylinders of coarse wire mesh implanted under the skin of rabbits. The animals were then placed in hypoxic, normoxic, and hyperoxic environments or subjected to enough trauma at a site away from the test wound to lower the central PO_2 at the wound. As noted in Figure 1-3, the clearance of bacteria was directly proportional to tissue oxygen supply.[7,8] The following experiments were designed to demonstrate whether this effect is likely to be helpful in clinical conditions.

Methods

E. coli, wild strain, or *S. aureus*, 502A, were placed on tryptose–blood agar base plates and incubated aerobically at 37°C for 24 hours. Ten separate colonies were selected and put into 10 ml of tryptose phosphate broth for 18 hours

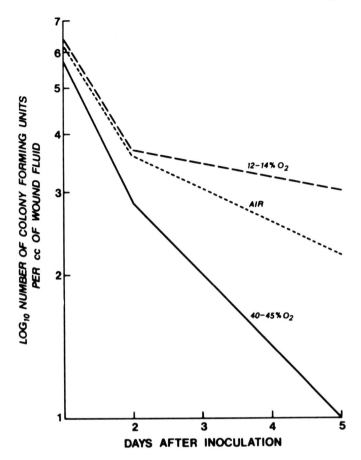

Fig. 1-3. Bacteria were placed in wounds caused by implanting wire mesh cylinders in rabbits, and the animals were placed in cages with regulated oxygen environments. Animals breathing enriched oxygen atmospheres cleared bacteria many times faster than those breathing low oxygen mixtures.

at 37°C. Part of the 1:2 diluted bacterial suspension was autoclaved in order to determine the influence of bacterial proteins on lesion size.[9]

Young adult female Hartley guinea pigs weighing 285 to 310 g were prepared for injection by removing the hair on their backs and sides with a commercial depilatory. This agent was carefully washed away, and care was taken to ensure uniform exposure of all animals. Before injection all animals were kept in room air, and after injection they were randomly assigned to test atmospheres. The bacteria were injected into the dermis of the guinea pigs' backs with an air injection gun designed for human mass immunization. The back of each animal was injected at 11 sites at 10 of which samples of approximately 10^8 organisms from the same culture were used. The eleventh was randomly chosen as a control site, and heat-killed bacteria in the same concentration were injected there. The injected guinea pigs were then placed in Plexiglas cages, four to a cage. One cage was ventilated with 45 percent oxygen, another with 12 percent oxygen, and a third with air. PCO_2 and humidity were kept in the normal range.

In the first set of experiments injected guinea pigs were divided into six groups. Group I was exposed to 12 percent oxygen for 48 hours. Group II was exposed to 45 percent oxygen for 1.5 hours, followed by 12 percent oxygen for 46.5 hours. Group III was exposed to 12 percent oxygen for 24 hours, followed by 45 percent oxygen for 48 hours, and group IV was exposed to 12 percent oxygen for 3 hours, followed by 45 percent oxygen for 45 hours. Group V was exposed to room air for 48 hours, and group VI was exposed to 45 percent oxygen for 48 hours. The guinea pigs were removed from the controlled environments at 24 and 48 hours, and the dimension of the infectious necrosis which developed at the inoculation site was measured. Necrosis was identified as the visibly infarcted and discolored skin centering on the injection site. The lesion diameter was recorded as the square root of Dd, where D and d are the lengths of the major and minor axes, respectively. Measurements were made to the nearest millimeter. Statistical analysis was performed by using the Wilcoxon rank sum to compare lesion diameters and chi-square analysis to assess differences in the incidence of necrosis.

In a further series of experiments using *E. coli*, half the animals were injected with ampicillin (8 mg intraperitoneally) at the same time that they were injected with bacteria. They were then placed in the same test environments. In these experiments *E. coli* 25922 (ATCC) were used, the 18-hour broth culture was diluted $1:2$ in tryptose phosphate broth, and the readings of both induration and necrosis were made with a Peak scale loupe ($7 \times$ magnification) to the nearest 0.1 mm.[9]

Results

Results for injection of *E. coli* are summarized in Figure 1-4. Obviously, the incidence and degree of necrosis were inversely proportional to the percentage of oxygen in the mixture breathed. Exposure to 45 percent oxygen for $1\frac{1}{2}$ hours before exposure to 12 percent for the rest of the observation period resulted in a 36 percent reduction in mean lesion diameter and a 48 percent reduction in the incidence of necrotic lesions. Exposure to 12 percent oxygen for 3 hours and then to 45 percent for 45 hours gave results similar to those obtained on initial exposure to 45 percent oxygen for $1\frac{1}{2}$ hours, followed by 12 percent oxygen for 46.5 hours. Longer (24 hour) exposure to 12 percent oxygen followed by 45 percent oxygen for 48 hours resulted in a 24 percent reduction in lesion size but only a 6 percent reduction in the number of necrotic lesions. When compared with 48-hour exposure to 12 percent oxygen, 48-hour exposure to 21 percent oxygen gave a 50 percent reduction in lesion size and a 30 percent reduction in their number. Exposure to 45 percent oxygen for 48 hours compared with 12 percent oxygen for 48 hours gave a 63 percent reduction in lesion

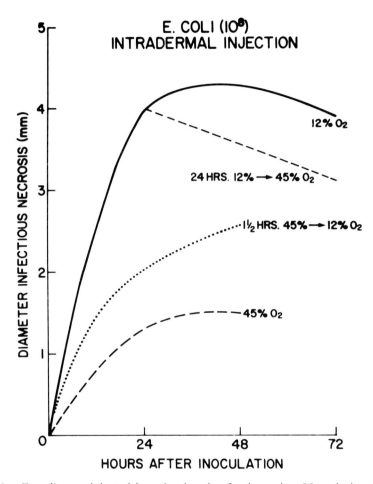

Fig. 1-4. *E. coli* were injected into the dermis of guinea pigs. Mean lesion diameter and incidence of infectious necrosis were greater in animals breathing hypoxic mixtures. The graphic analysis of the time sequences is illustrated. Correction of hypoxia exerted a beneficial effect even after 3 hours whereas antibiotics alone had little effect when given at 3 hours (as others have also shown).

diameter and a reduction of 57 percent in the number of necrotic lesions. Statistical analysis shows that all groups are significantly different in lesion size at $P < .010$ from the group exposed to 12 percent O_2 for 48 hours. The proportion of necrotic lesions was significantly less for groups exposed to 45 percent O_2 for 48 hours as compared with 12 and 21 percent oxygen exposure for 48 hours ($P < .001$).

Injections of *S. aureus* yielded similar data except that hyperoxia gave less improvement over normoxia. Nevertheless, both hyperoxic and normoxic groups were significantly improved as compared with the 12 percent oxygen group.

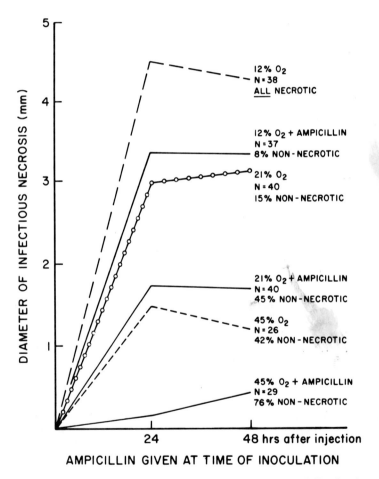

AMPICILLIN GIVEN AT TIME OF INOCULATION

Fig. 1-5.   Effect of oxygen and/or antibiotics on lesion diameter following intradermal injection of Escherichia coli bacteria into guinea pigs. Note that at every level oxygen adds to the effect of antibiotics and that raising O_2 in the breathing mixture from 12 to 20 percent or from 20 to 45 percent exerts an effect comparable with that of appropriately timed doses of antibiotics.

In the second series of experiments, in which a change in oxygen from 12 percent to 21 percent was compared with a timely, properly sized dose of specifically effective antibiotic, both the antibiotic group and the 21 percent-oxygen group had significantly fewer and smaller lesions than a group of animals breathing 12 percent oxygen. Significantly, the effect of raising the oxygen tension was marginally superior to that of giving antibiotics. Probably the most important finding was that hypoxia and antibiotics were additive, so that only rarely was any evidence of infection seen in animals treated with both, whereas every injection site became infected in hypoxic animals getting no antibiotics.[10,11]

Comment

The results clearly show that resistance to clinically important wound pathogens is proportional to the oxygenation of the tissues surrounding the area of inoculation. As opposed to antibiotics, whose effective period ends within about 3 hours of inoculation, the period of vulnerability to oxygen appears to last longer, with, however, the greatest effect exhibited in the first few hours. Furthermore, the effect of correcting tissue oxygenation from that produced by 12 percent oxygen-breathing to that corresponding to normal air was equivalent to the effect of an adequately sized, appropriately timed dose of specifically effective antibiotic (Fig. 1-5).

Silver has demonstrated that the injection of bacteria into tissue is followed by vasodilation and then vasospasm, with major corresponding changes in oxygen supply. The effects of changes in arterial PO_2 are passed on in terms of quantity of available oxygen at the site of infection.[12]

CANINE MODEL EXPERIMENTS, FIRST SERIES

The above experiments do not distinguish between local and systemic effects of hypoxia and hyperoxia. Experiments in which the whole animal is exposed to an artificial atmosphere are subject to some reservations about the role played by endocrine function, hemodynamics, catecholamines, etc. For the purpose of eliminating these effects we devised a dog model, in which a standard random pattern (RP) flap, in which tissue hypoxia is measurable, could be compared with a symmetrical, identically sized, simultaneously made musculocutaneous (MC) flap, whose circulation and oxygenation are demonstrably equal to those of nearby control tissues. A diagram of the experiment is presented in Figure 1-6.[6,13,14]

Methods

Flaps were raised in 12 animals as in Figure 1-6 and replaced immediately. The RP flap was dissected from the deeper tissue in a plane deep to the subcutaneous muscle, while the MC flap included the rectus abdominus muscle

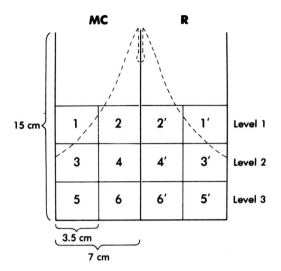

Fig. 1-6. Diagram of skin flap experiments. MC is the myocutaneous flap, which has a uniformly high tissue PO$_2$. The PO$_2$ of R, the random pattern flap, falls from normal at its base to about 15 mmHg at the tip.

but left intact its major vessels, namely the superficial epigastric artery and vein.

Oxygen tensions in the distal and proximal thirds of both flaps as well as in corresponding positions in the normal, unwounded tissue on each side were measured by the implanted Silastic sheath method.[5,6,14] Oxygen tension in the normal tissue and in both levels of the MC flap was approximately 50 mmHg. In contrast, oxygen tension in the distal aspect of the RP flap was approximately 20 mmHg, while the PO$_2$ in its proximal portion was approximately 40 mmHg.

Inoculations of 10^8 *S. aureus* were made by a tuberculin syringe with a 26-gauge needle, two in each level of each flap, with corresponding controls laterally. Lesion size was measured in the next 24 and 48 hours.

In a subset of experiments injections of *S. aureus* were made in the distal part of flaps raised in a set of three animals. Twenty four hours later 30 ml blood was withdrawn into acid citrate dextrose. The blood was sedimented with hydroxyethyl starch for 1 hour, and the supernatant was centrifuged slowly enough to separate granulocytes but not platelets. Granulocytes were resuspended in normal saline, and 0.3 mCi ^{111}indium oxine sulfate was added. After 15 min incubation, the cells were sedimented by low-speed centrifugation and resuspended in plasma, washed once, and injected in 10 ml plasma into a peripheral vein in the anesthetized donor animal.[15] Forty-eight hours after the flaps were raised, the dogs were killed. The flap was excised and imaged while calibrated against a known standard in a standard field scintillation camera interfaced to a DEC computer.[15] Counts were expressed as percent of the total dose of ^{111}In given (Table 1-1).

Table 1-1. Percent Injected Dose of ^{111}In–WBC

Normal Tissue	RP Flap	MC Flap
0.022 +/− 0.007[a]	0.062 +/− 0.020	0.020 +/− 0.006

[a] +/− Equals Standard Error of the Mean

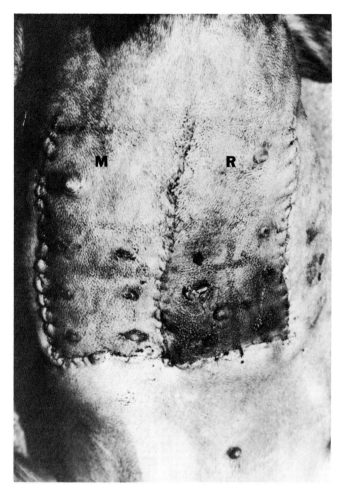

Fig. 1-7.   Illustration of infectious gangrene in the tips of the random pattern flap (right) as opposed to small abscesses in the myocutaneous flap (left).

Results

Results are illustrated in Figure 1-7. Infection of the distal (hypoxic) area of the RP flap resulted in confluent infectious gangrene. Histologic examination of the gangrenous tissue in the RP flap showed many white cells, some bacteria, no abscess formation, and considerable intravascular thrombosis. Lesions in the MC flap and control tissues were smaller than in the RP flap and were essentially similar to each other. Histological examination revealed abscess formation without gangrene and without intravascular thrombosis. Control flaps without injections survived in every case without necrosis. The amounts of radioactivity found in control and MC flap injections were essentially the same. For reasons that are not yet clear more cells appeared in the RP flap than in the normal tissue. Injection of turpentine instead of bacteria produced similar results.

Comment

Certain conclusions are already obvious. First, as predicted, ischemic, hypoxic tissue was far more than normally susceptible to infection. Infection in hypoxic tissue spread rapidly and seemed unlimited by the abscess formation, which hindered spread of infection in the immediately adjacent normal tissue and in the MC flap. Infection in the ischemic tissue caused intravascular thrombosis and infectious gangrene, which appeared indistinguishable from what we previously thought might be simple ischemic gangrene due to inadequate flap design.

As predicted by in vitro experiments, leukocytes enter the hypoxic tissue in greater numbers than they enter the control tissue. One must conclude, therefore, that the white cells which do arrive become inefficient in hypoxia. The oxygen tension of the hypoxic tissue in which these white cells function is well below the critical levels shown in Figure 1-2, and, as a first generalization, we submit that leukocytes probably lack sufficient oxygen to kill bacteria efficiently at the hypoxic site. Therefore, more leukocytes are recruited.

FINAL CANINE EXPERIMENTS

The above experiments exclude systemic variables, such as endocrine responses, which may have influenced the first set of studies. However, all that these experiments by themselves prove is that ischemia decreases local immunity in a pattern which corresponds to oxygen tension. The compelling fact is that the critical oxygen tensions for infection in this model correspond to that developed for oxygen deprivation of leukocytes by Hohn.[4] Therefore, a final set of experiments was done in which the oxygen content of ambient air was varied in the dog flap experiment to test the effect of addition or subtraction of this one substance on the extent of infection following a standard bacterial inoculation.

Methods

MC and RP flaps were elevated as described in 24 conditioned mongrel dogs, which were matched into groups of three according to weight. Immediately following resuture of the flaps *S. aureus* was injected in the same amount and pattern as above. During anesthesia and for the following 3 days, dogs chosen at random breathed a 12, 21, or 45 percent oxygen atmosphere, with gas mixtures fixed precisely as noted for guinea pig environments except that specially constructed individual cages were used. Experiments were done in

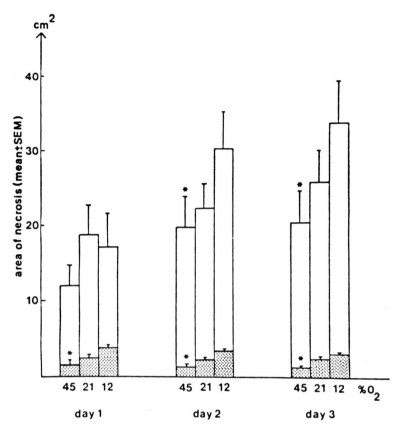

Fig. 1-8. Area of infectious necrosis in random pattern flaps (unfilled bars) and myocutaneous flaps (shaded bars) as influenced by amount of oxygen in the breathing mixture.

groups of three. Skin necroses were measured at 24, 48, and 72 hours. Differences in lesion size were compared by the Wilcoxon rank sum test.[10]

Results

The actual oxygen tensions achieved at the time of inoculation are described in Gottrup et al.[6] In brief, PO_2 at the tip of the RP flap was about 15 mmHg and could be raised only slightly by breathing 100 percent oxygen. The PO_2 at the base of the RP flap was about 40 mmHg, and the PO_2 of the entire MC flap and control skin was about 50 mmHg. Both of the latter PO_2 values could be raised by breathing oxygen.

The area of infectious necrosis was inversely proportional to the content of oxygen in the breathing mixture and corresponded quite precisely to the tissue PO_2 previously measured in the areas of inoculation. Results are summarized in Figure 1-8.[13]

Comment

With this experiment the cycle is complete. Hypoxia enhances infectability due to *S. aureus* and *E. coli*. Hyperoxia enhances immunity. According to in vitro tests this effect should extend to a variety of organisms, including *Proteus* spp, *Klebsiella, Salmonella*, and of course anaerobes such as *Bacteroides* spp and *Clostridia* spp.[1,2] We have also measured tissue oxygen tension in human tissue, including wound tissue.[5,16] Tensions in the range of 25 to 40 mmHg that were unresponsive to oxygen breathing have often been found. Patients in whom it has been studied have usually responded with increased PO_2 to expansion of blood volume with electrolyte solutions or blood transfusions. Patients with low arterial PO_2 have responded to respiratory therapy. It is unusual to have to be forced to accept a wound tissue PO_2 below 40 mmHg. Unfortunately, however, there are no clinical means which accurately predict tissue PO_2—one must measure it.

Discussion

Four major conclusions can be drawn from these data. The first, as predicted, is that well-oxygenated leukocytes are far more efficient than hypoxic leukocytes as killers of some major pathogens, particularly those involved in surgical infections. Second, degrees of hypoxia that are often reached in human and animal tissues under common physiologic conditions can seriously inhibit leukocyte function; and degrees of hyperoxia that are also easily reached under clinical conditions can facilitate leukocyte function. Third, bacterial killing can be increased to a degree which confers a benefit of approximately the same order of magnitude as that achieved by antibiotics. Fourth, the increased killing achieved by oxygen is additive to that of antibiotics.

Oxygen therapy has some problems. Simply having a patient breathe oxygen does not guarantee delivery to tissue; the only way to know that oxygen has reached tissue is to measure it there. Even subtle degrees of hypovolemia impair oxygen delivery, and current clinical skills are not sufficient to determine the extent to which oxygen reaches tissue. Therefore, to achieve the fullest use of the oxidative killing mechanism of leukocytes requires a technology to measure oxygen at the tissue level. We have developed several means of measuring it, and they will probably be generally available in a year or two. Meanwhile, the best way to assure that oxygen is delivered is to increase arterial PO_2 and give fluids aggressively enough to keep capillary return normal, peripheral skin warm, eyeball turgor normal, and mucous membranes moist and to ensure that there are no changes in vital signs on assuming erect posture.

In clinical use we have measured subcutaneous PO_2, which is particularly revealing because delivery of oxygen to subcutaneous tissue is the most vulnerable to vasoconstrictive influences such as the sympathetic discharge which occurs in hypovolemia. If subcutaneous tissue can be made hyperoxic by breathing oxygen at atmospheric pressure, all other tissues whose vascular anatomy is normal can probably be hyperoxygenated as well. In our first survey of patients leaving the recovery room after major abdominal surgery we found about 80 percent needlessly "tissue-hypoxic."[5] The hypoxia was almost always correctable with more aggressive fluid administration and increased oxygen in the breathing mixture. In a second (unpublished) survey the fraction of tissue-hypoxic patients was reduced to about half. Again, the condition was corrected in most patients with increased fluids and oxygen. In general, to oxygenate subcutaneous tissue, where most wound infections develop, we had to give fluids somewhat more aggressively than we were accustomed to doing. So far, in a survey of over 60 patients no well-oxygenated patient has become infected even after major contamination at operation. There is no obstacle to using oxygen in treatment of susceptible infections except that one must make sure that the oxygen breathed reaches tissue in the area of infection.

SUMMARY

Normal leukocytes kill some bacteria poorly in hypoxic tissue. Measurement of oxygen tension reveals that wounds are often hypoxic to a degree which compromises leukocyte function. This hypoxia is undetectable by conventional clinical means, but technology which can measure it has been developed. It is usually possible to raise tissue PO_2 above the critical zone, and the clinical benefits of doing so are roughly comparable in terms of infection to the effect of antibiotic administration. The effects of oxygen and antibiotics are additive.

REFERENCES

1. Klebanoff S: Oxygen metabolism and the toxic properties of phagocytes. Ann Intern Med 93:480, 1980
2. Mandell G: Bactericidal activity of aerobic and anaerobic polymorphonuclear neutrophils. Infect Immun 9:337, 1974
3. Hohn DC: Host resistance of infection: Established and emerging concepts. p. 264. In Hunt TK (ed): Wound Healing and Wound Infection: Theory and Surgical Practice. Appleton-Century-Crofts, New York, 1980
4. Hohn DC, MacKay RD, Halliday B, Hunt TK: The effect of O_2 tension on the microbicidal function of leukocytes in wounds and in vitro. Surg Forum 27:18, 1976
5. Chang N, Goodson WH III, Gottrup F, Hunt TK: Direct measurement of wound and tissue oxygen tension in postoperative patients. Ann Surg 197:470, 1983
6. Gottrup F, Firmin R, Hunt TK, Mathes SJ: Dynamic properties of tissue oxygen in healing flaps. Surgery 95:527, 1983
7. Hunt TK, Linsey M, Grislis G, et al: The effect of differing ambient oxygen tensions on wound infection. Ann Surg 181:35 (1975)

8. Connolly WB, Hunt TK, Sonne M, Dunphy JE: Influence of distant trauma on local wound infection. Surg Gynecol Obstet 128:713, 1969
9. Knighton DR, Halliday B, Hunt TK: Oxygen as an antibiotic: the effect of inspired oxygen on infection. Arch Surg 119:199, 1984
10. Knighton DR, Halliday B, Hunt TK: Oxygen as an antibiotic: a comparison of inspired oxygen concentration and antibiotic administration on in vivo bacterial clearance. Arch Surg (in press, 1985)
11. Hunt TK, Halliday B, Knighton DF, et al: Impairment of microbicidal functions in wounds: correction with oxygenation. p. 455. In Hunt TK, Heppenstall RB, Pines E, Rovee D (eds): Soft and Hard Tissue Repair. Biological and Clinical Aspects. Praeger Scientific, New York, 1984
12. Silver I: Tissue PO_2 changes in acute inflammation. Adv Exp Med Biol 94:769, 1978
13. Jonsson K, Hunt TK, Mathes SJ: Effect of environmental oxygen on bacterial-induced tissue necrosis in flaps. Surg Forum 35:589, 1984
14. Chang N, Mathes SJ: Comparison of the effect of bacterial inoculation in musculocutaneous and random-pattern flaps. Plast Reconstr Surg 70:1 1982
15. Price DC, Hartmeyer JA, Prager RJ, Lipton MJ: Evaluation of in vivo thrombus formation in dogs using indium-111-oxine labeled autologous platelets. p. 183. In Thakur ML, Gottschalk A (eds): Indium-111 Labeled Neutrophils, Platelets and Lymphocytes, Trivirum Publishing Co., New York, 1980
16. Goodson WH III, Andrews WS, Thakral KK, Hunt TK: Wound oxygen tension of large vs. small wounds in man. Surg Forum 30:93, 1979

2 | Adherence of Bacteria to Foreign Bodies: The Role of the Biofilm

J. William Costerton
Lee Watkins

The study of bacteria in nature has often been clouded by a fundamental misunderstanding of their mode of growth vis-à-vis surfaces. Since Pasteur, microbiologists have sampled the easily accessible floating (planktonic) bacteria in nature while ignoring the sessile bacteria, those that attach to surfaces and form thick, adherent biofilms. Sessile and floating bacteria are very different types of organisms. Because of their individual, floating nature, planktonic bacteria are essentially defenseless and make easy targets for antibacterial molecules and predatory cells. On the other hand, the attached, sessile bacteria, which are the most prevalent and often the most damaging bacteria in any system, whether natural, industrial, or medical, are much more resistant to these antibacterial agents.[1] When bacteria attach to a surface, they grow embedded in a hydrated fibrous matrix composed of their own exopolysaccharide glycocalyces, and these adherent bacteria will proliferate to produce adherent microcolonies that eventually coalesce to produce thick, matrix-enclosed biofilms. Once these biofilms have become well established, they show a strong resistance to antibacterial agents, and high concentrations must be used in order to penetrate down through the layers of bacteria to kill the innermost adherent cells. Often penetration is only partial and bacteria will begin to reestablish themselves on the remaining biofilm.[2] Thus, when antibacterial agents are proposed for use in industrial or medical systems in which bacterial

17

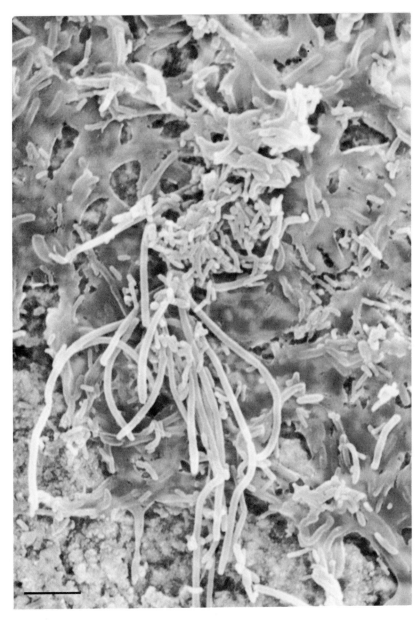

Fig. 2-1.   Scanning electron micrograph of a developing bacterial biofilm on a steel surface exposed to flowing industrial water for 4 days. Rod-shaped bacteria, some of which elongate in response to this sessile mode of growth, are seen to be buried to various extents in the amorphous, dehydrated residue of bacterial expolysaccharides that constitute the biofilm matrix. (Bar = 5 μm)

biofilms predominate, these agents must be tested against sessile bacteria if the test results are to bear any relationship to efficacy.[3]

For a number of years we have studied sessile bacteria in many different systems.[4] We have done extensive work in bacterial fouling of pipelines (Fig. 2-1), of water tanks, and of injection wells, and we have developed a good understanding of bacterial attachment and of its implications for industrial water systems. Recently we have begun to apply these findings to the human body, where we have examined the growth of autochthonous (native) bacteria on tissues and the effect on these bacteria of using foreign materials in close relationship to these tissues.

EARLY STUDIES

Our early studies examined the microbial ecology of skin. We found that autochthonous bacteria that are actively proteolytic naturally colonize this stratified squamous epithelium and penetrate progressively deeper into this tissue, breaking down cells as they "mine" deeper (Fig. 2-2). At the same time, skin cells which are working their way toward the surface of the epithelium are keratinized and subsequently consumed by these keratin-digesting bacteria. The proteolytic bacteria will feed on the keratinized skin cells and work their way downwards, so that by the time a cell is shed, it is "honeycombed" with bacteria—one of the most pervasive of these autochthonous skin bacteria is *Staphylococcus epidermidis*, which can be found at a depth of as much as six cells in the moist areas of skin (e.g., between the toes).

We removed the abdominal epidermis of experimental animals to determine how deeply the bacteria penetrated into the epithelium, and we used homogenization techniques to quantitate their autochthonous bacterial populations.[5] We prepped the animals with the standard povidine-iodine and hibitane techniques, excised the abdominal epidermis, homogenized it, and finally sonicated it in order to remove even the most adherent bacteria. We found that both preparations had killed the surface bacterial cells, many of which were gram-negative rods and fungi, but that the autochthonous *S. epidermidis* cells that were embedded deep within the skin remained unaffected by this treatment. Thus, most surgical procedures traverse a tissue (the skin) in which a large number of autochthonous colonizing bacteria have survived prepping procedures and are optimally located in the protein-rich inner layers of the epithelium.

We then examined sutures and staples, (obtained from an orthopedic practice) that had been placed across the skin for 3 to 7 days and then removed for examination by electron microscopy and quantitative recovery techniques.[6] The surfaces of these biomaterials were completely covered with a very extensive bacterial biofilm, in which gram-positive cocci predominated (Fig. 2-3). Skin cells associated with the devices were also very extensively colonized by cells of *S. epidermidis*. Interestingly, of the 100 sutures and staples studied, none of the devices was the focus of either inflammation or infection, although

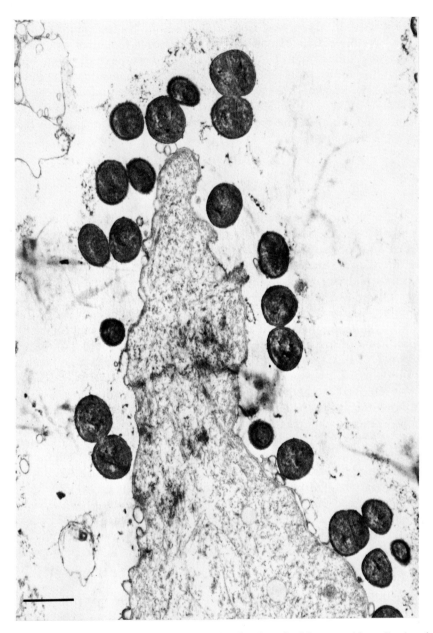

Fig. 2-2. Transmission electron micrograph of a detached human skin cell, showing the extent to which these epithelial cells are colonized by gram-positive cocci (notably *Staphylococcus epidermidis*) by the time they are detached at the surface of this stratified squamous tissue. (Bar = 1 μm)

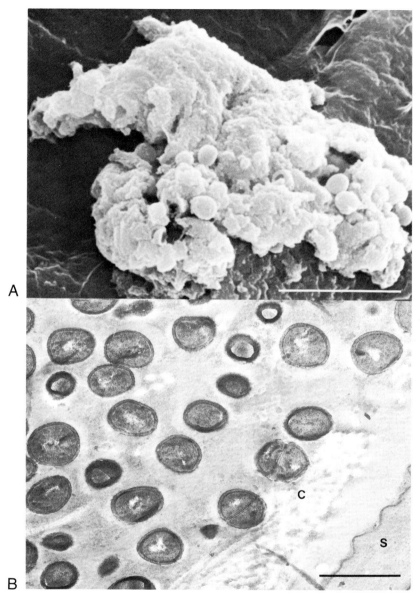

Fig. 2-3. Electron micrographs of the bacterial biofilm formed on the surface of a transcutaneous steel staple during the 5 days that this device was in place to close a surgical wound. (A) Scanning electron micrograph of the biofilm in which coccoid cells are buried to various extents in the amorphous dehydrated residue of the biofilm matrix. (Bar = 5 μm). (B) Transmission electron micrograph of a section of material scraped from the surface of the staple and stained with ruthenium red, showing gram-positive cocci in a matrix that also includes fragments of collagen (c) and some skin cells (s). (Bar = 1 μm)

the tract along the devices was virtually filled with bacteria and the body had virtually conceded this area to the native skin organism, no inflammation or infection is to be seen in Figure 2-3. In fact, the cells of *S. epidermidis* grow plaquelike as a "sleeve" along the surfaces of these biomaterials and keep much more pathogenic gram-negative organisms from penetrating these tracts and doing damage deeper in the skin. Thus, although there are extensive bacterial populations on these transcutaneous biomaterials, they have not penetrated more deeply than the skin and they have produced an essentially beneficial colonization. As long as the native skin population colonizing these materials is held in check by host defense mechanisms, it cannot be viewed as being pathogenic.

CATHETER BIOFILMS

Tenckhoff Catheter

Medical devices such as peritoneal (Tenckhoff) catheters constitute a much more massive intrusion into the body than do sutures and staples, and consequently their insertion into compromised patients has much more serious implications. We developed an animal model for peritoneal catheters, placing various devices into male New Zealand rabbits. Rabbits have their own autochthonous species of *S. epidermidis*, and their environment contains many species of bacteria, so we followed the colonization of the inserted catheters by both autochthonous and environmental organisms. In the control animals, which were not dialyzed, the subcutaneous tract of the catheter was completely colonized with *S. epidermidis* within 3 days of catheter insertion. However, this colonization did not extend beyond the peritoneal cuff within the first 3 weeks because host phagocytes were able to control the intraperitoneal surface of the catheter in the absence of dialysis and also because the outside of the peritoneal cuff was epithelialized sufficiently quickly to keep the bacterial cells firmly at bay. There was a small amount of inflammation around the exit site, but this was not a serious concern. Bacteria in the dialyzed rabbits, however, were not restricted to the subcutaneous tract. With dialysis, fluid is constantly being fed and drained in and out of the peritoneal cavity so that the activity of peritoneal phagocytes may be reduced. Bacteria in the dialysis fluid adhere and form biofilms on the luminal surfaces, and repeated irrigation washes many of these organisms into the peritoneum, where they eventually form biofilms[7] on the external surfaces of these peritoneal catheters (Fig. 2-4). When this happens, as it inevitably does in these compromised patients, a severe peritonitis can develop when sufficient planktonic cells can be mobilized from the protected biofilms on the catheter surfaces to overwhelm the host defense systems of the peritoneum (phagocytes, antibodies). Resolution of the peritonitis, using standard antibiotic therapy, leaves many living bacteria within the biofilms,[2] and these sessile populations constitute a continuing nidus of

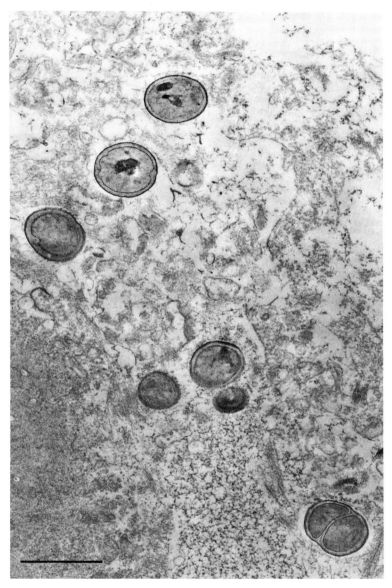

Fig. 2-4. Transmission electron micrograph of a section of a ruthenium red–stained preparation of material scraped from the external surface of the intraperitoneal segment of a Tenckhoff catheter used by a patient for 8 months, for chronic ambulatory peritoneal dialysis (CAPD). Large numbers of Gram-positive cocci are seen within a very extensive fibrous biofilm matrix which is composed of bacterial exopolysaccharides and polymers and debris of host origin. (Bar = 1 μm).

potential disseminated infection since the planktonic population can again form and overwhelm the host defenses.

Hickman Catheter

An equally massive intrusion of biomaterials through the skin and deep into human organ systems is typified by the Hickman catheter, which is placed into the heart and retained in place for periods of up to 18 months. In Figure 2-5 we see the heavy bacterial biofilm on the luminal surface of a Hickman catheter which had been in place in the heart for $4\frac{1}{2}$ months. The cardiac tip of this catheter was virtually occluded by a large mass composed primarily of cells of *Candida albicans* and *S. epidermidis*—this particular patient had had previous episodes of infections with both these bacteria.[8] The mass was so large that it acted as a valve, allowing fluid down into the heart but not out of it. We found that when patients in this situation were treated with the conventional doses of antibiotics, we found that the disseminating organisms were effectively killed, but the nidus of the infection, the bacterial biofilm on the luminal surface, remained and eventually led to recurring infections.

Urinary Catheters

We then looked at the insertion of biomaterial devices into the urinary system. The urinary tract is interesting because it has a very protective native bacterial population, which forms a continuous blanket over the cells in the distal third of the human female urethra.[9] If an extraneous bacterium such as *Escherichia coli* is to penetrate from the external environment, it must first overcome this natural bacterial "barrier" population. Using the microbial ecology methods, we tried to determine how catheter-associated infection would develop—whether pathogens ascend the outside of the catheter in the periurethral space or whether they ascend the lumen of the whole drainage system as a biofilm and thus become established in the bladder.

When a catheter is first placed up the urethra, it scrapes off a large number of autochthonous bacteria, and bacteria are subsequently present in the bladder, although these native organisms rarely cause serious infections. We selected a uropathogenic strain of *E. coli* containing genetic markers and placed it either on the meatus of the catheterized rabbit or at the end of the drainage tube of the urine bag. After 7 days the pathogenic organisms placed on the meatus had achieved only a 60 percent passage up into the bladder. There was obviously a route for infection on the outside of the catheter, but it was relatively slow. In contrast, the organisms placed on the drainage tube of the urine bag had developed a biofilm up through the lumen of the whole drainage system and into the bladder in just over 2 days (Fig. 2-6), and this biofilm closely resembled that seen on urinary catheters recovered from patients.[10] These results suggested that control of the biofilm by antibacterials should center around

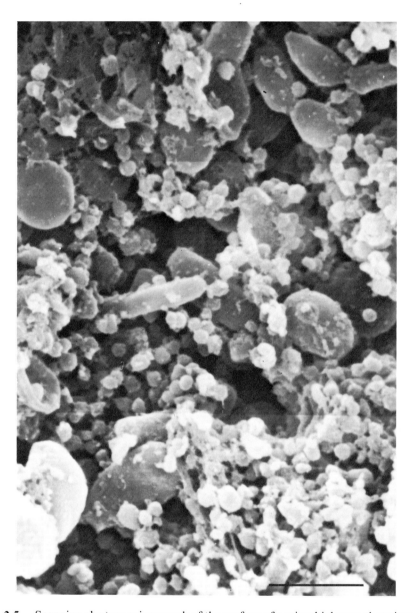

Fig. 2-5. Scanning electron micrograph of the surface of a microbial mass that virtually occluded the cardiac end of a Hickman catheter in place in a cancer patient for 18 weeks. This macroscopic mass was seen to be composed of coccoid bacterial cells and of the larger hyphal cells of fungi. *S. epidermidis* and *Candida albicans* were recovered from this device; the patient had suffered repeated bacteremias and fungemias involving these organisms. (Bar = 5 μm).

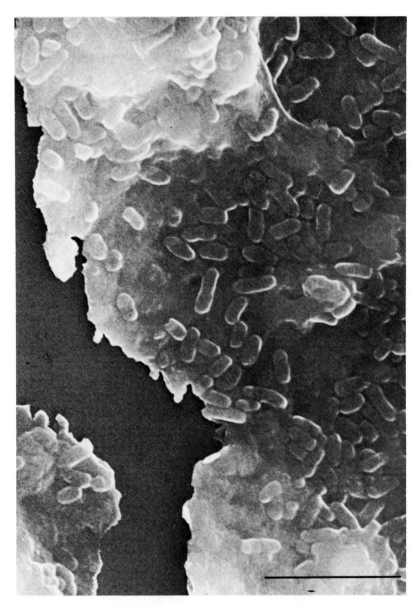

Fig. 2-6. Scanning electron micrograph of the bacterial biofilm that developed on the luminal surface of a conventional urine drainage system after catheter insertion into a male rabbit. Cells of a "genetically marked" uropathogenic strain of *E. coli* were applied to the drainage spout; a well-defined biofilm developed progressively from this distal element, through the collection bag, up the catheter, and into the bladder, so that a catheter-associated urinary tract infection was established within 28 hours. Rod-shaped bacterial cells are seen to be buried to various degrees within the residue of the biofilm matrix, which is radically condensed and cracked by dehydration. (Bar = 5 μm).

the distal elements of the urine drainage system, where the bacterial biofilm was most prevalent and infection most likely.

Bladder Infection Control: Initial Experiments

In our initial search for a means to control catheter-associated bacterial infections of the bladder, we examined the efficacy of conventional antibiotics (e.g., tobramycin) against bacteria in the biofilms. In vitro tests were done with a modified Robbins device, which is a linear rectangular acrylic pipe with a series of sampling ports located symmetrically along its upper surface. Studs are placed in these sampling ports so that the sides and the back of each individual stud are kept sterile, while the face of the stud is exposed to the test materials. We attached latex catheter material onto the sterile faces of the studs and pumped urine down through the modified Robbins device while bacteria were placed at the exit site of the device and the upward progress of their colonization on the studs was monitored. In a subsequent experiment we flowed artificial urine, containing cells of a uropathogenic strain of *Pseudomonas aeruginosa*, down through the device in order to establish a biofilm on the latex catheter material. Figure 2-7 shows the latex surfaces of studs at various stages of biofilm development. At 8 hours the latex surface was no longer visible but was covered by a biofilm 12 to 15 cells thick. This biofilm was treated with an aminoglycoside antibiotic[3]; the results were very similar to those we have seen previously in industry.[3]

The floating organisms were killed by 40 μg/ml of tobramycin, a standard minimal bacterial concentration (MBC) for this pathogenic strain, whereas the corresponding organisms on the bottom of the biofilm were still active after 12 hours of exposure to 1,000 μg/ml of tobramycin. The antibiotic was simply not penetrating to, or affecting, the lowest organisms in the biofilm. This penetration limit for antibiotics suggested to us that it would make sense, rather than trying to kill an established biofilm on the catheter, to develop a catheter which had an antibacterial already polymerized into it.[11] If the material could emit an antibacterial into the system immediately upon its insertion, an organism would be killed before it could attach to the catheter surface and begin the colonization process.

Infection-Control Urine Drainage System

C. R. Bard Inc. has recently developed a catheter bag with an antimicrobial drainage tube, and we have tested it with excellent results. The antimicrobial material is located in the outlet tube of the catheter, distal to the clamp and not in the urine bag itself, and this ensures that there is no reflux back into the patient. We installed these infection control units into male rabbits and regularly inoculated the outlet tubes with live cultures of an auxotrophically marked uropathogenic strain of *E. coli*. In the control animals a biofilm quickly de-

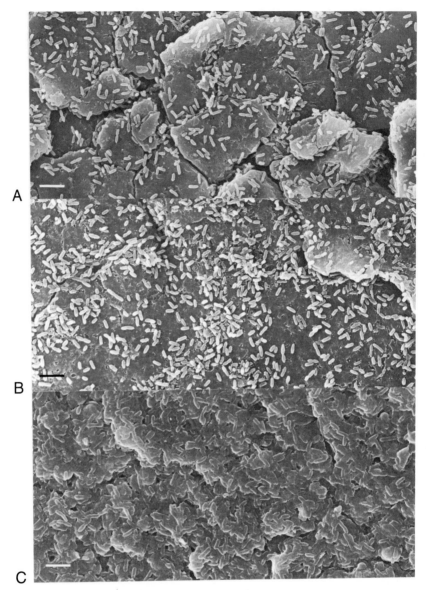

Fig. 2-7. Scanning electron micrographs showing the progressive colonization of the surfaces of latex catheter material by cells of a uropathogenic strain of *Pseudomonas aeruginosa* flowed past these surfaces in artificial urine. (A) The sparse colonization of the platelike latex surface after 5 minutes of exposure to the bacteria-laden artificial urine is shown. (B & C) The developing bacterial biofilm after 2 and 8 hours of exposure is shown. Note that at 8 hours the latex surface is virtually occluded by a very thick biofilm, in which rodlike bacterial cells are buried in the amorphous residue of the biofilm matrix. (Bars = 5 μm).

veloped at the drainage tube of the urine bag, moved up the bag, through the catheter, and into the bladder within 2 days. Once established, cells within the biofilm resisted any attack by antibiotics. In the test animals there was a shower of bacteria into the bladder when the catheter was inserted and a minimal colonization of the catheter tip with species from native population. However, the antimicrobial element in the drainage tube of these infection-control catheters successfully prevented colonization of the urine drainage system by this genetically marked strain of *E. coli*. Over the 8-day test period there were six cases in which no bacteria reached the bladder or colonized the proximal drain system, six in which organisms other than the test strain colonized the system in 2 to 5 days, and only four in which the marked *E. coli* strain was found in large numbers in the drainage system after 6 to 8 days. Thus, the infection-control catheters remained relatively sterile over this short period of time, while control catheters were all heavily colonized by the test strain within 2 to 5 days. Because the antimicrobial material kills bacteria trying to attach to the catheter surface but does not have the capacity to remove the subsequent dead bacteria, this form of infection control is only a temporary measure. For patients with long use of indwelling catheters such as those with spinal cord injuries this new drainage set will not be able to control the inevitable infections, which will continue to recur as long as a colonized catheter is in place. For short-term (1 to 7 day) catheterization, however, it should reduce catheter-associated infections.

SUMMARY AND CONCLUSIONS

In summary, we have used the direct observation and quantitative recovery methods developed in our industrial work[5] to show that bacteria growing in association with the surfaces of the biomaterials used in medical devices grow in adherent biofilms, within which individual cells are embedded in a matrix of their own extracellular polysaccharides.[15] Like the biofilms found in natural and industrial water systems, these biofilms on medical biomaterials constitute a protected mode of growth, in which individual cells are protected from phagocytes, antibodies, and antibiotics[13] and often escape detection when the fluid samples or swabs fail to remove bacteria from their dental plaque–like accretions.

The surfaces of biomaterials that traverse the skin are rapidly colonized by autochthonous skin bacteria (e.g., *S. epidermidis*), which grow deep in this stratified squamous tissue and easily survive preoperative preparation. This colonization of transcutaneous biomaterials may not pose an infection problem in devices that only penetrate the skin and/or are indwelling for short periods of time. However, both autochthonous skin organisms and introduced environmental organisms eventually form biofilms on the surfaces of more invasive devices (e.g., Tenckhoff and Hickman catheters), and these biofilms constitute protected bacterial niduses from which repeated disseminated infections can originate if host defense mechanisms fail to contain the colonizing bacteria.

We have confirmed the current clinical consensus that conventional antibiotic therapy often fails to kill the bacteria within biofilms on biomaterials, and our data suggest that the removal of the colonized device and/or very high dose antibiotic chemotherapy will be more effective[14] in the treatment of biomaterial-related infections.

We report the success of a new infection-control urine drainage system, which incorporates an antimicrobial element into its distal drainage tube and materially delays the colonization of the proximal catheter in patients with urinary catheters. This incorporation of antimicrobial biomaterials into medical devices show some promise in the prevention of the bacterial infections that presently limit the usefulness of these potentially very exciting products of modern biomedical engineering.

REFERENCES

1. Costerton JW: The role of bacterial exopolysaccharides in nature and disease. Dev Ind Microbiol 26:249, 1985
2. Nickel JC, Ruseska I, Costerton JW: Tobramycin resistance of cells of *Pseudomonas aeruginosa* growing as a biofilm on urinary catheter material. Antimicrob Agents Chemother 27:619, 1985
3. Costerton JW, Lashen ES: Influence of biofilm on the efficacy of biocides on corrosion-causing bacteria. Mater Performance 23:13, 1984
4. Costerton JW, Marrie TJ, Cheng KJ: Phenomena of bacterial adhesion. p. 3. In Savage DC, Fletcher M (eds): Bacterial Adhesion. Plenum Press, New York, 1985
5. Costerton JW, Nickel JC, Ladd TI: Suitable methods for the comparative study of free-living and surface-associated bacterial populations. p. 49. In Poindexter ES, Ledbetter ER (eds): Bacteria in Nature. Plenum Press, New York (1986)
6. Gristina AG, Price JL, Hobgood CD, et al: Bacterial colonization of percutaneous sutures. Surgery 98:12, 1986
7. Marrie TJ, Noble MA, Costerton JW: Examination of the morphology of bacteria adhering to intraperitoneal dialysis catheters by scanning and transmission electron microscopy. J Clin Microbiol 18:1388, 1983
8. Tchekmedyian NS, Newman K, Moody MR, et al: Special studies of the Hickman catheter of a patient with recurrent bacteremia and candidemia. Am J Med Sci 291:419, 1986
9. Marrie TJ, Lam J, Costerton JW: Bacterial adhesion to uroepithelial cells—a morphologic study. J Infect Dis 142:239, 1980
10. Nickel JC, Gristina AG, Costerton JW: Electron microscopic study of an infected Foley catheter. Can J Surg 28:50, 1985
11. Costerton, JW: The formation of biocide-resistant biofilms in natural, industrial and medical systems. Dev Ind Microbiol 25:363, 1984
12. Gristina, AG, Costerton JW: Bacterial infection and the glycocalyx, and their role in musculoskeletal infection. Orthop Clin North Am 15:517, 1984
13. Costerton JW: The etiology and persistence of cryptic bacterial infections: a hypothesis. Rev Infect Dis 6:s608, 1984
14. Costerton JW: Biofilm formation and inherent antibiotic resistance in prosthesis-related and chronic bacterial infections. p. 137. In Sande M (ed): Current Topics in Infectious Diseases. 1985, University of California, San Francisco, San Francisco
15. Gristina AG, Costerton JW: Bacteria-laden biofilms—a hazard to orthopedic prostheses. Infect Surg 3:655, 1984

3 | Pus: Friend or Foe?

Richard E. Bryant

This rhetorical question is relevant to the important host defense functions of abscess fluid and is especially relevant to the understanding of the importance of surgical management of suppurative infection. For purposes of this discussion, pus will be defined as the neutrophil-rich inflammatory exudates that are turbid, viscous, and below pH 7.0. Both the early and late phases of the suppurative process will be considered, as will the beneficial and potentially harmful properties of pus. This analysis will focus on:

1. The pathophysiological basis for the adequacy of the early and late host response to infection
2. The clinical assessment of the efficacy of pus as a host defense function in closed-space infections
3. Factors in pus that may limit local host defenses
4. Factors in pus that may injure the host
5. The perspective of the potentially helpful and harmful effects of pus

THE PATHOPHYSIOLOGICAL BASIS FOR THE ADEQUACY OF THE EARLY AND LATE HOST RESPONSE TO INFECTION

The initial stages of local infection represent a critically timed conflict between the ability of bacteria to grow in tissues or body fluids and the ability of the cellular and humoral host defenses to destroy them. The importance of the rapid delivery of a number of normally functioning polymorphonuclear leukocytes (PMNs) that is adequate to contain bacterial infection and to prevent tissue injury has been demonstrated in a number of classic studies.[1-7] Miles, Miles, and Burke[1] and Burke[2] demonstrated that tissue injury at sites of intradermal injection of bacteria into guinea pigs was directly related to the logarithm

31

Table 3-1. The Effects of Suppressing Leukocyte Delivery or Function or Bacterial Growth during the Decisive Period of Infection on the Size of *S. aureus* Skin Lesions in Guinea Pigs

Variable Tested	Lesion Size (% of Control at 24 Hours) after Application of Variable at Time after Injecting *S. aureus*			
	1 Hour	2 Hours	4 Hours	6 Hours
Ischemia (local adrenalin)	143	~100	~100	~100
Shock (dehydration)	149	105	~100	~100
Liquoid (anticomplementary)	231	176	145	100
Penicillin	58	81	94	98

(Data from Miles A, Miles E, Burke J: The value and duration of defense reactions of the skin to the primary lodgement of bacteria. Br J Exp Pathol 38:79, 1957; also from Burke J: Wound infection and early inflammation. Monogr Surg Sci 1:301, 1964.)

of the dose (log-dose) of injected bacteria and inversely proportional to the adequacy of PMN delivery and function in infected tissues. Their elegant studies established that measures that inhibited local delivery or function of neutrophils were associated with an increased size of the local inflammatory lesion when measured 20 to 24 hours after injection.[1,2] Their studies of dermal infection with *Staphylococcus aureus* are illustrated in Table 3-1.

The same authors helped to establish the concept of the decisive period during the first 2 to 4 hours after infection as the time during which lesions are most susceptible to modifications that could help or harm the host. Their studies also confirmed the relative immutability of the course of infection after the first 4 to 6 hours. These studies were supported by the observations of Andriole and Lytton, who found that increased tissue pressure during the decisive period of infection enhanced subsequent tissue injury.[3] Andriole and Lytton corroborated the importance of the decisive period of infection by observing that lesions subjected to pressure for longer than 4 hours were not significantly different from the lesions treated for 4 hours. Increased tissue pressure appeared to suppress local delivery of leukocytes and serum to sites of *S. aureus* injection in guinea pigs and enhanced local tissue injury.

These findings were corroborated also by Cohn's elegant studies of *S. aureus* peritonitis in mice.[4-6] Modification of host defenses that impaired leukocyte delivery during the decisive early period of infection led to overwhelming infection and death of the animals. This occurred with leukopenia caused by irradiation or systemic endotoxin injection, with delayed delivery of neutrophils to peritoneal fluid caused by hydrocortisone, and with metabolic inhibitors of leukocyte function.[4-6] Survival of animals was enhanced if the peritoneal leukocyte counts were elevated by intraperitoneal injection of endotoxin 48 hours before bacterial challenge.[5] These findings are summarized in Table 3-2.

Increased antimicrobial susceptibility of bacteria during the early period of infection was established by Eagle's classic studies of group A streptococcal myositis in mice (Table 3-3).[7] Animals treated during the first 6 hours of in-

Table 3-2. Animal Models Documenting the Key Role of Impaired Leukocyte Delivery or
Function during the Decisive Early Period of Infection

Methods of Demonstration	Authors
1. Ischemia, hypotension, and suppressed complement activity	Miles et al.[1]; Burke[2]
2. Increased tissue pressure	Andriole et al.[3]
3. Leukopenia from x-ray or systemic endotoxin, delayed diapedesis from hydrocortisone, and metabolic inhibition of PMN function	Cohn[4-6]

fection had rapid reduction of bacteria in tissues, but animals treated thereafter did not. The mechanism of antimicrobial refractoriness was shown to be independent of bacterial numbers because high inocula 7 to 8 [$\log_{10}$ of the number of colony-forming units (CFU)] were quite susceptible to antibiotics if treated immediately after initiation of infection.[7]

Mechanisms limiting the efficacy of the early inflammatory process in certain tissues were clarified by the landmark studies of W. Barry Wood, Jr. and his collaborators.[8-11] Those authors examined the inability of PMNs to contain the early phase of encapsulated pneumococcal or *Klebsiella* infection in the murine lung and lymph nodes.[8,9] Their studies demonstrated a marked delay in PMN delivery to infected tissue and described the ineffectiveness of host defense function prior to development of specific immunity that would delay bacterial multiplication and enhance phagocytosis. Early in infection phagocytosis in tissues was rendered ineffective by the small number of PMNs and relatively large volumes of fluid that precluded effective phagocytosis.[8] Wood and co-workers described a "primordial" capability of PMNs to ingest encapsulated bacteria prior to development of specific immunity if the tissue environment permitted leukocytes to trap bacteria against surface membranes of the host.[8,10,11] Those studies were carried out both in vitro and in vivo, and demonstrated conclusively that PMNs can ingest even the most well-encapsulated bacteria if given the proper surface against which to trap them. This was demonstrated in a variety of fresh and fixed tissues and on a variety of artificial surfaces such as filter paper.[8] Conversely, smooth surfaces with no means to prevent bacteria from "slipping away" from migrating PMNs failed

Table 3-3. Effect of Delayed Treatment and Concentration of Bacteria in Tissues on Antibiotic
Susceptibility of Group A Streptococci Causing Murine Myositis

Delay in Therapy	Bacteria in Tissue ($\log_{10}$ CFU)	Reduction of Bacteria in Tissues 8 Hours after Therapy ($\log_{10}$ CFU)
0 hour	3	3
3 hours	4	4
6 hours	5	5
12 hours	~7	1
24 hours	~8	1
0 hour	~7.5	~7

(Data from Eagle H: Experimental approach to the problem of treatment failure with penicillin. Am J Med 13:389, 1952.)

Table 3-4. Effect of Alveolar Fluid on Lethality of Inhaled Pneumococci after Intrabronchial Injection of Serum or Saline in the Mouse

Intrabronchial Injection	Died	Survived
Serum	35	5
Saline	9	13
None	1	17

$P < .001$ (Saline–None bracket)
$P < .001^a$ (overall bracket)

^{a} Chi square test
(Adapted from Harford C, Hara M: Pulmonary edema in influenzal pneumonia of the mouse and the relation of fluid in the lung to the inception of pneumococcal pneumonia. J Exp Med 91:245, 1950.)

to permit surface phagocytosis.[8] By convention this phenomena is termed *surface phagocytosis*, but in fact it represents surface-enhanced phagocytosis.

It has been learned subsequently that the alternate complement pathway facilitates surface phagocytosis and that specific immunity and the classical complement pathway are required for optimal facilitation of phagocytosis by agglutination of bacteria and adhesion of bacteria to host surfaces.[12,13] The studies of the qualitative and quantitative effects of various antibody classes and complement components in the phagocytic process and related host defenses will not be described in greater detail than to emphasize their considerable importance in clearance of bacteria from the body tissues and the bloodstream.[14–16]

Effective phagocytosis requires contact between PMNs and bacteria. This is significantly affected by the ratio of PMNs to bacteria and by the volume of fluid in which the PMNs and bacteria are diluted. In relatively large volumes there is little chance of contact, whereas the likelihood of contact is greatly enhanced in small volumes. The concept of the adverse effect of a large volume of distribution of the phagocytic system was cited as the key factor predisposing mice with viral influenza to lethal infection with experimentally induced pneumococcal pneumonia.[17,18] Harford demonstrated that fluid-filled alveoli enhanced the lethality of bacterial pneumonia in mice by 15-fold and could be induced by endobronchial injection of either serum or saline (Table 3-4).[18] The critical feature of bacteria "floating away to safety" on a wave of edema fluid represents a picturesque characterization of the mechanisms responsible for enhanced susceptibility of the fluid-filled lung.[8–11,18] Efficient phagocytosis can not take place in the lung or any other fluid-filled tissue space until that space is literally packed with PMNs.

THE CLINICAL ASSESSMENT OF THE EFFICACY OF PUS AS A HOST DEFENSE FUNCTION IN CLOSED-SPACE INFECTION

If adequate delivery and function of PMNs in infected tissue are thwarted by a response that is "too little and too late," infection spreads to adjacent body tissues or fluid and an infection of greater severity occurs. This is the

Table 3-5. Mortality of Meningitis Prior to the Antibiotic Era

Bacteria	Author (year)	Patients (No.)	Antiserum $(+,-,\pm)$	Mortality (%)
S. pneumoniae	Finland[19] (1938)	99	$\pm$	100
H. influenzae	Fothergill[20] (1937)	78	$-$	98
N. influenzae	Fothergill[20] (1937)	201	$+$	85
N. meningitidis	Flexner[21] (1913)	1,500	$-$	75
N. meningitidis	Flexner[21] (1913)	1,294	$+$	31

point at which overt quantities of pus will be seen. Serious disease occurs when vital structures such as the meninges, pleura, pericardium, or joint spaces develop suppurative infection. Efficacy of phagocytosis in those areas is impaired by large volumes of fluid, by a relative lack of structural elements to enhance surface phagocytosis, by a rich source of nutrients for bacterial growth, and possibly by a lack of sufficient opsonins. Similar observation can be made of infected hematomas after trauma or seromas after surgery.

Infections of the meninges, pleura, pericardium, or joints have a poor prognosis if left untreated. This is put into perspective by studies of the mortality of such infections prior to the antibiotic era. As shown in Table 3-5, meningitis had an extraordinarily high mortality in the first part of this century.[19-21] Although removal of spinal fluid had been used to reduce increased intracranial pressure associated with meningitis, it was not until the availability of antiserum therapy that significant reduction in mortality was observed.[19-22] Table 3-5 provides insight into the ability of the suppurative process to control infection in the spinal fluid if augmented by antiserum therapy. Of the three types of meningitis considered, meningococcal meningitis is the most readily amenable to antiserum therapy. Phagocytosis appears to occur in the spinal fluid of patients with meningococcal meningitis, as judged by demonstration of intracellular gram-negative diplococci in stained smears of infected spinal fluid prior to treatment. PMNs in spinal fluid of patients with pneumococcal meningitis do not contain intracellular pneumococci unless the patient has pneumococcal endocarditis or chronic pneumococcal infection prior to development of meningitis.[19]

Finland and co-workers noted that the cure rate of patients with pneumococcal meningitis was enhanced when sulfonilamide was used concomitantly with intrathecal antiserum.[19] Although few patients were cured with that regimen, spinal fluids became sterile almost immediately after cerebrospinal fluid (CSF) antibody titers were raised to a level of 1:2. They were unable to detect antibody titers in the CSF of untreated patients. The scientific community apparently lost interest in antiserum therapy of meningitis after penicillin became available.

Mortality of bacterial empyema prior to and during the antibiotic era is shown in Table 3-6. Finland's review makes a strong statement concerning management of empyema. Surgical drainage was and is the primary modality responsible for successful treatment of bacterial empyemas, and the techniques for surgical drainage were well known in 1935.[23] Therefore it is not surprising that there has been little change in mortality of that disease from 1935 to 1965.[23]

Table 3-6. Mortality of Bacterial Empyema at Boston City Hospital

Year	Community-Acquired		Hospital-Acquired	
	(No.)	Mortality (%)	(No.)	Mortality (%)
1935	107	36	18	50
1955	19	37	26	62
1965	25	44	34	53

(Adapted from Finland M, Barnes M: Changing ecology of acute bacterial empyema: occurrence and mortality at Boston City Hospital during 12 selected years from 1935 to 1972. J Infect Dis 137:274, 1978.)

Admittedly, factors such as bacterial virulence, the extent of infection, the severity of the patient's underlying disease, and the patient's age are not reflected in such a table, and therefore modest changes in improved medical care would not be reflected in improved survival. The mortality of undrained empyemas must be high but cannot be determined precisely because drainage has become a universally accepted principle of treatment for that disease.

The mortality of purulent pericarditis was 38 to 65 percent prior to the antibiotic era and represents another well-established indication for surgical drainage.[24] In 1939 it was recognized that the only hope of survival from pneumococcal pericarditis lay in successful surgical drainage of the pericardium.[24] In 1902 the mortality of pneumococcal arthritis was cited as 65 percent, but it was recognized that most patients died of complications of infection involving other organs.[25] Pneumococcal arthritis responded well to surgical drainage if it was carried out prior to joint destruction by the inflammatory process.[25]

FACTORS IN PUS THAT LIMIT HOST DEFENSES

There are few reports defining the composition of pus, but the contribution of pus constituents to the containment of infection and the inflammatory process has received increased attention.

As shown in Table 3-7, pus is an acidic fluid with increased concentrations of intracellular ions such as potassium and phosphate and concentrations of sodium and chloride that are slightly lower than those of serum.[26] To my knowledge there are no definitive studies of the PO_2 of human pus despite the awareness that hypoxia may be responsible for suppressed PMN function in abscesses. Wood hypothesized that the PO_2 of pus should be low because of limited diffusion of oxygen from capillary membranes.[27] Hayes and Mandel found the PO_2 of experimentally induced staphylococcal abscesses ranged from 13 to 71 mmHg.[28] Mader et al. found the PO_2 of osteomyelitic bone to be 20.9 $\pm$ 1.7 mmHg; they observed enhanced PMN function when leukocytes that had been exposed to hypoxic environments were exposed to the higher oxygen tension produced by hyperbaric oxygen therapy.[29] Not surprisingly, oxydation-reduction potential, (the eH) of polymicrobic anaerobic abscesses has been found to be as low as -200 to -400.[30] Values of eH or PO_2 of abscesses caused by *S. aureus* or gram-negative aerobic bacilli are, to my knowledge, not available.

Table 3-7. Constituents of Abscess Fluid

Assay	Value	Range	Units
pH	6.17	5.5–6.8	
Osmolality	402	207–535	mOsm/kg H_2O
Ionic strength	0.131	0.075–0.198	[a]
Sodium	119	92–134	mEq/L
Potassium	18.5	10–33.5	mEq/L
Chloride	87.9	60–109	mEq/L
Calcium	6.2	2.8–9.3	mg/dl
Phosphate	14.5	62–28.2	mg/dl

[a] Expressed relative to solutions of NaCl of known ionic strength.
(Adapted from Bryant R: Effect of the suppurative environment on antibiotic activity. p. 313. In Root RK (ed): Contemporary Issues in Infectious Diseases. Vol. 1. Churchill Livingstone, New York, 1984.)

The microbial content of empyema and abscess fluid has been surprisingly constant. Bartlett and also Onderdonk, Weinstein and co-workers found that pus contained 10^7 and 10^9 CFU of aerobic or anaerobic bacteria per milliliter of abscess fluid.[31,32] We found similar concentrations of bacteria in abscesses of patients with polymicrobic anaerobic abscesses or with staphylococcal abscesses.[26] Wood found that experimentally induced pneumococcal lesions contained $\geq 10^8$ CFU of pneumococci per milliliter.[27] The fact that clinically encountered abscesses and experimentally induced abscesses have similar numbers of aerobic or anaerobic organisms suggests that the regulation of bacterial concentrations in abscesses is under tight biologic control.[32] In fact, it is surprising that the numbers are in such good agreement in view of the fact that patients with abscesses may be treated for variable periods with antibiotics before surgical drainage is performed and bacteria can be counted.

The concentration of PMNs in empyema fluid has been studied by Waldvogel and by Suter and co-workers.[33,34] Abscess fluid from three patients contained 4×10^7 to 1.5×10^8 leukocytes per milliliter, of which 95 percent were PMN's and 60 to 90 percent were viable by dye exclusion studies.[33] Empyema fluid from 10 patients had a protein content of 29.9 $\pm$ 12.6 g/L and contained 5.0 $\pm$ 6.2 $\times 10^8$ leukocytes per milliliter. The phagocytic and bactericidal capability of PMNs in pus has yet to be defined.

The concentration of immunoglobulin and complement in empyema fluid is shown in Tables 3-8 and 3-9. Levels of immunoglobulins and of C_3 and C_4 were considerably below those found in normal serum.[35] There was evidence that both immunoglobulins and complement were degraded by the proteolytic, enzyme-rich environment of abscess fluid.[35] Breakdown products of IgG were found in 11 of 14 patients with culture-positive pleural fluid; this finding confirmed the studies of Waller, who demonstrated hydrolysis of IgG in abscess fluid.[35,36] Subsequent studies by Lew and co-workers demonstrated a predictable association between pleural fluid concentrations of complement breakdown components and the presence of an empyema (Table 3-10).[37] It was not altogether clear that low complement levels were solely attributable to degradation by PMNs or PMN breakdown products because the authors had pre-

Table 3-8. Immunoglobulin Levels of Infected Pleural Fluids

Immunoglobulin	Culture Positive[a]	Sterile[a]
IgG (mg/dl)	425 ± 321	711 ± 210
IgA (mg/dl)	175 ± 146	159 ± 104
IgM (mg/dl)	40 ± 24	64 ± 25
IgG breakdown products by immunoelectrophoresis	11/14	0/14

[a] mean ± S.D.
(Adapted from Lew P, Perrin L, Waldvogel F et al: Demonstration of a local exhaustion of complement components and of an enzymatic degradation of immunoglobulins in pleural empyema: a possible factor favouring the persistence of local bacterial infections. Clin Exp Immunol 42:506, 1980.)

viously demonstrated that pneumococci, *S. aureus*, and gram-negative aerobic bacilli in concentrations likely to be present in empyema fluid, i.e., 5×10^7 to 2×10^8 CFU/mL, could reduce hemolytic complement CH 50 units by 50 percent in 1 hour under conditions likely to affect both the classic and the alternate complement pathway.[38]

Table 3-9. Complement Activity in Infected Pleural Fluid[a]

Complement Activity	Culture-Positive	Sterile
Alternate pathway Mediated opsonic activity (%)[b]	4.1 ± 34	47 ± 58
Total C_4 (%)[c]	46 ± 34	56 ± 48
Hemolytic C_4 (%)	3 ± 7	26 ± 29
Total C_3 (%)[c]	66 ± 46	57 ± 44
Native C_3 (%)[c]	6 ± 14	38 ± 23
C_3d fragment (%)[d]	50 ± 44	26 ± 24

[a] mean ± S.D.
[b] Measured by uptake of endotoxin coated paraffin (percent of values observed in normal pooled serum).
[c] Percent of values with normal pooled plasma.
[d] Percent of normal sera pool activated with insulin.
(Adapted from Lew P, Perrin L, Waldvogel F et al: Demonstration of a local exhaustion of complement components and of an enzymatic degradation of immunoglobulins in pleural empyema: a possible factor favouring the persistence of local bacterial infections. Clin Exp Immunol 42:506, 1980.)

Table 3-10. Complement Breakdown Products in Infected or Sterile Pleural Fluid

Type of Fluid (No.)	C3d Fragment[a]	Ba Fragment	CH50[b]
Empyema (13) (culture-positive)	50 ± 51	122 ± 102	11 ± 19
Postpneumonic (13) (sterile)	20 ± 11	41 ± 10	50 ± 12

[a] C3d, Ba fragments: small breakdown product expressed as percent values with insulin-activated normal serum.
[b] CH50 total complement hemolytic activity expressed as percent of normal pooled plasma.
(Adapted from Lew P, Perrin L, Waldvogel F et al: Loculated pleural empyema: Identification of complement breakdown products in contiguous sterile pleural fluid Scand J Infect Dis 14:225, 1982.)

There has been speculation as to whether the lack of bactericidal or opsonic activity in cerebrospinal fluid (CSF) might be partially responsible for the susceptibility of patients to meningitis[39,40]. Simberkoff et al. found that spinal fluid was devoid of appreciable opsonic activity.[39] Zwahlen and co-workers found that normal patients and those with viral meningitis had undetectable levels of complement-mediated opsonic activity. However, they found that some patients with meningitis had detectable opsonic antibody titers.[40] All the patients with detectable titers survived, but 7 of 12 patients with undetectable levels died.[40] It is difficult to be sure whether increased opsonic titers in CSF represent an epiphenomenon, reflecting that patients with less severe infection would have an increased likelihood of a vigorous immunologic response. Similarly, it may be difficult to demonstrate antibody titers when bacteria are still present in spinal fluid, and there is a known association between high CSF concentrations of bacteria and death. The differences in demonstration of CSF opsonic antibody titers probably reflect the differences in techniques used to measure them. Simberkoff et al. looked for opsonic antibody against the strains of bacteria causing meningitis, and Zwahlen et al. studied opsonic antibody directed against a Wood 46 strain of *S. aureus* that had nothing to do with the patient's infection.[39,40]

The efficacy of serum therapy of meningitis prior to the antibiotic era as shown in Table 3-5 makes it difficult to feel that CSF antibody titers are irrelevant.[19-21] In certain patients with meningitis it seems probable that opsonin-enhanced phagocytosis in the CSF may play a significant, albeit small, role in recovery. This may give patients time to manifest their disease and seek medical help prior to development of irremediable disease, despite the fact that the majority will die unless more effective measures are used. This represents an outstanding, but slightly speculative, testimonial to the beneficial effects of white cells in pus in a setting where it is usually considered to be deleterious to host defenses. The early studies by Petersdorf and Luttrell demonstrated that leukopenic animals survived experimental meningitis longer than normal animals and reasoned that the suppurative process was harmful to the host.[41] Similarly Sande and co-workers demonstrated that growth of bacteria in the CSF was the same in normal and leukopenic animals in the early period of experimental meningitis, thus verifying both the impact of delayed leukocyte mobilization and the ineffective leukocyte function in the cerebrospinal fluid.[42]

There are fairly convincing associations between the presence of dead tissue, or pus, in patients and the development of hypocomplementemia with subsequent sepsis or further tissue injury.[43,44] It is not clear whether local or systemic consumption of complement, suppression of complement production, or both account for these observations. Nor is it clear whether bacteria in ischemic tissue may contribute to these findings, but the association of abscesses, low levels of complement, and subsequent bacteremia or development of the acute respiratory distress syndrome are at least consonant with clinical observations.[43,44] Whether the low levels of serum complement contribute to reduction of complement in abscess and whether that has a significant impact on the host defense function in abscesses is conjectural.

Table 3-11. Factors in Pus That May Limit Host Defenses or Therapy of Abscesses

Milieu suboptimal for phagocytosis or bactericidal activity:
Lacks or may destroy opsonins
Lacks structure for surface phagocytosis
Bad ratio of bacteria to PMN's, volume of distribution
Reduced PO_2, pH, and eH (by inference)
Dead tissue or foreign bodies
Concentration of microbial enzymes and/or toxins injurious to PMN's, IgG, complement, proteinase inhibitors
Milieu may inhibit antibiotic activity by:
Altering bacterial metabolism (and susceptibility)
Enzymatic destruction of antibiotics (β-lactamase)
Altering membrane transport of aminoglycosides

The encapsulation process associated with abscesses has the potential of localizing microbial enzymes or toxins injurious to the host. Some of those bacterial products are known to inactivate proteinase inhibitors and may contribute indirectly to degradation of immunoglobulin and complement by inhibiting the proteolytic enzyme inhibitors that normally limit degradation of opsonins and complement.[45,46]

It must have been a great disappointment to investigators in the early days of antibiotic research to learn that antibiotic therapy did not change the need for drainage of focal collections of pus. It was clearly appreciated that bacteria in abscesses were relatively indifferent to antibiotics and that focal collections of pus still had to be drained.[7,27]

The suppressed growth rate of bacteria in abscesses is probably the key determinant affecting their diminished antibiotic responsiveness in this environment. We are still in the process of defining the mechanisms responsible for this observation.[47] It has also been recognized that the abscess environment may suppress activity of β-lactamase-susceptible β-lactam antibiotics via enzymatic degradation of those antibiotics and may also suppress activity of aminoglycoside antibiotics based on the pH, osmolality, ionic strength, and PO_2 of pus and on the binding of aminoglycosides by purulent sediment of pus.[26] Diminished aminoglycoside activity in abscesses is probably due to the suppressive effect of the abscess milieu on aminoglycoside uptake by bacteria.[48]

Table 3-11 summarizes a list of factors in the suppurative milieu that impair host defenses or antibiotic activity against bacteria in abscesses. Studies to expand our knowledge in this area are needed.

FACTORS IN PUS THAT ARE HARMFUL TO THE HOST

It is generally accepted that suppurative processes associated with pus are destructive to tissues. Most of us have experienced the heat, swelling, and pain associated with a staphylococcal abscess that will erupt spontaneously unless drained surgically. Clinicians have had the experience of observing erosion of lung, bone, brain, or of the visceral organs of the body by abscesses and are

Table 3-12. Granulocyte Collagenase, Elastase, and Protease Inhibitors in Human Pus

Material	Value	Range	Units
Collagenase	0.17	(0.05–0.34)	mg/ml
Elastase	0.19	(0.07–0.41)	mg/ml
α_1 Antitrypsin	0.55	(0.22–0.83)	mg/ml
α_2 Macroglobulin	0.32	(0.13–0.46)	mg/ml

(Delshammar M, Ohlsson K: Granulocyte collagenase and elastase and the plasma protease inhibitors in human pus. Surgery 83:323, 1978.)

aware that there are no tissues that are insusceptible to destruction by suppurative involvement. Thus it is commonly thought that abscesses and pus are injurious to tissues.

A number of studies have verified the potent tissue-destroying capacity of abscess fluid. Aside from the toxins produced by bacteria or the injury secondary to ischemia associated with infection, there is a considerable body of evidence linking tissue injury to the PMN-derived abscess constituents. The potentially noxious properties of PMNs in pus were noted by Opie in 1905, but most information has been reported during the last 20 years.[49] Studies by Delshammar and Ohlsson have described the collagenase, elastase, and antiprotease content of pus (Table 3-12).[52] Curtiss and Klein repeated a classic earlier experiment of Phemister by demonstrating that pus incubated with cartilage at 55°C was capable of dissolving it in 2 to 3 days (Table 3-13).[50,51] Control studies with buffer or *S. aureus* cultures or suspensions had no effect on cartilage integrity. Although denaturation by heat may have played a role in enhancing susceptibility of cartilage to degradation, the experiment conclusively proves the noxious capability of pus.[50]

The capabilities of neutral proteases and cathepsins to injure tissues have received a great deal of attention (Table 3-14). They have been shown also to degrade complement, fibrinogen, and the clotting cascade.[53,54] Granulocyte-derived neutral proteases have been proposed as potential contributors to the respiratory distress syndrome in neonates and to airway damage in patients with cystic fibrosis.[55,56] There is an interesting link between the oxidants derived from PMNs, which may activate α_{-1} proteinase inhibitor and thereby

Table 3-13. Effect of Pus and *S. aureus* on Bovine Articular Cartilage

Incubation Fluid	Effect on Cartilage	
	37°C	55°C
Buffer	None	None
Pus	None	Dissolved 2–3 days
S. aureus culture	None	None
S. aureus suspension	None	None

(Curtiss P, Klein L: Destruction of articular cartilage in septic arthritis. I. In vitro studies. J Bone Joint Surg 45A:797, 1963.)

Table 3-14. Factors in Pus That May Be Injurious to the Host

Chemical milieu
    Direct injury
        Neutral proteases: elastase, collagenase, cathepsins
        Polyunsaturated fatty acids–affecting brain cell edema
        Oxidative injury: superoxide, H_2O_2, OH^-
        Aldehydes
        Reduced nutrients
        Bacterial enzymes or toxins
    Indirect injury
        Microbial enzymes that degrade α_1 proteinase inhibitor
        Oxidative suppression of α_1 antiproteinase
Physical factors
    Reduced pH, eH, PO_2
    Increased tissue pressure
    Mechanical injury

lead to relatively unopposed activity of the neutral proteases, and a vicious cycle of enzyme-mediated tissue destruction perpetuated in pus.[57–59]

There is a large body of evidence linking oxidants generated during phagocytosis to tissue injury, especially in the lung.[60] This has been confirmed by experiments noting enhanced lung injury after infusion of Fe^{3+} ion, which was presumed to enhance lipid peroxidation, and by experiments showing reduced injury after use of potent hydroxyl radical scavengers such as dimethylthiourea.[61,62] Similarly, cationization of catalase and peroxidase, which permitted persistence of those enzymes in joints subjected to antigen-induced arthritis, markedly suppressed the arthritis, whereas cationic superoxide dismutase or native catalase or peroxidase had no effect.[63]

Other factors in purulent exudates that are capable of causing tissue injury include polyunsaturated fatty acids which can cause edema of brain tissue[64,65] and aldehydes.[66] None of the aforementioned factors shown in Table 3-14 operates in isolation, and production of tissue injury is probably a composite effect of chemical and physical injury applied in concert with microbial enzymes and toxins, reduced nutrients, and increased tissue pressure. There are several opportunities for oxidants and host and bacterial enzymes to induce a vicious cycle of tissue damage.

THE PERSPECTIVE OF THE POTENTIALLY HELPFUL AND HARMFUL EFFECTS OF PUS

With the "rogues' gallery" of potentially toxic factors available in pus, it is miraculous that abscess walls are able to contain those factors and sequester them away from nearby vital structures. Herein lies the key to consideration of the host defense function of pus—it can not be considered separately from the abscess wall that contains it nor should we expect a milieu capable of containing the growth of a myriad of virulent pathogens to be a totally innocuous media.

Table 3-15. Effect of Antibiotic Therapy at the Time of Subcutaneous Injection of 8–9 $\log_{10}$ CFU of *E. coli* and *B. fragilis* in Sterile Stool on Mortality and Abscess[a] Formation in Mice

Treatment	Previous Injection	Outcome (Lived/Total)
None	−	0/10
None	+	10/10
Amakacin (125 mg/kg × 1)	−	9/10

[a] Abscess content day 5 > 8 $\log_{10}$ CFU/ml of *E. coli* and *B. fragilis*.

Pus has been given an undeservedly bad reputation. Pus was once given the term *laudable* and was felt to represent an exemplary host defense function. Understandably this perspective was lost when science demonstrated that the suppurative response associated with pus frequently reflected a host defense that arrived too late, did too little in the early stages of infection, and later contributed to persistent tissue injury that could be characterized as too much or too long. This was highlighted by the immutability of the downhill clinical course of patients with multiple organ failure secondary to sepsis whose abscesses were not or could not be adequately drained. Experienced physicians have been aware of the association between deep-seated, antibiotic-unresponsive abscesses and persistent chills and fever that may progress to multiple organ failure.[67,68]

These associations have fostered a guilt-by-association linkage between the presence of pus and the cause of disease. Pus is generally judged to be a coparticipant in disease, is occasionally regarded as a traitorous host response, and at the least is generally considered disgusting. Although it is laudable to drain pus because that is likely to cure the patient, it is proper to view suppurative material as the life-saving host defense that it truly is.

This perspective is supplied by consideration of the host defenses of mice against subcutaneous polymicrobic anaerobic infection using a modification of the model of Joiner et al.[69] Animals were inoculated with a mixture containing 10^8 CFU/ml of *Escherichia coli* grown in trypticase soy broth (Becton Dickinson and Co., Cockeysville, Maryland), 10^8 CFU/ml of *Bacteroides fragilis*, grown in cooked meat media (PML Microbiologicals, Tualatin, Oregon), and one-third volume of sterile stool in isotonic saline. Each animal received four subcutaneous injections of 0.25 ml. As shown in Table 3-15, animals virtually all died from *E. coli* sepsis if they did not receive antibiotics after initiation of this overwhelming infection (E. Gardner, personal communication). However, animals receiving only one injection of 125 mg/kg of amikacin at the time of inoculation survived their initial bacteremia. They formed abscesses that by 48 to 96 hours contained 10^8 to 10^9 CFU of both *E. coli* and *B. fragilis* and formed lesions that matured to well-formed abscesses, which ultimately drained spontaneously without overt impairment of the animal's health. This experiment demonstrates the other end of the suppurative process after the animal has survived the critical early period of infection. Once formed, the local suppurative process is able to contain quantities of bacteria that would kill the host if they were not sequestered locally. Animals previously inoculated with such mixtures while receiving amikacin could withstand repeated injection without antibiotics. The exact mechanisms by which this occurs are poorly understood but undoubtedly represent an orchestration of defenses associated with the rapid early delivery of leukocytes, local tissue necrosis, development of a walled abscess, which limits further dissemination of bacteria, and finally spontaneous drainage of the abscess with ultimate cure.

This beautifully coordinated series of host defense functions has built-in mechanisms for containing and then disposing of bacteria and postinflammatory debris by spontaneous drainage. The totality of factors capable of injuring tissues appears to provide the capability of destroying enough adjacent tissue to permit drainage of the abscess. This has been documented for rodents with *S. aureus, B. fragilis, Streptococcus pneumoniae*, and polymicrobic abscesses and is well known in the clinical practice of medicine.[27,54,69] Unassisted abscess drainage is both slow and painful and is fortuitously assisted by surgery. Nevertheless the abscess has the capability of metaphorically fighting the battle and cleaning up debris. This has been described by some as equivalent to landscape sculpturing with the finesse of an artillary barrage,[60] but for the most part pus formation is roughly equivalent to the need for local containment. Consider how much more frequent pimples are than boils. Even boils represent a superior alternative to the fulminant sepsis they may prevent. It is only when suppurative infection is inopportunely located or occurs at sites where encapsulation and sequestration are prevented that abscesses and pus fail their ordinarily heroic function. Viewed in this light, suppuration and pus play elegant roles in host defenses, with an overall function that is usually efficient and vital to survival.

Our dependence on this process has been obscured by artifacts associated with our current medical knowledge and practices. Clearly, the suppurative process in general and pus in particular deserve a reinstatement of their reputation as laudable components of our host defenses.

REFERENCES

1. Miles A, Miles E, Burke J: The value and duration of defense reactions of the skin to the primary lodgement of bacteria. Br J Exp Pathol 38:79, 1957
2. Burke J: Wound infection and early inflammation. Monogr Surg Sci 1:301, 1964
3. Andriole V, Lytton B: The effect and critical duration of increased tissue pressure on susceptibility to bacterial infection. Br J Exp Pathol 46:308, 1964
4. Cohn Z: Determinants of infection in the peritoneal cavity: I. Response to and fate of *Staphylococcus aureus* and *Staphylococcus albus* in the mouse. Yale J Biol Med 35:12, 1962
5. Cohn Z: Determinants of infection in the peritoneal cavity: II. Factors influencing the fate of *Staphylococcus aureus* in the mouse. Yale J Biol Med 35:29, 1962
6. Cohn Z: Determinants of infection in the peritoneal cavity: III. The action of selected inhibitors on the fate of *Staphylococcus aureus* in the mouse. Yale J Biol Med 35:48, 1962

7. Eagle H: Experimental approach to the problem of treatment failure with penicillin. Am J Med 13:389, 1952
8. Wood WB Jr: Studies on cellular immunology of acute bacterial infections. Harvey Lect 47:72, 1951
9. Smith MR, Wood WB Jr: Cellular mechanisms of antibacterial defense in lymph nodes: I. Pathogenesis of acute bacterial lymphadenitis. J Exp Med 90:555, 1949
10. Wood WB Jr, Smith MR, Perry W, et al: Studies on the cellular immunology of acute bacteremia: I. Intravascular leukocytic reaction and surface phagocytosis. J Exp Med 94:521, 1951
11. Smith M, Perry W, Berry J, et al: Surface phagocytosis in vivo. J Immunol 67:71, 1951
12. Winkelstein J, Shin H, Wood W: Heat liable opsonins to pneumococcus: III. The participation of immunoglobulins and of the alternate pathway of C3 activation. J Immunol 108:1681, 1972
13. Smith M, Shin H, Wood WB Jr: Natural immunity to bacterial infections: the relation of complement to heat-liable opsonins. Proc Natl Acad Sci USA 63:1151, 1969
14. Guckian J, Christensen G, Fine D: The role of opsonins in recovery from experimental pneumococcal pneumonia. J Infect Dis 142:175, 1980
15. Hosea S, Brown E, Frank M: The critical role of complement in experimental pneumococcal sepsis. J Infect Dis 142:903, 1980
16. Brown E, Hosea S, Hammer C, et al: A quantitative analysis of the interactions of antipneumococcal antibody and complement in experimental pneumococcal bacteremia. J Clin Invest 69:85, 1982
17. Harford C, Leidler V, Hara M: Effect of the lesion due to influenza virus on the resistance of mice to inhaled pneumococci. J Exp Med 89:53, 1949
18. Harford C, Hara M: Pulmonary edema in influenzal pneumonia of the mouse and the relation of fluid in the lung to the inception of pneumococcal pneumonia. J Exp Med 91:245, 1950
19. Finland M, Brown J, Rauh A: Treatment of pneumococcic meningitis: a study of ten cases treated with sulfanilamide alone or in various combinations with specific antipneumococcic serum and complement, including six recoveries. N Engl J Med 218:1033, 1938
20. Fothergill L: *Hemophilus influenzae* (Pfeiffer bacillus) meningitis and its specific treatment. N Engl J Med 216:587, 1937
21. Flexner S: The results of the serum treatment in thirteen hundred cases of epidemic meningitis. J Exp Med 17:553, 1913
22. Tauber M, Sande M: The impact of penicillin on treatment of meningitis. JAMA 251:1877, 1984
23. Finland M, Barnes M: Changing ecology of acute bacterial empyema: occurrence and mortality at Boston City Hospital during 12 selected years from 1935 to 1972. J Infect Dis 137:274, 1978
24. Heffron R: Pneumonia. The Commonwealth Fund, New York, 1937
25. Herrick J: Pneumococcic arthritis. Am J Med Sci 124:12, 1902
26. Bryant R: Effect of the suppurative environment on antibiotic activity. p. 313. In Root RK (ed): Contemporary Issues in Infectious Diseases. Vol. I. Churchill Livingstone, New York, 1984
27. Wood B, Smith M: An experimental analysis of the curative action of penicillin in acute bacterial infections: I the relationship of bacterial growth rates to the antimicrobial effects of penicillin. J Exper Med 509:487, 1956

28. Hays R, Mandell G: PO_2, pH, and redox potential of experimental abscesses. Proc Soc Exp Biol Med 147:29, 1974
29. Mader J, Brown G, Guckian J, et al: A mechanism for the amelioration by hyperbaric oxygen of experimental staphylococcal osteomyelitis in rabbits. J Infect Dis 142:915, 1980
30. Tally F: Factors affecting antimicrobial agents in an anaerobic abscess. J Antimicrob Chemother 4:299, 1978
31. Bartlett J: Anaerobes survive in clinical specimens despite delayed processing. J Clin Microbiol 3:133, 1976
32. Onderdonk A, Weinstein WM, Sullivan NM, et al: Experimental intra-abdominal abscesses in rats: quantitative bacteriology of infected animals. Infect Immun 10:1256, 1974
33. Waldvogel F: Pathophysiological mechanisms in pyogenic infections: two examples—pleural empyema and acute bacterial meningitis. p. 115. In Majno G, Cotran R, Kaufman N (eds): Current Topics in Inflammation and Infection. Williams & Wilkins, Baltimore, 1982
34. Suter S, Nydegger U, Roux L, et al: Cleavage of C3 by neutral proteases from granulocytes in plural empyema. J Infect Dis 144:499, 1981
35. Lew P, Despont J, Perrin L, et al: Demonstration of a local exhaustion of complement components and of an enzymatic degradation of immunoglobulins in pleural empyema: a possible factor favouring the persistence of local bacterial infections. Clin Exp Immunol 42:506, 1980
36. Lew P, Perrin L, Waldvogel F, et al: Loculated pleural empyema: identification of complement breakdown products in contiguous sterile pleural fluid. Scand J Infect Dis 14:225, 1982
37. Waller, M: IgG hydrolysis in abscesses. I. A study of the IgG in human abscess fluid. Immunology 26:725, 1974
38. Lew P, Zubler R, Vaudaux P: Decreased heat-labile opsonic activity and complement levels associated with evidence of C3 breakdown products in infected pleural effusions. J Clin Invest 63:326, 1979
39. Simberkoff M, Moldover N, Rahal J: Absence of detectable bactericidal and opsonic activities in normal and infected human cerebrospinal fluids. J Lab Clin Med 95:362, 1980
40. Zwahlen A, Nydegger U, Vaudaux P, et al: Complement-mediated opsonic activity in normal and infected human cerebrospinal fluid: early response during bacterial meningitis. J Infect Dis 145:635, 1982
41. Petersdorf R, Lutterell C: Studies of the pathogenesis of meningitis. I. Intrathecal infection. J Clin Invest 41:311, 1962
42. Ernst J, Decazes J, Sande M: Experimental pneumococcal meningitis: role of leukocytes in pathogenesis. Infect Immun 41:175, 1983
43. Heideman M: A shared effect of abscesses and nonviable tissue influencing the development of sepsis and acute respiratory distress syndrome. Acta Chir Scand [Suppl] 508:295, 1982
44. Heideman M, Saravais C, Clowes G: Effect of nonviable tissue and abscesses on complement depletion and the development of bacteremia. J Trauma 22:527, 1982
45. Moskowitz R, Heinrich G: Bacterial inactivation of human serum alpha-1 antitrypsin. J Lab Clin Med 77:777, 1971
46. Morihara K, Tsuzuki H, Hoda K: Protease and elastase of *Pseudomonas aeruginosa*: inactivation of human plasma α_1 proteinase inhibitor. Infect Immun 24:188, 1979

47. Kim K, Anthony B: Importance of bacterial growth phase in determining minimal bactericidal concentrations of penicillin and methicillin. Antimicrob Agents Chemother 19:1075, 1981
48. Bryan L, Van Den Elzen H: Effects of membrane energy mutations and cations on streptomycin and gentamicin accumulation by bacteria: a model for entry of streptomycin and gentamicin in susceptible and resistant bacteria. Antimicrob Agents Chemother 12:163, 1977
49. Opie E: Enzymes and antienzymes of inflammatory exudates. J Exp Med 7:316, 1905
50. Curtiss P, Klein L: Destruction of articular cartilage in septic arthritis. I. In vitro studies. J Bone Joint Surg 45A:797, 1963
51. Phemister D: The effect of pressure on articular surfaces in pyogenic and tuberculous arthritides and its bearing on treatment. Ann Surg 70:481, 1924
52. Delshammar M, Ohlsson K: Granulocyte collagenase and elastase and the plasma protease inhibitors in human pus. Surgery 83:323, 1978
53. Janoff A, Carp H: Proteases, antiproteases, and oxidants: pathways of tissue injury during inflammation. p. 62. In Majno G, Cotran R, Kaufman N (eds): Current Topics in Inflammation and Infection. Williams & Wilkins, Baltimore, 1982
54. Havemann K, Janoff A (eds): Neutral Proteases of Human Polymorphonuclear Leukocytes. Urban & Schwarzenberg, Baltimore, 1978
55. Merritt T, Cochrane C, Holcomb K, et al: Elastase and α_1-proteinase inhibitor activity in tracheal aspirates during respirator distress syndrome: role of inflammation in the pathogenesis of bronchopulmonary dysplasia. J Clin Invest 72:656, 1983
56. Suter S, Schaad U, Roux L, et al: Granulocyte neutral proteases and *Pseudomonas* elastase as possible causes of airway damage in patients with cystic fibrosis. J Infect Dis 149:523, 1984.
57. Campbell E, Senior R, McDonald J, et al: Proteolysis by neutrophils: relative importance of cell-substrate contact and oxidative inactivation of proteinase inhibitors in vitro. J Clin Invest 70:845, 1982
58. Carp H, Janoff A: Potential mediator of inflammation: phagocyte-derived oxidants suppress the elastase-inhibitory capacity of $alpha_2$-proteinase inhibitor in vitro. J Clin Invest 66:987, 1980
59. Johnson D, Travis J: The oxidative inactivation of human α-1-proteinase inhibitor: further evidence for methionine at the reactive center. J Biol Chem 254:4022, 1979
60. Babior B: Oxidants from phagocytes: agents of defense and destruction. Blood 64:959, 1984
61. Ward P, Till G, Kunkel R, et al: Evidence for role of hydroxyl radical in complement and neutrophil dependent tissue injury. J Clin Invest 72:789, 1983
62. Fox R: Prevention of granulocyte-mediated oxidant lung injury in rats of hydroxl radical scavenger, dimethylthiourea. J Clin Invest 74:1456, 1984
63. Schalkwijk J, van den Berg W, van de Putte L, et al: Cationization of catalase, peroxidase, and superoxide dismutase: effect or improved intraarticular retention on experimental arthritis in mice. J Clin Invest 76:198, 1985
64. Chan P, Fishman R: Brain edema: induction in cortical slices by polyunsaturated fatty acids. Science 201:358, 1978
65. Fishman R, Sligar K, Hake R: Effects of leukocytes on brain metabolism in granulocytic brain edema. Ann Neurol 2:89, 1977
66. Stelmaszynska T, Zgliczynski J, Chlobowska Z: Detection of some aldehydes in pus. Mater Med Pol 6:257, 1974

67. Polk H, Shields C: Remote organ failure: a valid sign of occult intra-abdominal infection. Surgery 81:310, 1977
68. Fry D, Pearlstein L, Fulton R, et al: Multiple system organ failure. Arch Surg 115:136, 1980
69. Joiner K, Onderdonk A, Gelfand J, et al: A quantitative model for subcutaneous abscess formation in mice. Br J Exp Pathol 61:97, 1980

4 | Alterations in Host Resistance in Surgical Patients

Christopher C. Baker

As surgical skills have improved over the last several decades, surgeons have operated upon and cared for increasingly critically ill patients. Despite major advances in a number of areas, the problems of infection and sepsis continue to plague us. Although neurologic injury continues to account for approximately 50 percent of deaths following major trauma, sepsis has been identified as a cause of death in 75 percent of late nonneurologic deaths.[1] If a patient survives inhalation injury following a major burn, sepsis constitutes the most significant threat to life thereafter.[2] In these two high-risk groups, sepsis is associated with a 50 percent mortality, which is increased to 75 percent if multiple organ failure supervenes.[3] Infectious complications also constitute a significant risk in patients following major elective surgery (abdominal aortic surgery, hepatic resections, colorectal surgery, etc.) Despite major advances in surgical techniques, pre- and postoperative care, anesthetic and intensive care unit management, blood bank technology, and antibiotics, surgical sepsis remains a challenge.

A number of factors must be considered when evaluating the risk of sepsis for a surgical patient. This review will attempt to highlight some of these considerations by summarizing classical concepts and material from the recent literature on host defense along with predictions of future directions. Areas that will be covered include *normal host resistance; patient factors* that must be considered in determining risk for sepsis; *specific surgical conditions*, such as trauma and burns, in which the risk of sepsis is high; and *future directions for therapy* directed at preventing and/or treating sepsis. The area of host resistance and immunology has been rapidly changing, significant advances having been made over the past few years. Because of the complexity of this area and the controversial nature of some of the data in the current literature, this review will attempt to aid the reader in developing a basic understanding of the foundations of this field and a knowledge of what is currently accepted.

NORMAL HOST RESISTANCE

Normal host resistance is an extremely complex defense system with multiple subsystems. Some of the basic principles involved in host defense depend upon systems which work in sequence (e.g., the complement and coagulation systems), while others depend upon interactive cellular responses deriving from the integration and balance of stimulatory and regulatory activities (e.g., the specific immune system). Host factors involved in defense against bacterial infection have classically been divided into nonspecific and specific factors. A brief outline of these factors is offered below.

Nonspecific Factors

The nonspecific factors that are involved in host defense are legion; a partial list is included in Table 4-1. Owing to limitations of space, only phagocytosis and complement will be discussed in detail.

Both *phagocytosis* and the *complement cascade* are systems in which a series of well-defined steps follow one upon another. What makes these two systems unique is that they interrelate very importantly not only to each other

Table 4-1. Nonspecific Factors in Host Defense

Mechanical Barriers
    Skin
    Mucous membranes
        Gastrointestinal tract
      Respiratory tract
        Genitourinary tract
Complement
Chemotactic factors
Phagocytosis
Fever (pyrogen)
Interferon
Inflammatory mediators (e.g., prostaglandins, leukotrienes)
Acute-phase reactants (e.g., opsonins)
Coagulation; fibrinolytic system
Hormonal factors (e.g., steroids)
Nutrition
Heredity
Age
Normal indigenous microflora

Table 4-2. Steps in Phagocytosis

I. Chemotaxis (complement, other factors)
II. Opsonization (complement, immunoglobulin)
III. Bacterial ingestion
    A. Alterations in cellular morphology
    B. Alterations in cellular metabolism
IV. Bacterial killing
    A. Oxygen-dependent mechanisms
    B. Oxygen-independent mechanisms

but to other systems involved in host defense (e.g., the coagulation and specific immune systems). Phagocytosis is the process by which bacteria and other organisms are ingested and killed by polymorphonuclear leukocytes, monocytes, and macrophages. This is a complex system involving a number of steps which occur in series (Table 4-2); therefore there are several ways in which this system can fail. In the initial phase of phagocytosis, known as *chemotaxis*, phagocytes are drawn into the area of bacterial infection by several chemotactic agents, which cause them to migrate outside the capillary. Interestingly, one of the complement fragments (C5a) is a powerful chemotactic agent. Its formation may be triggered by gram-negative lipopolysaccharide. A number of other microbial substances such as the formylated peptides, which are closely related to compounds released by bacteria, have also been found to be powerful chemotactic agents. Finally, products of the metabolism of arachidonic acid by the 5-lipoxygenase pathway (in particular leukotriene B4) are chemotactic. The ability of white cells to migrate toward a stimulus can be measured in several in vitro systems. Chemotaxis has been shown by several investigators to be abnormal in patients undergoing major surgery or who have suffered major trauma.[4]

The next step in the phagocytic process is *opsonization*, the process by which bacteria are made more susceptible to ingestion (cf. Greek *opsonein* "to prepare to eat"). Most pathogenic bacteria require opsonization before ingestion by phagocytes and development of specific antibodies. Opsonization occurs primarily by the attachment of the Fab portion of immunoglobulin (IgG), which binds to the bacterial surface, allowing the Fc portion to bind with Fc receptors on the plasma membranes of macrophages and neutrophils. In the absence of specific antibodies, other opsonic agents include the bound cleavage fragments of C3 (C3b and C3bi). These fragments may be generated and bound to the bacterial surface by activation of either the classical or the alternative complement pathway.[5]

During phagocytosis the neutrophil undergoes major alterations in morphology and sends pseudopodia around the bacteria to form the phagocytic vacuole. During this interesting feat, neutrophil glycolytic and oxidative metabolism increases markedly. Specific glycoproteins on the neutrophil and monocyte/macrophage cell surface play an important role in both chemotactic and phagocytic responses by promoting adherence to endothelial cells and other surfaces as well as interleukocytic adherence (aggregation) reactions. When these proteins are missing from cells, these adherence reactions and all other secondary dependent events are markedly impaired. The result is a genetically determined syndrome of severe cutaneous and soft tissue infections caused by normally pyogenic bacteria (but without pus), a chronic circulating leukocytosis, and severe periodontal disease.[6]

Killing of bacteria occurs in several ways. Initially, lysosomes from within the neutrophil fuse with the phagocytic vacuole and discharge their potent bactericidal substances into the vacuole. Some of the lysosomal substances that have bactericidal characteristics include myeloperoxidase, lactoferrin, specific cationic proteins, and lysozyme.[7] Concomitantly with these metabolic changes, the pH within the vacuole drops significantly, which also promotes bacterial killing. Therefore, it is conceivable that metabolic alkalosis, which might counteract this intracellular acidosis, may account for some decrease in phagocytic capabilities. Similarly, hypophosphatemia, which decreases the process of phosphorylation and the production of ATP, may cause decreases in phagocytosis. In addition to the above-mentioned oxygen-independent factors, there are a number of oxygen derivatives which are very potent microbicidal agents: hydrogen peroxide (H_2O_2), hydroxyl ion (OH^-), superoxide (O_2^-), and singlet oxygen ($^1O_2^-$). The metabolism of H_2O_2 by the enzyme myeloperoxidase in the presence of Cl^- ion leads to the formation of $HOCl$, a potent oxidizing microbial agent. Although avoidance of hypoxia and hypotension is a straightforward issue for anesthesiologists, it is clear that surgeons must make efforts to provide adequate levels of oxygen to tissues in order to maintain normal phagocytic activity. Hohn and co-workers have previously shown that neutrophils in a hypoxic environment will be able to ingest bacteria but will not be able to kill them.[8]

Other phagocytic cells include the mononuclear leukocytes and fixed macrophages. These cells are critical in recognizing and processing bacterial antigen, as will be discussed in more detail below. The entire process of phagocytosis is complex; it has been well summarized in a recent review by Cates.[9] Clearly the neutrophil plays a major role in phagocytic defenses. The clinical correlate of this is the markedly increased incidence of bacteremia in granulocytopenic patients.[10] With increasing numbers of patients on chemotherapy requiring surgery, surgeons should remember that patients with an absolute peripheral neutrophil count of less than 500 cells per cubic millimeter are at high risk for sepsis. Under certain circumstances they may benefit from granulocyte transfusions.[11]

The *complement* system functions primarily as a biologically active cascade over initial activation. Because of its complexity it will not be covered here in detail. Several points, however, should be emphasized. The major split products C3a and C5a are powerful anaphylatoxins, which cause capillary dilatation and smooth muscle contraction and lead to histamine release from mast cells. C5a is a potent chemoattractant and causes fusion of neutrophil-specific granules with the plasma membrane as well as activation of oxidative metabolism. C3b, which is the larger of the split products of the C3, functions primarily as a bacterial opsonin for both the classical and the alternative complement pathway. In addition, C3b stimulates B cell antibody production and antibody-dependent cell-mediated cytotoxicity. Surgeons should be aware of the fact that C5a causes leukocyte aggregation, which may be related to the adult respiratory distress syndrome (ARDS).[12] Finally, the assembly of C3b6789 on bacterial cell walls can lyse gram-negative bacteria. Interested readers are directed to an excellent review by Frank.[13]

Specific Factors

Understanding of the specific immune system has increased exponentially in the last 10 years. Both specific antibody formation and cell-mediated immunity may play important antimicrobial roles. The complexity of the specific immune system is such that the old dichotomy between humoral and cellular elements of the immune system is no longer relevant. The major cellular components of the specific immune system are as follows: the bursa-equivalent (B) cells, which arise in the bone marrow, differentiate to plasma cells, and are primarily responsible for the production of immunoglobulins, or antibody; the thymus-derived (T) cells, which are responsible for cell-mediated interactions between macrophages and B cells and for cell-mediated cytotoxicity; and the population of accessory adherent cells consisting of wandering and fixed *macrophages* (Mϕ), which have a diverse number of functions. All these cells produce humoral components and have cellular interactions that are extremely complex. In-depth analysis is beyond the scope of this review, but an excellent recent summary by Paul et al.[14] is available.

With respect to the specific immune defenses against bacteria, it is probably most appropriate to begin with the Mϕ population. These cells have a diverse number of functions and have at least two subpopulations. A stimulatory or facility population of Mϕ has been identified that can be inhibited by prostaglandin E$_2$, steroids, and T suppressor cells. The facility Mϕ interact with T helper cells, bear immune response antigen (Ir) on their surface, and produce a number of monokines or serum substances. Some of the serum substances produced by facilitory Mϕ include interleukin 1, several complement products, and plasminogen activator. These cells are critical in the recognition of bacterial antigen and in processing this antigen for subsequent interactions in the specific immune system. Facilitory Mϕ are balanced by inhibitory Mϕ, which interact with T suppressor cells, are activated by prostaglandin E$_2$, are resistant to steroids, and are Ir-negative. These cells also interact with the coagulation-fibrinolytic system by producing tissue thromboplastin.

The population of *T cells* is heterogenous and has been demonstrated to have at least four specific subsets (T helper, T suppressor, T effector, and T amplifier). T helper cells have Fc receptors on their surface and produce a number of lymphokines, including interleukin 2. The production of interleukin 2 by T helper cells in response to production of interleukin 1 by Mϕ leads to B cell differentiation and antibody production. T helper cells are sensitive to steroids and can be inhibited by prostaglandin E$_2$. Other lymphokines that are produced by T cells include chemotactic factors, macrophage-inhibiting factor, and macrophage-activating factor. T suppressor cells lack the Fc receptor on their surface, are resistant to steroids, and regulate cell-mediated cytotoxicity. In humans, T helper cells normally constitute 60 to 70 percent of T cells and have generally been identified by the monoclonal antibody OKT4. The T suppressor cells constitute approximately 20 percent of T cells in humans, and these cells have generally been identified by the monoclonal antibody OKT8.

The final step in the specific immune system is the differentiation of B cells to plasma cells with subsequent elaboration of immunoglobulin or antibody. This occurs following the recognition of antigen by Mϕ, the production of interleukin 1 by Mϕ, and the stimulation of T cells to produce interleukin 2, which in turn stimulates B cell differentiation along with B cell growth factor. B cells generally constitute 15 percent of peripheral blood lymphocytes and are found most commonly in lymph nodes, spleen, blood, and bone marrow. They produce five classes of immunoglobulin, but IgG, IgM, and IgA are the antibodies with specific activity against microorganisms.

Cell-mediated immunity (CMI), frequently measured as delayed cutaneous hypersensitivity, is a complex integration of several aspects of the specific immune system. This system attempts to provide maximum recognition and destruction of antigen with minimal damage to tissues through intercellular communication. Effector T cells, through interleukin 2, lead to T lymphocyte–B lymphocyte interactions in antigen-antibody responses. Macrophages appear to regulate CMI both by their initiation of T cell activation and by interaction with suppressor T cells. Meakins et al.[4] have correlated sepsis with DCH, but the complex nature of CMI makes evaluation of such studies difficult.

PATIENT FACTORS

Despite the increasing challenge of sepsis and the increasing complexity of surgical procedures being performed on critically ill patients, there is an old adage regarding complications in surgery which still holds true. Major complications in surgery generally result from one of three factors: (1) errors in judgment; (2) errors in technique; and/or (3) the patient's disease. The former two factors have been well covered in the literature, and this section will discuss some of the factors intrinsic to the patient that affect the risk for sepsis following surgery or major injury. The two areas that will be discussed here are the importance of paying attention to the patient's premorbid status and the importance of various surgical risk factors in assessing the risk for sepsis.

Premorbid Status

It is critical for the surgeon to evaluate carefully the various medical diseases that affect host resistance. It is beyond the scope of this paper to deal with these in detail, but several things should be highlighted. There are a number of diseases that depress neutrophil function and therefore tend to inhibit phagocytosis. These range from such rare congenital disorders as chronic granulomatous disease, in which neutrophils are capable of ingesting bacteria but unable to kill catalase-positive organisms due to a defect in the production of O_2^- and $H_2O_2^-$, to such common diseases as diabetes mellitus and chronic renal failure, in which the increased risk of sepsis is probably due to multiple factors. Patients with major traumatic or thermal injury have been shown to have an increased risk of sepsis due to defects in neutrophil function[4] as well as abnormalities in T cell and Mϕ function.[16] As mentioned previously, chemotherapeutic agents that result in granulocytopenia put patients at a significantly increased risk for infection. Renal transplantation patients, with their associated immunosuppression, are also at increased risk.

Certain diseases that may have an impact on the ability of various mechanical barriers to repel bacteria include chronic obstructive pulmonary disease (ciliary dysfunction), achlorhydria and gastric outlet obstruction, prolonged stasis in the GI tract in such conditions as scleroderma, and breaks in cutaneous integrity ranging from local wounds to major thermal injury. Other conditions that may impinge negatively on the ability of patients to tolerate a septic insult include atherosclerotic cardiovascular disease with local ischemia to tissues, malnutrition, with its multiple defects in host resistance, and irradiation, which often depresses local and systemic defense mechanisms.

Although the term *reticuloendothelial system* has become relatively outmoded, the system of fixed and wandering monocyte Mϕ is still critical in host defense. Obviously splenectomy leads to abnormalities in this area, particularly in children,[17] and recent studies have suggested a monocyte defect following splenectomy.[18] Patients with diseases such as lymphoma, sarcoidosis, sickle cell disease, various autoimmune diseases, previous irradiation to the lymphoid system, and intracellular parasites are all susceptible to defects in phagocytic function in the Mϕ system. These patients should be treated with special care when undergoing surgery.

Surgical Risk Factors

In addition to the above premorbid factors, there are a number of other factors involved in surgical patients that will decrease host resistance (Table 4-3). Local wound factors that interfere with host resistance include necrotic tissue, inadequate wound perfusion or oxygenation, retained foreign body or suture material, and undrained hematoma or seroma. In general these factors interfere with host resistance either by inhibiting the delivery of neutrophils to the wound site or by inhibiting their function in the wound. Opsonic factors have been shown to be decreased in a number of wounds, which supports this concept. It follows that the surgeon must be gentle with tissue, maximize debridement of necrotic tissue, and optimize oxygenation and perfusion of surgical wounds. Although the clinical suspicion that shock places patients at risk for sepsis has been held for some time, there are only a few studies that doc-

Table 4-3. Factors in the Surgical Patient at Risk

I. Promorbid factors Diabetes COPD ASCVD Malnutrition	II. Septic challenge Inoculum Bacterial virulence Tissue trauma
III. Host resistance Primary defenses Specific immune Mφ T cells B cells Lymphokines Monokines	IV. Iatrogenic factors Antibiotic abuse Steroids Chemotherapy Nutrition Untreated shock Inadequate debridement Undrained pus

ument this.[19] Further work in this area will be necessary. Aggressive resuscitation of trauma patients with minimization of shock has led to a decrease in the incidence of sepsis and multiple organ failure.[3] Recent data on sublethal hemorrhage in a rat model suggest that decreased survival was due to an inhibition of the acute peritoneal inflammatory response.[20]

As mentioned above, intracellular alkalosis and hypoxia have a profound depressive effect on the killing actions of neutrophils and should be avoided. Steroids inhibit the ability of leukocytes to participate in the inflammatory response and have been associated with increased mortality from sepsis in several settings. The abandonment of steroids in the treatment of inhalation injury and of severe head injury in many centers is testimony to the fact that decreases in "iatrogenesis imperfecta" can improve results in critically ill surgical patients. Fibrin debris associated with disseminated intravascular coagulation may also affect phagocytic function either in neutrophils or in Mφ by impairing reticuloendothelial function. Splenectomy not only decreases reticuloendothelial function by removing 15 to 30 percent of fixed phagocytes but also has been shown to have other deleterious effects on host defense in a well-controlled rat model.[21] Dextran, stroma-free hemoglobin, fibrin debris, and transfusion reactions may also inhibit the function of fixed phagocytic cells. As mentioned above, prostaglandin E_2 stimulates inhibitory Mφ and inhibits facilitory Mφ and T helper cells. This regulatory effect may not be bad, but premature efforts to utilize prostaglandin inhibitors to prevent sepsis in patients at risk may be unwise without further study. This will be discussed in greater detail in the section on future directions.

There are a number of bacteriologic considerations that affect the surgical patient at risk. Since these have been covered well in the literature, I will only mention certain generic points. It is critical when evaluating a patient with surgical sepsis to obtain adequate cultures and to culture for anaerobes. It may even be necessary to consider laparotomy for diagnosis and microbial isolation when patients fail to improve on adequate antimicrobial therapy. Appropriate culture and sensitivity determinations will allow the surgeon to minimize the blind use of antibiotics. In addition, in our present environment, with a large number of immunosuppressed patients, it is critical to be suspicious of "non-pathogens" (e.g., *Staphylococcus epidermidis*, saprophytic fungi, and viruses). One must try to predict what bacteria will be present based on the known flora of a given portion of the GI tract or other areas of the body and select antibiotic therapy appropriately. It is critical to use an appropriate antibiotic at an adequately high dosage. For example, patients with major burns have been shown to have increased volume of distribution and increased clearance of aminoglycoside antibiotics; thus dosages used in normal patients will often result in subtherapeutic levels. In general, most patients must be monitored with aminoglycoside levels in order to ensure dosages in the therapeutic range and to prevent toxicity. It is important to repeat cultures since the flora may change.

An important thing to consider in critically ill patients is to set a *prospective* time limit for the use of antibiotics and to terminate antibiotics at this time, or sooner if possible. If the patient develops recurrent signs of infection, appropriate culturing techniques and a search for abscesses is usually more productive than changing antibiotics (what I call the "mergy-go-round phenomenon"). To every good surgeon it is anathema to rely on antibiotics for treatment of abscesses when incision and drainage constitute the treatment of choice and antibiotics often are not required.

Although a great deal has been written about prophylactic antibiotics, a few summary statements are in order. Prophylactic antibiotics have been abused to a large extent and have been responsible for the selection of resistant bacteria in numerous hospitals. Prophylactic antibiotics should be used only when the benefit/risk ratio is high. The antibiotic must be administered preoperatively and used for the anticipated flora in an appropriate concentration. Most importantly, these antibiotics must be discontinued promptly, preferably within 24 to 48 hours.[22]

Many of the successes of modern surgical care have been tied to major advances in nutritional therapy over the last 20 years. Total parenteral nutrition, as initially pioneered by Dudrick, has led to a reduction in mortality for gastrointestinal fistulae from 60 to 15 percent and has allowed a number of critically ill surgical patients to survive previously life-threatening illnesses.[23] A number of authors have looked at the interaction of host resistance, sepsis, and nutritional status.[4] Meakins and his group have shown that anergy occurs frequently in elective surgical patients and that this defect in delayed hypersensitivity can be either partially or completely reversed by aggressive nutritional support preoperatively.[24] In other studies, depressed immunocompetence of patients with protein calorie malnutrition was reversed with nutritional repletion.[23] In certain conditions, such as major thermal injury, major trauma, and sepsis, requirements may be as high as 5,000 kcal/day. Aggressive nutritional support with a combination of parenteral and enteral nutrition is critical to decrease the risk of sepsis and its associated mortality. Preoperative assessment of nutritional status in patients undergoing elective major surgery should be performed. Data in the literature would suggest that postponing elective surgery while nutritional repletion is undertaken may decrease patient morbidity and mortality.[23] More recent developments, such as the use of branched-chain amino acids in trauma patients, show some promise, but further work needs to be done in this area. An excellent review of this entire field is available for those who wish to pursue this matter further.[25]

In addition to the problems associated with certain premorbid factors, several well-documented patterns have been described in surgical patients. The association of pulmonary infection with intra-abdominal abscess has been well described. Critically ill surgical patients who develop pneumonitis should also be evaluated for intra-abdominal sepsis. The etiology of this association is not known, but it is suggested that intra-abdominal sepsis leads to a defect in pulmonary Mɸ function, which then increases the risk of pulmonary infection.[26] Various nosocomial factors that increase the risk of sepsis must be considered in all surgical patients. Prolonged utilization of foley catheters leads to a high incidence of bacteriuria with subsequent urinary tract infections. Patients on ventilatory support for more than 5 days have a high incidence of colonization of the upper respiratory tract with the attendant risk of pneumonia and ARDS. If the latter complication develops, mortality approaches 50 percent.[3]

The occurrence of infections in patients with intravenous catheters has been documented extensively in the literature. Surgical patients are particularly at risk for the complication of septic phlebitis with a septic thrombus in the vein. In a study we performed several years ago, I.V. devices were responsible for development of septic phlebitis in 54 out of 100 patients. The overall number of patients with septic emboli was 20 (17 of these had I.V.s).[27] Patients with septic phlebitis often have high fever (103.5°F or higher) in the absence of an obvious source. In this setting the index of suspicion for septic phlebitis should be high, and presently and recently cannulated veins should be examined. Excision of the vein along with antibiotic therapy appears to be the treatment of choice. Finally, it must be reiterated that failure of asepsis and antibiotic abuse contribute to nosocomial infections with bacteria that are resistant to multiple antibiotics. Careful attention to sterile technique and minimization of antibiotic abuse will go a long way toward decreasing the risk of sepsis in surgical patients.

SPECIFIC SURGICAL CONDITIONS

Extensive studies have been performed over the last several years on the interrelationship of host defenses and various surgical conditions. For instance, depression of phagocytosis in an experimental peritonitis model in dogs was recently demonstrated, but this depression could be reversed following proper surgical therapy.[18] The largest body of data on host resistance is from patients who have suffered major trauma or major thermal injury and therefore some brief comments will be made regarding these two situations.

Major Thermal Injury

It has been well documented that patients with burns are among the most susceptible to sepsis and have the largest number of abnormalities in host resistance.[29] Obviously, a major burn leads to disruption in the skin as a mechanical barrier, but problems in phagocytosis with decreased cellular immobilization and intracellular killing of bacteria have been demonstrated. In addition, levels of IgG and IgE are decreased and delayed hypersensitivity is depressed; more recently defects in specific immune function have been identified. Recently, using a murine burn model in our laboratory, we have been able to demonstrate both the elaboration of a suppressor effector factor by T cells and depressed production of interleukin 1 by Mφ.[30,31] Utilizing some fairly simple immunologic tests, it may eventually be possible to predict those burn patients at risk for life-threatening sepsis.[32]

Major Trauma

Studies of immunologic function and host resistance in major trauma patients have not progressed as rapidly as in major burn patients because of the heterogeneity of the trauma patient population. Nonetheless, several abnormalities have been identified, which suggest that further study is warranted in this area. Abnormalities in chemotaxis and neutrophil function have been associated with serum inhibitory substances, which appear to be immunosuppressive polypeptides.[34] As previously mentioned, abnormalities of T cell function arising in patients 2 weeks after splenectomy appear to be due to an inhibitory Mφ.[16,18] Also, Miller has recently identified decreases in the production of plasminogen activator and increases in production of tissue thromboplastin factor in trauma patients.[33] The exact meaning of these abnormalities is not yet clear. In recent studies in our laboratory the mitogenic responses of lymphocytes to phytohemagglutinin (PHA) from trauma patients were measured. Patients with depressed cellular PHA responses had a much higher risk of sepsis, but this abnormality could be reversed with indomethacin in vitro.[35] The possibilities for future therapy in trauma patients based on these data are exciting, but it is premature to contemplate such studies at this point without further understanding of the complex immune abnormalities following major trauma.

FUTURE DIRECTIONS

Numerous possibilities loom on the horizon for further research and possible therapeutic intervention in the critically ill surgical patient at risk for sepsis. Some modalities have already been tested in humans, whereas others have only been tested in animals or are conceptual possibilities. One very real therapeutic application of the above-mentioned data is the increasing trend to conserve the spleen whenever possible or to autotransplant splenic tissue in patients following splenic injury. There is good experimental support for this approach,[36] and a small body of data is accumulating in humans. Following splenectomy in an animal model, glucan, a nonspecific immunostimulant, has been shown to have a protective effect.[37] Glucan has also had a protective effect in a model of *Staphylococcus aureus* bacteremia associated with enhancement in serum lysosome activity.[38]

Significant interest has been generated by efforts to utilize antisera to *Escherichia coli* J5 as a vaccine. Enhanced opsonization and systemic clearance of bacteria resulted in improved survival in an animal model,[39] and suggestive evidence has been presented utilizing this modality in humans.[40] The possibility of improving opsonic function by utilization of cryoprecipitate to reverse deficiencies in opsonic α_2-surface binding glycoprotein has been tested in trauma patients with some success,[40] but the exact role of this therapy is undetermined as yet.

Controversies surround efforts to manipulate the immune response with agents such as thymosin (stimulator of T cell production), indomethacin (prostaglandin inhibitor), H_2 blockers (inhibitors of surface membrane H_2 receptors on suppressor cells), low-dose cyclophosphamide (inhibitor of T suppressor cell proliferation), scavengers of free radicals, levamisole, and plasmapheresis. Some of these techniques have been utilized only on experimental animals, whereas encouraging results have been obtained in certain clinical situations (e.g., plasmapheresis following major thermal injury). Perhaps the most important caveat that needs to be made regarding immunotherapy is that the host resistance system is very delicately balanced. Efforts to stimulate the immune system may result in autoimmune or inflammatory abnormalities, which might be just as deleterious to the critically ill patient as the negative regulatory effects of immunosuppression. Although exciting advances have been made in this field in the last 10 years, our knowledge is still incomplete, and therapeutic modulation of the immune system in humans must proceed with great caution.

REFERENCES

1. Baker CC, Oppenheimer L, Lewis FR, et al: The epidemiology of trauma deaths. Am J Surg 140:144, 1980
2. Polk HC: Consensus summary on infection. J Trauma 19:894, 1979
3. Baker CC, Degutis LC, DeSantis J, et al: The effect of a trauma service on trauma care in a university hospital. Am J Surg 149:453, 1985
4. Meakins JL, Christou NV, Shizgal HM, et al: Therapeutic approaches to anergy in surgical patients. Ann Surg 190:286, 1979
5. Newman SL, Johnson RB Jr: Role of binding through C3b and IgG polymorphonuclear neutrophil function: studies with trypsin-generated C3b. J Immunol 123:1839, 1979
6. Anderson DC, Schmalsteig FC, Finegold MJ et al: The severe and moderate phenotypes of heritable Mac-1, LFA-1 deficiency: their quantitative definition and relation to leukocyte dysfunction and clinical features. J Infect Dis 152:668, 1985
7. Klebanoff SJ: Antimicrobial mechanisms in neutrophilic PMN leukocytes. Semin Hematol 12:117, 1975
8. Hohn DC, MacKay RD, Halliday B, Hunt TK: Effect of O_2 tension on microbicidal function of leukocytes in wound and in vitro. Surg Forum 27:18, 1976
9. Cates KL: Host factors in bacteremia. Am J Med 75(1B):19, 1983

10. Bodey GP, Rodriquez V, Chang H, et al: Fever and incidence of infection in leukemia patients. Cancer 41:1610, 1978
11. Strauss RG, Connett JE, Gale RP, et al: A controlled trial of prophylactic granulocyte transfusions during initial induction chemotherapy for acute myelogenous leukemia. N Engl J Med 305:597, 1981
12. Jacob HS, Craddock PR, Hammerschmidt DE, et al: Complement-induced granulocyte aggregation. N Engl J Med 302:789, 1980
13. Frank MM: The complement system in host defense and inflammation. Rev Infect Dis 1:483, 1979
14. Paul WE, Fathman CG, Metzger H: Annual Review of Immunology. Vol 1. Annual Reviews, Inc., Palo Alto, Calif. 1983
15. Janeway C, Jason J: How T-lymphocytes recognize antigen. CRC Crit Rev Immunol 1:133, 1980
15a. Gallin JI, Fauci AS. Chronic granulomatous disease. Adv. Host Defense Mech 1:1, 1983
16. Baker CC, Miller CL, Trunkey DD, et al: Identity of mononuclear cells which compromise the resistance of trauma patients. J Surg Res 26:478, 1979
17. Singer DB: Post-splenectomy sepsis. Perspect Pediatr Pathol 1:285, 1973
18. Miller CL, Baker CC: Development of inhibitory macrophages (Mφ) after splenectomy. Transplant Proc 11:1460, 1979
19. Baker CC, Miller CL, Trunkey DD: Correlation of traumatic shock with immunocompetence and sepsis. Surg Forum 30:20, 1979
20. Fink MP, Gardiner M, MacVittie TJ: Sublethal hemorrhage impairs the acute peritoneal inflammatory response in the rat. J Trauma 25:234, 1985
21. Chaudry IH, Tabata Y, Schleck S, et al: Effect of splenectomy on reticuloendothelial function and survival following sepsis. J Trauma 20:649, 1980
22. Nichols RL: Postoperative wound infection. N Engl J Med 307:1701, 1982
23. Law DK, Dudrick SJ, Abdou NI: Immunocompetence of patients with protein-calorie malnutrition: the effects of nutritional repletion. Ann Intern Med 79:545, 1973
24. Pietsch JB, Meakins JL, MacLean LD: The delayed hypersensitivity response: application in surgery. Surgery 82:349, 1977
25. Suskind RW (ed): Malnutrition and the Immune Response. Vol 7. Raven Press, New York, 1977
26. Richardson JD, DeCamp MM, Garrison RN, Fry DE: Pulmonary infection complicating intra-abdominal sepsis: clinical and experimental observations. Ann Surg 195:732, 1982
27. Baker CC, Peterson SR, Sheldon GF: Septic phlebitis: a neglected disease. Am J Surg 138:97, 1979
28. Palmer MA, Bornside GH, Nance FC: Sepsis-induced depression of phagocytosis in experimental canine peritonitis. Ann Surg 48:520, 1982
29. Baxter C: The current status of burn research. J Trauma 14:1, 1974
30. Kupper TS, Baker CC, Ferguson TA, Green DR: A burn induced Ly-2 suppressor T cell lowers resistance to bacterial infection. J Surg Res 38:606, 1985
31. Kupper TS, Green DR, Durum SK, Baker CC: Defective antigen presentation to a cloned T helper cell by macrophages from burned mice can be restored with interleukin 1. Surgery 98:199, 1985
32. Baker CC, Trunkey DD, Baker WJ: A simple method of predicting severe sepsis in burn patients. Am J Surg 139:513, 1980
33. Miller SE, Miller CL, Trunkey DD: The immune consequences of trauma. Surg Clin North Am 63:167, 1982

34. Christou NV, Meakins JL: Neutrophil function in surgical patients: two inhibitors of granulocyte chemotaxis associated with sepsis. J Surg Res 26:355, 1979
35. Faist E, Kupper TS, Baker CC, et al: Depression of cellular immunity after major injury: its association with post-traumatic complications and its restoration with immunomodulating agents. Arch Surg (in press)
36. Likhite VV: Protection against fulminant sepsis in splenectomized mice by implantation of autochthonous splenic tissue. Exp Int 6:433, 1978
37. Browder W, Rakinic J, McNamee R, et al: Protective effect of nonspecific immunostimulation in post-splenectomy sepsis. J Surg Res 35:474, 1983
38. Kokoshis PL, Williams DL, Cook JA, DiLuzio NR: Increased resistance to *Staphylococcus aureus* infection and enhancement in serum lysozyme activity by glucan. Science 199:1340, 1978
39. Dunn DL, Ferguson RM: Immunotherapy of gram-negative bacterial sepsis: enhanced survival in a guinea pig model by use of rabbit anti-serum to *Escherichia coli* J5. Surgery 92:212, 1982
40. Saba TM, Blumenstock FA, Scovill WA, Bernard H: Cryoprecipitate reversal of opsonic α_2-surface binding glycoprotein deficiency in septic surgical and trauma patients. Science 201:622, 1978

5 | Strategies to Counteract Antimicrobial Resistance

Christine C. Sanders

Certain aspects of infectious diseases are analogous to war. The microbes are the enemy, the hospital a major battlefield, and antimicrobial agents the primary weapons. In this analogy microbial drug resistance must represent the fallout from the use of these weapons. When antibiotics were relatively small weapons of narrow spectrum, the fallout was fairly easy to deal with—the strategy to counteract this resistance primarily involved the design of bigger, broader-spectrum weapons. Now that the weaponry has progressed from rifles and cannons to "the bomb," the fallout from the use of antimicrobial weapons is much more difficult to control.

To adequately assess strategies to counteract resistance to antimicrobial agents one must consider the mechanisms responsible, as well as the clinical settings in which resistance has been encountered. Strategies that have back-fired must also be identified before newer, more successful approaches can be designed.

STRATEGIES BASED ON MECHANISM OF RESISTANCE

Altered Drug Targets

One of the three major mechanisms whereby microorganisms may resist antimicrobial agents involves alteration of the drug's target so that it is no longer susceptible to the action of the drug (Table 5-1).[1] The drug's target is often an

Table 5-1. Approaches to Counteract Resistance Due to an Altered Drug Target

Antibiotic	Altered Target	Countermeasure	Example
Nalidixic acid	DNA gyrase	Newer quinolones	Ciprofloxacin, norfloxacin
Sulfonamides	Dihydropteroate synthetase	Synergistic combination	Sulfamethoxazole/ trimethoprim
Penicillins	Penicillin-binding proteins	?	

enzyme, and its alteration usually involves a mutation within the chromosome, although resistance mediated via this mechanism can also be conferred by a plasmid. Owing to the specificity of the interaction between the drug and its target, this mechanism usually causes a relatively narrow spectrum of resistance, which is confined to some, but not all, related agents within the same class.

There are numerous examples of antibiotics for which this type of resistance has drastically reduced the clinical settings in which they can be used effectively (Table 5-1). Resistance to nalidixic acid due to an altered DNA gyrase[2] may be counteracted by any of a number of newer quinolone antibiotics,[3,4] which appear to penetrate the bacterial cell better and have a higher affinity for DNA gyrase than does nalidixic acid. Results of initial clinical trials suggest that these new quinolones may help to solve many of the problems posed by nalidixic acid–resistant bacteria.[5–11] Resistance to the sulfonamides due to an altered target dihydropteroate synthetase has limited the usefulness of this family of drugs in the treatment and prevention of many infections, including that due to the meningococcus.[12,13] To counteract this resistance the combination of sulfamethoxazole/trimethoprim has been designed; this produces a synergistic double blockade on the folic acid synthetic pathway, even in certain sulfonamide-resistant strains.[14]

Resistance to various β-lactam antibiotics mediated by alterations in the drugs' primary targets—the penicillin-binding proteins—is being increasingly recognized in clinical isolates.[1] This mechanism appears to be responsible for much of the penicillin resistance encountered in clinical isolates of *Neisseria gonorrhoeae*[15] and *Streptococcus pneumoniae*,[16,17] as well as for methicillin resistance in *Staphylococcus aureus*.[18–22] To date there has been no effective approach designed to specifically counteract this mechanism of resistance.

Inactivating Enzymes

A second mechanism of resistance involves the ability of microorganisms to inactivate an antibiotic.[12,23,24] This mechanism is by far the one most frequently encountered among clinical isolates and can be mediated by either plasmid or chromosomal genes. Depending upon the substrate specificity of

Table 5-2. Approaches to Counteract Resistance Due to Inactivating Enzymes

Antibiotic	Enzymes	Countermeasure	Examples
Aminoglycosides	Acetylases, phosphorylases, nucleotidylases	Enzyme-resistant drugs	Amikacin, netilmicin
β-Lactams	β-Lactamases	β-Lactamase-resistant drugs	Penicillinase-resistant penicillins; second- and third-generation cephalosporins
		Enzyme inhibitor + enzyme-labile drug	Augmentin

the inactivating enzyme, this mechanism can confer either narrow- or broad-spectrum resistance among similar drug classes.

The production of inactivating enzymes is probably the single most important mechanism of resistance to the aminoglycosides and β-lactam antibiotics (Table 5-2). This mechanism has been successfully counteracted in many instances through the design of new drugs that are not susceptible to inactivation by these enzymes.[24-29] Examples of enzyme-stable aminoglycosides currently available for clinical use in the United States are amikacin and netilmicin. Among the β-lactam drugs, the penicillinase-resistant penicillins, such as methicillin, nafcillin, and the isoxazolyl penicillins, were the first enzyme-stable drugs of this class.[27] They have proved invaluable for treatment of infections due to penicillinase-producing *S. aureus*. Several of the newer second- and third-generation cephalosporins are significantly less affected by the plasmid-mediated β-lactamases of gram-negative bacteria.[28,29] Also, enzyme inhibitors such as clavulanic acid and sulbactam, used in combination with an enzyme-labile drug, appear to be able to block resistance due to many of the plasmid-mediated β-lactamases.[30,31] Unfortunately, neither of these strategies has been very successful in counteracting resistance due to certain chromosomally mediated β-lactamases. This problem will be addressed in the next section.

Impermeability

This third major mechanism of antimicrobial resistance is the least well studied or understood.[25,32-34] It usually involves a chromosomal mutation, which effects a change within the outer structure of the microorganism; this in turn diminishes the ability of antibiotics to penetrate or to be transported into the microbial cell. In gram-negative bacteria this often involves a change in outer membrane proteins, or porins, through which the drugs normally enter the cell. Since many dissimilar drugs may use the same route of entrance, this mechanism can result in a very broad spectrum of resistance, which involves many drugs of unrelated classes. To date no strategy has been designed that

Table 5-3. Chromosomal, Inducible β-Lactamases

Characteristically Found in	Antibiotics Affected by
Enterobacter spp	Second-generation cephalosporins
Citrobacter freundii	Cephamycins
Serratia spp	Third-generation cephalosporins
Indole-positive *Proteus*	Broad-spectrum penicillins
Providencia spp	Monobactams
Pseudomonas aeruginosa	
Other nonfermenters	

would predictably counteract this type of resistance. Unfortunately, this mechanism is responsible for resistance to aminoglycosides, β-lactams, and quinolone antibiotics in an increasing number of clinical isolates.[35–39]

STRATEGIES THAT HAVE BACKFIRED

The newer-generation cephalosporins were designed to enhance the antibacterial spectrum of this drug class through improved potency and decreased susceptibility to hydrolysis by β-lactamases. As mentioned, these agents have proved effective against many bacteria that possess plasmid-mediated β-lactamases; however, unanticipated problems have arisen in using them against bacteria possessing chromosomally mediated β-lactamases.[40,41] These problems include rapid development of resistance, which can occur during therapy, even with seemingly appropriate doses of the drugs. This resistance usually involves multiple antibiotics within the β-lactam family.

Numerous therapeutic failures associated with the development of multiple β-lactam resistance have been documented for the newer enzyme-stable β-lactam antibiotics.[40–54] The drugs involved have included the newer second- and third-generation cephalosporins as well as aztreonam, a new monobactam. In most instances the patient either failed to respond to therapy or relapsed despite apparent sensitivity of the initial isolate to the drug. The organisms most commonly involved have been *Enterobacter* spp, *Serratia* spp, and *Pseudomonas aeruginosa*. The use of combination therapy has not prevented this emergence of resistance.[35,46,54]

In the cases examined to date the infecting strain which developed resistance has possessed an inducible, chromosomally mediated β-lactamase. This enzyme is primarily a cephalosporinase, although it will inactivate the penicillins.[23] It is characteristically found in a number of gram-negative bacteria (Table 5-3). Development of resistance has been found to be due to the induction of β-lactamase in the infecting strain. Once induced, the enzyme is capable of mediating resistance to a number of diverse β-lactams, including those previously thought to be enzyme-stable (Table 5-3).[40]

How frequently are clinical problems with this type of resistance encountered? From several of the larger clinical trials with the newer cephalosporins it appears that emergence of resistance in *P. aeruginosa* may occur in approximately one-third of patients.[40] Although precise figures for all organisms possessing inducible β-lactamases are not yet available, the potential size of the problem can be estimated. On the basis of data provided by the most recent Study on the Efficacy of Nosocomial Infection Control Project Report[55] and the 1983 National Nosocomial Infections Study,[56] there could be as many as 760,000 patients per year in U.S. hospitals with nosocomially acquired infections due to *Enterobacter* spp, *Serratia* spp, or *P. aeruginosa*, three of the most commonly encountered bacteria with inducible β-lactamases. If one of the newer enzyme-stable β-lactams is used to treat these infections and if failure due to induction of β-lactamase occurs in 10 to 30 percent of patients, then emergence of resistance could potentially be encountered in 76,000 to 250,000 patients in a single year.

There are also data indicating that these multiply resistant organisms are spreading within the hospital.[40,56-58] There have been outbreaks of nosocomial infections due to multiply resistant *Enterobacter cloacae* and *P. aeruginosa* in burn and intensive care units during periods of heavy use of the newer β-lactam drugs. Surveillance programs in a number of hospitals, both in the United States and abroad, have documented significant decreases in the susceptibility of organisms with inducible β-lactamases to the newer generation of β-lactam drugs.[40,56-58] Similar changes have not been observed for organisms lacking these enzymes.

Can this resistance associated with the use of the newer cephalosporins be avoided? Probably not entirely. To date the only strategy available for avoiding this resistance involves judicious use of the drugs, which includes avoidance of their use in surgical prophylaxis and empiric therapy. These drugs should be used only in those few clinical settings wherein they have been proved more effective than older antibiotics. When resistance does occur, strict adherence to infection control procedures should help to limit its spread.

FUTURE STRATEGIES

Only through a thorough knowledge of the mechanisms responsible for antimicrobial resistance can effective strategies be designed to counteract this resistance. The newer cephalosporins backfired in the case of inducible β-lactamases because the strategy was based upon the assumption that in vitro enzyme stability was all that was necessary to produce an effective drug. This assumption was valid for β-lactamases of gram-positive but not gram-negative bacteria. It is now quite clear that in gram-negative bacteria β-lactamases are much more efficient in mediating resistance than any in vitro assay ever predicted. This is due to the fact that these enzymes, in situ within the periplasmic space of the organisms, can achieve a concentration greatly in excess of the drug concentration; such conditions are not simulated in any assay performed in vitro. Thus, strategies to overcome resistance mediated by β-lactamases in gram-negative bacteria must now be redesigned to take into account the newly described conditions that can occur within the milieu of the bacterial cell.

In the war against infection one must use weapons cautiously and plan strategies carefully. It is all too clear that merely designing bigger "bombs" is no longer an effective strategy for counteracting antimicrobial resistance—this approach will only make the fallout much more difficult to handle.

REFERENCES

1. Reynolds, PE: Resistance of the antibiotic target site. Br Med Bull 40:3, 1984
2. Cozzarelli NR: The mechanism of action of inhibitors of DNA synthesis. Annu Rev Biochem 46:641, 1977
3. Smith JT: Mutational resistance to 4-quinolone antibacterial agents. Eur J Clin Microbiol 3:347, 1984
4. Inoue S, Ohue T, Yamagishi J, et al: Mode of incomplete cross-resistance among pipemidic, piromidic, and nalidixic acids. Antimicrob Agents Chemother 14:240, 1978
5. Haase DA, Harding GKM, Thomson MJ, et al: Comparative trial of norfloxacin and trimethoprim-sulfamethoxazole in the treatment of women with localized, acute, symptomatic urinary tract infections and antimicrobial effect on periurethral and fecal microflora. Antimicrob Agents Chemother 26:481, 1984
6. Ramirez CA, Bran JL, Mejia CR, Garcia JF: Open, prospective study of the clinical efficacy of ciprofloxacin. Antimicrob Agents Chemother 28:128, 1985
7. Thomas MG, Ellis-Pegler RB: Enoxacin treatment of urinary tract infections. J Antimicrob Chemother 15:759, 1985
8. Eron LJ, Harvey L, Hixon DL, Poretz DM: Ciprofloxacin therapy of infections caused by *Pseudomonas aeruginosa* and other resistant bacteria. Antimicrob Agents Chemother 27:308, 1985
9. Leigh DA, Emmanuel FXS: The treatment of *Pseudomonas aeruginosa* urinary tract infections with norfloxacin. J Antimicrob Chemother 13:suppl B, 85, 1984
10. Reeves DS, Lacey RW, Mummery RV, et al: Treatment of acute urinary infection by norfloxacin or nalidixic acid/citrate: a multi-centre comparative study. J Antimicrob Chemother 13:suppl B, 99, 1984
11. Vogel R, Deaney NB, Round EM, et al: Norfloxacin, amoxycillin, cotrimoxazole and nalidixic acid. A summary of 3-day and 7-day therapy studies in the treatment of urinary tract infections. J Antimicrob Chemother 13:suppl B, 113, 1984
12. Benveniste R, Davies J: Mechanisms of antibiotic resistance in bacteria. Annu Rev Biochem 42:471, 1973
13. Smith JT, Amyes SGB: Bacterial resistance to antifolate chemotherapeutic agents mediated by plasmids. Br Med Bull 40:42, 1984
14. Hitchings GH: Mechanism of action of trimethoprim-sulfamethoxazole. J Infect Dis, suppl 128:S433, 1973
15. Dougherty TJ, Koller AE, Tomasz A: Penicillin-binding proteins of penicillin-susceptible and intrinsically resistant *Neisseria gonorrhoeae*. Antimicrob Agents Chemother 18:730, 1980
16. Hakenbeck R, Tarpay M, Tomasz A: Multiple changes of penicillin-binding proteins in penicillin-resistant clinical isolates of *Streptococcus pneumoniae*. Antimicrob Agents Chemother 17:364, 1980
17. Zighelboim S, Tomasz A: Penicillin-binding proteins of multiply antibiotic-resistant South African strains of *Streptococcus pneumoniae*. Antimicrob Agents Chemother 17:434, 1980

18. Hayes MV, Curtis NAC, Wyke AW, Ward JB: Decreased affinity of a penicillin-binding protein for β-lactam antibiotics in a clinical isolate of *Staphylococcus aureus* resistant to methicillin. FEMS Microbiol Lett 10:119, 1981
19. Brown DFJ, Reynolds PE: Intrinsic resistance to beta-lactam antibiotics in *Staphylococcus aureus*. FEBS Lett 122:275, 1980
20. Hartman B, Tomasz A: Altered penicillin-binding proteins in methicillin-resistant strains of *Staphylococcus aureus*. Antimicrob Agents Chemother 19:726, 1981
21. Rossi L, Tonin E, Cheng YR, Fontana R: Regulation of penicillin-binding protein activity: description of a methicillin-inducible penicillin-binding protein in *Staphylococcus aureus*. Antimicrob Agents Chemother 27:828, 1985
22. Ubukata K, Yamashita N, Konno M: Occurrence of a β-lactam-inducible penicillin-binding protein in methicillin-resistant staphylococci. Antimicrob Agents Chemother 27:851, 1985
23. Sykes RB, Matthew M: The β-lactamases of gram-negative bacteria and their role in resistance to β-lactam antibiotics. J Antimicrob Chemother 2:115, 1976
24. Davies J, Smith DI: Plasmid-determined resistance to antimicrobial agents. Annu Rev Microbiol 32:469, 1978
25. Phillips I, Shannon K: Aminoglycoside resistance. Br Med Bull 40:28, 1984
26. Davies J, Courvalin P: Mechanisms of resistance to aminoglycosides. Am J Med 62:868, 1977
27. Richmond MH: β-Lactam antibiotics and β-lactamases: two sides of a continuing story. Rev Infect Dis 1:30, 1979
28. Neu HC: Factors that affect the *in-vitro* activity of cephalosporin antibiotics. J Antimicrob Chemother 10:suppl C, 11, 1982
29. Fisher J: β-Lactams resistant to hydrolysis by the β-lactamases. p. 33. In Bryan LE (ed): Antimicrobial Drug Resistance. Academic Press, Inc., New York, 1984
30. Cole M: β-Lactams as β-lactamase inhibitors. Philos Trans R Soc Lond [Biol] 289:207, 1980
31. Wise R: β-Lactamase inhibitors. J Antimicrob Chemother 9(Suppl B):31, 1982
32. Costerton JW, Cheng KJ: The role of the bacterial cell envelope in antibiotic resistance. J Antimicrob Chemother 1:363, 1975
33. Chopra I, Ball P: Transport of antibiotics into bacteria. Adv Microb Physiol 23:183, 1982
34. Yoshimura F, Nikaido H: Diffusion of beta-lactam antibiotics through the porin channels of *Escherichia coli* K-12. Antimicrob Agents Chemother 27:84, 1985
35. Preheim LC, Penn RG, Sanders CC, et al: Emergence of resistance to β-lactam and aminoglycoside antibiotics during moxalactam therapy of *Pseudomonas aeruginosa* infections. Antimicrob Agents Chemother 22:1037, 1982
36. Goldstein FW, Gutmann L, Williamson R, et al: In vivo and in vitro emergence of simultaneous resistance to both beta-lactam and aminoglycoside antibiotics in a strain of *Serratia marcescens*. Ann Microbiol (Paris) 134A:329, 1983
37. Gutmann L, Williamson R, Moreau N, et al: Cross-resistance to nalidixic acid, trimethoprim, and chloramphenicol associated alterations in outer membrane proteins of *Klebsiella, Enterobacter* and *Serratia*. J Infect Dis 151:501, 1985
38. Mirelman I, Nuchamowitz Y, Rubinstein E: Insensitivity of peptidoglycan biosynthetic reactions to β-lactam antibiotics in a clinical isolate of *Pseudomonas aeruginosa*. Antimicrob Agents Chemother 19:687, 1981
39. Irvin RT, Govan JWR, Fykfe JAM, Costerton JW: Heterogeneity of antibiotic resistance in mucoid isolates of *Pseudomonas aeruginosa* obtained from cystic fibrosis patients: role of outer membrane proteins. Antimicrob Agents Chemother 19:1056, 1981

40. Sanders CC, Sanders WE Jr: Microbial resistance to newer generation beta-lactam antibiotics: clinical and laboratory implications. J Infect Dis 151:399, 1985
41. Collatz E, Gutmann L, Williamson R, Acar JF: Development of resistance to beta-lactam antibiotics with special reference to third-generation cephalosporins. J Antimicrob Chemother 14:Suppl B, 13, 1984
42. File TM Jr, Tan JS, Salstrom SJ: Clinical evaluation of ceftriaxone. Clin Ther 5:653, 1984
43. Rapp RP, Young B, Foster TS, et al: Ceftazimide versus tobramycin/ticarcillin in treating hospital acquired pneumonia and bacteremia. Pharmacotherapy 4:211, 1984
44. Benn RAV, Kemp RJ: Effect of antibiotic use on the incidence of cephalosporin resistance in two Australian hospitals. J Antimicrob Chemother 14:suppl B, 71, 1984
45. Reitberg DP, Cumbo TJ, Schentag JJ: Cefmenoxime in the treatment of nosocomial pneumonias in critical care patients. J Antimicrob Chemother 14:suppl B, 81, 1984
46. Winston DJ, Barnes RC, Ho WG, et al: Moxalactam plus piperacillin versus moxalactam plus amikacin in febrile granulocytopenic patients. Am J Med 77:442, 1984
47. DeMaria A, McCabe WR: A clinical study of moxalactam in the treatment of infections due to gram negative bacilli. Scand J Infect Dis 16:83, 1984
48. Scully BE, Neu HC: Ceftriaxone in the treatment of serious infections, particularly after surgery. Am J Surg 148(4A):35, 1984
49. Bradsher RW, Snow RM: Ceftriaxone treatment of skin and soft tissue infections in a once daily regimen. Am J Med 77(4C):63, 1984
50. Nichols L, Gudmundsson S, Maki DG: Experience with cefsulodin therapy for lower respiratory tract infections caused by *Pseudomonas aeruginosa* in adults without cystic fibrosis or granulocytopenia. Rev Infect Dis 6:suppl 3, S711, 1984
51. Caplan DB, Buchanan CN: Treatment of lower respiratory tract infections due to *Pseudomonas aeruginosa* in patients with cystic fibrosis. Rev Infect Dis 6:suppl 3, S705, 1984
52. Bergin CJ, Phillips P, Chan RMT, et al: Treatment of *Pseudomonas* and *Serratia* infections with ceftazidime. J Antimicrob Chemother 15:613, 1985
53. Dworzack DL, Bartelt MA, Baily R Jr, Fitzgibbons RJ Jr: Emergence of resistance to aztreonam. Clin Pharmacol 3:467, 1984
54. Jarlier V, Philippon A, Nicolas MH, et al: *Enterobacter cloacae*: émergence *in vivo* d'un variant résistant aux nouvelles β-lactamines lors d'un traitement par lamoxactam-gentamicine. Pathol Biol (Paris) 32:399, 1984
55. Haley RW, Culver DH, White JW, et al: The nationwide nosocomial infection rate: a new need for vital statistics. Am J Epidemiol 121:159, 1985
56. Centers for Disease Control: Nosocomial infection surveillance, 1983. In CDC Surveillance Summaries 33 (No. 2SS):9SS, 1984
57. Benn RAV, Kemp RJ: Effect of antibiotic use on the incidence of cephalosporin resistance in two Australian hospitals. J Antmicrob Chemother 14:suppl B, 71, 1984
58. Jarlier V, Bismuth R, Nicolas MH, et al: Survey of the phenotypes of susceptibility to β-lactams in Enterobacteriaceae at the Pitie-Salpetriere Hospital. J Antimicrob Chemother 14:suppl B, 59, 1984

6 | Selected Recent Advances in the Therapy of Central Nervous System Infections

Ralph G. Dacey, Jr.

NEUROSURGICAL INFECTIONS RELATED TO TRAUMA

One of the major objectives in the treatment of patients with open or penetrating craniocerebral trauma is the prevention of later central nervous system (CNS) infection (see Fig. 6-1). Much of the data on such injuries has come from military neurosurgeons, and the importance of extensive debridement has been emphasized because of the nature of wartime injuries.[1,2] Recent civilian experience has provided a somewhat different approach, which relies on rapid availability of neurosurgical care, computed tomographic (CT) scanning, and parenterally administered antibiotics.

Fractures of the skull base sometimes cause cerebrospinal fluid (CSF) fistulae, providing a route for access of bacteria to the subarachnoid space. These fistulae become clinically apparent as CSF rhinorrhea or otorrhea. Most post-traumatic leaks cease spontaneously within days, but treatment is indicated for those that persist beyond 2 weeks. Although the incidence of meningitis or brain abscess after basilar skull fracture is low, 5 to 25 percent of

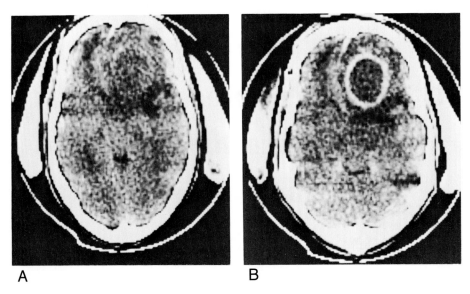

A   B

Fig. 6-1. Frontal brain abscess complicating trauma. This patient sustained a frontal impact during an automobile accident and suffered multiple facial fractures; the patient appeared clinically to have sustained a basilar skull fracture, but no CSF fistula and no comminuted fractures communicating with the sinuses were apparent. (A) Unenhanced scan showed irregular areas of high density. (B) An enhanced scan showed a well-encapsulated brain abscess, which responded to systemic antibiotics and multiple burr hole drainage procedures. Cultures eventually confirmed a polymicrobial infection with mixed aerobic and anaerobic streptococci.

patients with *persistent* CSF leaks will develop meningitis.[3-5] *Streptococcus pneumoniae* is the most common organism isolated in this setting.

Computed tomographic metrizamide cisternography has dramatically facilitated accurate preoperative localization of CSF fistulae. Metrizamide in low concentrations is introduced into the lumbar cistern, and a combination of axial and coronal scans is obtained to demonstrate the first site of appearance of metrizamide in the paranasal sinuses or middle ear. This study has permitted more restricted procedures to be performed for direct repair of dural defects after head injury.

The great potential for post-traumatic meningitis to cause adverse outcomes has prompted the use of prophylactic antibiotics in patients with basilar skull fracture with and without CSF leak. Ignelzi and VanderArk studied 129 patients with basilar skull fracture.[6] Two groups were studied sequentially; one group received antibiotic prophylaxis with ampicillin or cephalothin, and the other received none. No difference was found in the low incidence of infection in the two groups. Similarly, Hoff et al. found no infections in 160 patients with basilar skull fracture treated either with placebo or penicillin in a randomized clinical trial.[7] In another randomized trial Klastersky et al. found that penicillin had no effect on the incidence of meningitis in this situation. Haines has concluded that a reasoned approach based on current data would be to withhold antibiotics from patients with basilar skull fracture and no overt CSF leak while conducting a large randomized trial to determine if prophylaxis is useful in those patients with CSF leak.[8]

With adequate and rapid debridement contaminated cranial wounds can be managed with a low infection rate, irrespective of whether antibiotics are used or not.[9] Primary replacement of cranial fragments at the time of depressed fracture debridement has been accomplished without an increased incidence of infection, although most neurosurgeons administer antibiotics in this situation.[10-12]

SUBDURAL EMPYEMA

Subdural empyema is an extremely serious intracranial infection, which usually occurs as a complication of frontoethmoidal sinusitis. A critical delay in diagnosis of this disease often occurs because the need for surgical drainage of the collection is not immediately appreciated, since the manifestations of the disease may be similar to those of meningitis or viral encephalitis.[13] As experience accumulates with the CT appearances of subdural empyema, rapid diagnosis should be facilitated. The early appearance of subdural empyema

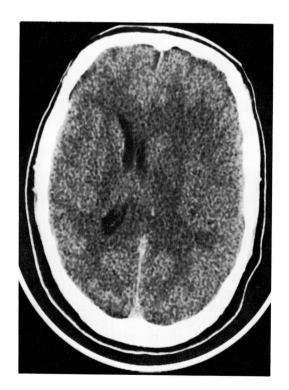

Fig. 6-2. CT appearance of subdural empyema. This enhanced CT scan shows effacement of the left lateral ventricle and shift of the pineal gland and septum pellucidum from left to right. At craniotomy the patient proved to have a large liquid subdural empyema. No extracranial source for the infection was found.

may consist solely of a mass effect, with shift of midline structures and effacement of the lateral ventricle without an apparent extracerebral collection (Fig. 6-2).[14,15] Subdural pus collections frequently occur in subfrontal and interhemispheric locations.[16]

Medical management of subdural empyema should be directed at anaerobic organisms and is crucial in halting the progression of the infection. Surgical drainage is required in almost all cases, since the infection occurs in a relatively avascular plane between the arachnoid and dura.

The surgical management of subdural empyema must be individualized to provide optimal drainage. Multiple burr holes may be sufficient in some cases when accompanied by copious irrigation. However, most patients will require an osteoplastic craniotomy to provide adequate access to frontal and interhemispheric regions. The pus is frequently tenacious and may extend across superficial layers of the arachnoid, making it difficult to remove from the cortical sulci. Closed system drains may be left in the subdural space for 24 to 48 hours.

BRAIN ABSCESS

Recently a number of factors has led to changes in the presentation and therapy of patients with brain abscess. More immunocompromised patients are presenting with complex neurologic illnesses requiring new approaches to diagnosis and treatment. New antibiotics and improved diagnostic neuroimaging modalities have allowed selected patients to be managed without neurosurgical procedures, but these developments have not simplified the management of patients with brain abscess. If anything, more collaboration between the physician and the neurosurgeon is now needed for the successful management of these patients.

Pathogenesis of Brain Abscess

Brain abscess usually occurs as a result of direct spread from a contiguous paranasal sinus infection or metastatic spread from a distant infection, usually in the chest. Less frequently, brain abscess complicates cranial trauma in which a dural opening has occurred. The mechanism whereby bacteria gain access to the brain from the paranasal sinus and mastoid air cells is thought to involve inflamed or thrombosed diploic veins which traverse the subarachnoid space in the frontal and temporal areas. Metastatic brain abscess usually develops in the distribution of the middle cerebral artery after hematogenous spread from pulmonary, dental, or cardiac sources.[17–19]

Experimental models of brain abscess have provided much information about the components of the cerebral response to bacterial inoculation in animals. For most models direct injection of bacteria in agar or of some other foreign material is required to produce an abscess. Molinari et al. were able

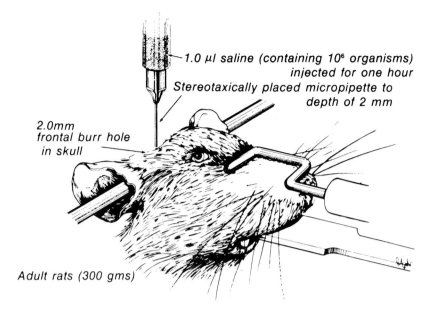

1.0 µl saline (containing 10⁶ organisms)
injected for one hour
Stereotaxically placed micropipette to
depth of 2 mm

2.0mm
frontal burr hole
in skull

Adult rats (300 gms)

Fig. 6-3. Production of experimental brain abscess in the rat. In this model, developed by Winn et al., a stereotaxic microinjection of 1 L of isotonic saline containing 10⁶ bacteria reproducibly causes brain abscess in the frontal lobe of the rat without associated meningitis or the need for a foreign body to be implanted. (Winn HR, Mendes M, Moore P et al: Production of experimental brain abscess in the rat. J Neurosurg 51:685, 1979.)

to produce brain abscess in dogs by the intra-arterial injection of silicone rubber cylinders coated with bacteria.[20] Winn et al. developed a model of brain abscess in the rat by injecting high concentrations of bacteria in small volumes of saline at very slow rates through a stereotaxic needle (Fig. 6-3).[21] These studies indicate that significant host defense mechanisms exist to prevent the establishment of brain abscess. For an abscess to occur these mechanisms must be overcome by the presence of a foreign body or very high bacterial inocula. The studies of Winn et al. indicate that brain is relatively more susceptible to bacterial infection than is skin (Fig. 6-4).[22]

The cellular response in cerebral infection begins almost immediately. Winn et al. noted mass effect and collapse of the ipsilateral ventricle within 48 hours after infection. At 2 days the lesions were characterized by a coalescent inflammatory response and cerebral necrosis. Collagen in the abscess wall was first detected at 10 days, although a glial reaction surrounding the inflammatory exudate was noted at 4 days. Britt et al. reported similar findings in their abscess model in dogs,[23,24] noting the appearance of fibroblasts with surrounding reticulin as early as 4 days after injection; mature collagen appeared at 10 days, with increasing numbers of macrophages and fibroblasts. Thus, the brain rapidly mounts a cellular response to bacterial infection, consisting of an initial

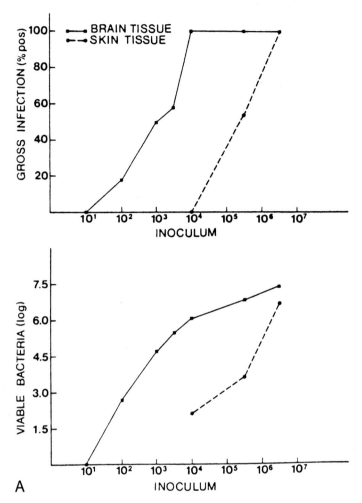

Fig. 6-4. Relative susceptibility of brain and skin to bacterial infection. (A) Tissue response of brain and skin 4 days after challenge with different inocula of *Staphylococcus aureus*. (*Figure continues.*)

cerebritis stage followed within several days by a glial and fibroblastic response, which serves to encapsulate the abscess (Fig. 6-5).

Corticosteroids appear to change the cellular response in brain abscess. Encapsulation is impaired in experimental animals given steroids during the early development of brain abscess. However, when administered simultaneously with antibiotics to which the causative organisms are sensitive, steroids were effective in reducing mass effect due to periabscess edema without significantly increasing tissue destruction or abscess size.[25]

Antibiotic therapy may abort the development of brain abscess if given at the time of bacterial implantation in the brain. Haley et al. demonstrated that the development of brain abscess could be prevented by penicillin and chlor-

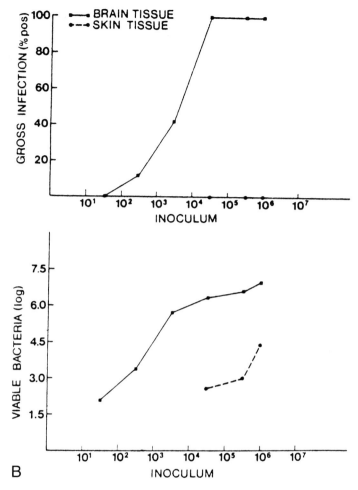

Fig. 6-4. (*Continued*) (B) Tissue response of brain and skin 4 days after challenge with different inocula of *Escherichia coli*. (Mendes M, Moore P, Wheeler CB et al: Susceptibility of brain and skin to bacterial challenge. J Neurosurg 52:772, 1980.)

amphenicol administered immediately after bacterial inoculation, but if antibiotic therapy was delayed by 48 hours, no effect on abscess development could be seen (Fig. 6-6). These experimental studies indicate that once encapsulation has begun, the abscess appears to be more resistant to cure by medical therapy alone, at least with the antibiotics employed.

Clinical Findings and Diagnosis of Brain Abscess

The clinical characteristics of the nonimmunosuppressed patient with brain abscess have been well described. Most patients present with findings referable to an intracranial mass lesion, and 45 to 50 percent of patients will have fever.

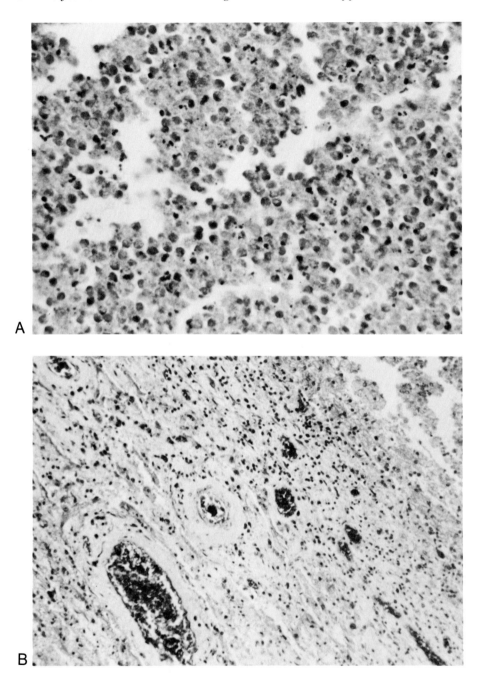

Fig. 6-5. Brain abscess encapsulation. (A) During the cerebritis stage of cerebral infection, the histological response consists of sheets of polymorphonuclear leukocytes. (B) As encapsulation proceeds, fibroblasts elaborate bands of collagen, which serve to wall off the inflammatory response.

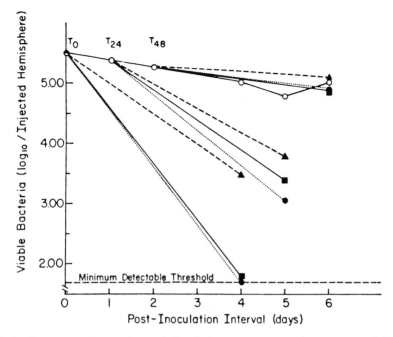

Fig. 6-6. Response of experimental *Staphylococcus aureus* abscess to penicillin and chloramphenicol treatment. At various times after intracerebral injection of bacteria, rats were treated with penicillin (●), penicillin plus chloramphenicol (■), or chloramphenicol alone (▲), or were not treated (○). When therapy was initiated at the time of contamination, "cure" of brain abscess was achieved in this model system. (Haley EC Jr, Costello GT, Rodeheaver GT et al: Treatment of experimental brain abscess with penicillin and chloramphenicol. J Infect Dis 148:737, 1983.)

Most will have a diminished level of consciousness, about half will have focal neurologic deficits, and 25 percent will have seizures. Eighty percent of patients will be found to have an extracranial predisposing condition (Table 6-1), the recognition of which may aid in determining the probable etiologic organism(s).[27,28]

Computed tomographic findings in nonimmunosuppressed patients with bacterial brain abscess depend upon the age of the abscess. In mature, well-encapsulated lesions the contrast-enhanced scan usually shows a relatively thin, regular area of contrast enhancement surrounding a hypodense or isodense central core (Figs. 6-1, 6-7). Varying degrees of low attenuation of periabscess due to edema can be noted and may significantly contribute to mass effect.

Britt et al. made a significant recent contribution to the management of brain abscess by carefully correlating the histological stages of brain abscess with CT appearance (Table 6-2).[29] They determined that in the early cerebritis stage irregular, patchy contrast enhancement may occur within an area of low density. During the late cerebritis stage thick and irregular ring enhancement

Table 6-1. Brain Abscess: Predisposing Conditions and Bacteriology

Predisposing Condition[a]	Site of Abscess	Usual Bacterial Isolate from Abscess
Contiguous site of primary infection		
Otitis media and mastoiditis	Temporal lobe or cerebellar hemisphere	Streptococci (anaerobic or aerobic), *Bacteroides fragilis*, Enterobacteriaceae
Frontoethmoidal sinusitis	Frontal lobe	Predominantly streptococci; *Bacteroides*, Enterobacteriaceae. *S. aureus*, and *Haemophilus* species
Sphenoidal sinusitis	Frontal or temporal lobe	Same as in frontoethmoidal sinusitis
Dental sepsis	Frontal lobe	Mixed *Fusobacterium*, *Bacteroides*, and *Streptococcus* species
Penetrating cranial trauma or postsurgical infection	Related to wound	*S. aureus*; streptococci, Enterobacteriaceae, clostridia
Distant site of primary infection		
Congenital heart disease	Multiple abscess cavities: middle cerebral artery distribution common but may occur at any site	Viridans, anaerobic, and microaerophilic streptococci; *Haemophilus* species
Lung abscess, empyema, bronchiectasis	Same as in congenital heart disease	*Fusobacterium, Actinomyces, Bacteroides*, streptococci, *Nocardia asteroides*
Bacterial endocarditis	Same as in congenital heart disease	*S. aureus*, streptococci
Compromised host (immunosuppressive therapy or malignancy)	Same as in congenital heart disease	Toxoplasma, fungi, Enterobacteriaceae
Acquired Immunodeficiency Syndrome	Any location	Toxoplasma, Cryptococcus, Candida albicans, CMV encephalitis (consider Kaposi's sarcoma and primary lymphoma)

[a] Predisposing conditions identified in approximately 80 percent of cases.
(Modified from Dacey RG Jr., Winn HR: Brain abscess and perimeningeal infections. p. 1213. In Stein JH, Cline MJ, Daly WJ et al (eds): Internal Medicine. Little Brown, Boston, 1987, 2nd ed.)

occurs, with increasing diffusion of the contrast material on delayed (30- to 60-min) scans. As encapsulation develops, the ring enhancement becomes thinner and more regular, with decay of contrast enhancement on delayed scans.

The CT diagnosis of intracranial infection in the compromised host is more complex. The appearance of intracerebral infection in such patients depends on the causative organism (i.e., fungus, parasite, or bacterium) and the tissue response of the host. The variety of CT appearances is shown in Figures 6-8 through 6-10. Because neuroradiologic studies do not yield enough specific

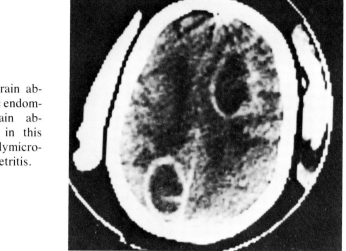

Fig. 6-7. Multiple brain abscess due to anaerobic endometritis. Multiple brain abscesses were noted in this elderly woman with polymicrobial anaerobic endometritis.

information about the causative organism in compromised hosts, the etiologic agent is best determined by surgical aspiration in these patients.

Treatment of Brain Abscess

Significant changes have recently occurred in the management of brain abscess; it has become clear that selected patients can be managed successfully without surgical intervention. This new alternative makes management decisions more complex because a patient treated without surgery may precipitously deteriorate while under observation and because antibiotic choice cannot be based on culture data. Most patients with brain abscess will require at least one surgical procedure.

Medical Management

Although antibiotic therapy has been an important part of the treatment of brain abscess since penicillin first became available, mortality from this condition has not significantly changed with the addition of newer antibiotics to treatment regimens. Nevertheless, Heineman was among the first to report that some patients with brain abscess, especially in the early (cerebritis) stage, could be managed without surgery on a regimen of antibiotics alone.[30,31] As CT scanning became available, more and better documented cases of successful medical management were reported. The CT scanner made it possible to follow the progression of brain abscess (either improvement or deterioration) in some

Table 6-2. Staging of Brain Abscess Using Computerized Tomography

Stage of Brain Abscess	Pre-Contrast Scan	Pattern of Contrast Enhancement (10 min)	Delayed Contrast Scan (30–60 min)
Early cerebritis	Irregular area of low density	May or may not show contrast enhancement; enhancement may be nodular, patchy, or ring-like	No significant decrease in contrast enhancement if present; further diffusion of contrast often occurs
Late cerebritis	Larger area of low density	Typical ring enhancement; ring is often diffuse and thick, however, it may be thin; if lesion is small, it will appear as a solid nodule; if lesion is larger, a lucent center remains	No significant decrease in contrast enhancement; further diffusion of contrast often occurs
Early capsule	Developing capsule delineated as a possible faint ring surrounding a lower-density necrotic center; area of low density (edema) surrounds developing capsule	Ring enhancement; may be thinner on ventricular or medial surface	Decay in contrast enhancement
Late capsule	Capsule visualized as a faint ring	Thin to moderately thick dense ring of contrast enhancement	Decay in contrast enhancement
Healed abscess	Collagen capsule commonly isodense with surrounding brain	May appear as nodular contrast enhancement for 4 to 10 weeks after completion of antibiotic treatment; no contrast enhancement if cured	

(Britt RH, Enzmann DR: Clinical stages of human brain abscess on serial CT scans after contrast infusion. Computerized tomographic, neuropathological, and clinical correlations. J Neurosurg 59:972, 1983.)

relatively asymptomatic patients before a change in their neurologic findings could be noticed.

Antibiotic therapy must be chosen empirically when the abscess is not to be aspirated. Anaerobes are the predominant isolates in most brain abscesses, and as Ouvis and others have shown, *Staphylococcus aureus* is also commonly seen.[27] An antibiotic regimen of chloramphenicol and penicillinase-resistant penicillin is the usual first choice.[32] Metronidazole is widely used outside the United States because of its excellent brain penetration and efficacy against anaerobes.[33]

Medical therapy alone is contraindicated in patients who show progressive neurologic deficits or altered level of consciousness. Abscesses larger than 2.0

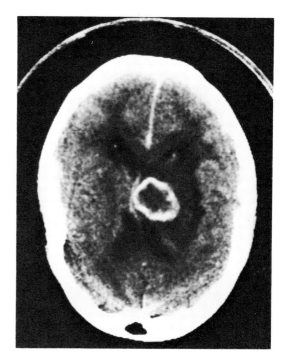

Fig. 6-8. Tuberculosis. This large, well-encapsulated lesion adjacent to the body of the right lateral ventricle proved to contain *Mycobacterium tuberculosis*.

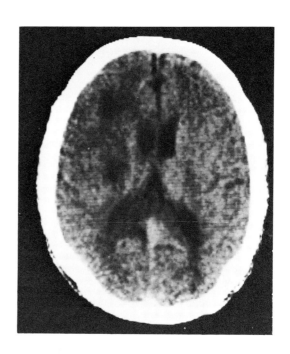

Fig. 6-9. Progressive multifocal leukoencephalopathy. This patient with Hodgkin's disease was found on brain biopsy to have progressive multifocal leukoencephalopathy of the right hemisphere.

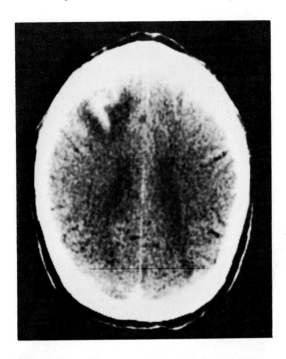

Fig. 6-10. Cerebral toxoplasmosis in a patient with AIDS. This patient with acquired immunodeficiency syndrome (AIDS) was found to have cerebral toxoplasmosis at brain biopsy after he presented with confusion and lethargy.

cm or those associated with significant mass effect should not be treated with medical therapy alone.[34] Abscesses seen to progressively enlarge on followup CT scans should be aspirated or excised (Fig. 6-11).

Surgical Management

The two most commonly used surgical procedures in the treatment of brain abscess are needle aspiration and excision. Needle aspiration for lobar brain abscess is usually accomplished via a single burr hole. The procedure can be done under local anesthesia, and subsequent reaspirations can be performed via the same approach if necessary. Adequate drainage can usually be accomplished with a large-bore needle, which allows simultaneous decompression and etiologic diagnosis. Aspiration has the disadvantage of providing only incomplete removal of the pus and no removal of the capsule.

Total excision is most successful with accessible lobar or cerebellar abscesses that are relatively well encapsulated. Abscesses which are refractory to repeated aspiration and antibiotic therapy are also best treated by total excision. Fungal or parasitic brain abscesses which harbor organisms resistant to antimicrobial chemotherapy should be considered for excision.

The recent resurgence of interest in stereotaxic techniques and their widespread availability, especially for approaching deep lobar or diencephalic brain tumors, has been extended to the treatment of brain abscess. The Brown-Roberts-Wells technique uses an externally applied ring to localize the target

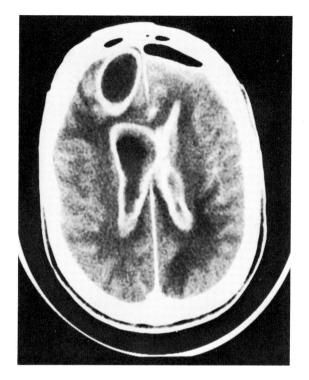

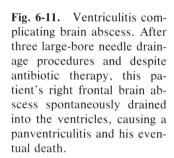

Fig. 6-11. Ventriculitis complicating brain abscess. After three large-bore needle drainage procedures and despite antibiotic therapy, this patient's right frontal brain abscess spontaneously drained into the ventricles, causing a panventriculitis and his eventual death.

abscess in the x, y, and z dimensions on the preoperative CT scan. The three-dimensional data are then transformed by a microcomputer into a format which allows the target to be accessed by an arc system mounted on the ring. The development of these stereotaxic techniques has facilitated accurate aspiration of lesions that previously could only be approached with the risk of significant neurologic morbidity. These techniques also allow the surgeon to aspirate more than one lesion during the same operative procedure if necessary to achieve decompression.

TREATMENT OF CEREBRAL CONTRAST-ENHANCING LESIONS IN PATIENTS WITH AIDS

The increasing incidence of acquired immunodeficiency syndrome (AIDS) has made the management of contrast-enhancing cerebral lesions in high-risk-group patients very complex. This disease has been demonstrated to be associated with human immunodeficiency virus (HIV) infection and is characterized by a decrease in helper/inducer T-cell function, causing an increased incidence of lymphoma, Kaposi's sarcoma, and opportunistic infections in homosexual or bisexual men, intravenous drug abusers, Haitians, and hemophiliacs.[35,36] Neurologic deficits are seen in 30 to 40 percent of patients with

AIDS, and about 30 percent of these (10 percent of all AIDS patients) have presented with neurologic symptoms.[37]

The neurologic complications of AIDS are associated with a wide variety of viral and nonviral infections, as well as with neoplasms and vascular lesions. Therefore it is extremely difficult to predict on the basis of clinical and CT findings which patients have opportunistic infections or the nature of the etiologic organism for these infections (Figs. 6-8, 6-9).

Toxoplasma gondii is the most common of the relatively localized, nonviral infections that may present as intracerebral contrast-enhancing lesions on CT scan (see Fig. 6-10).[36] These infections usually present with focal deficits or seizures, and single or multiple contrast-enhancing lesions are seen on CT. Magnetic resonance imaging may be helpful in demonstrating additional or more accessible lesions for biopsy. Although serologic means of diagnosis are available for toxoplasmosis, the rate of false negatives may be as high as 20 percent in the AIDS patient.[38] The lack of reliable serologic tests and the lack of specificity of CT scanning in this group have lead Levy et al. to recommend diagnostic biopsy in AIDS patients with CNS mass lesions.[36] Despite pyrimethamine-sulfadiazine treatment, their mortality is greater than 50 percent.[39] *Candida albicans* and aspergillus brain abscesses may also present as localized infections in AIDS. Central nervous system cryptococcosis, coccidioidomycosis, and mycobacterial infection may present as localized infection but usually cause meningitis. Primary and secondary lymphoma, Kaposi's sarcoma, and intracerebral hemorrhage or infarction are also differential considerations in the AIDS patient with a neurologic deficit.

Since therapy for each of the numerous causes of contrast-enhancing lesions in the AIDS patient varies according to the diagnosis, a biopsy should be seriously considered. The surgical team should be particularly careful to employ standard infection-control procedures to reduce exposure to blood and other body fluids while caring for AIDS patients. Since aerosolization and conjunctival splash accidents can occur with the use of high-speed drills and bone-cutting instruments, protective eyewear is also recommended.[40] However, to date no health care worker in the United States has acquired the AIDS virus while conducting surgery on an AIDS patient.

INFECTIONS OF CSF SHUNTS AND CSF DRAINAGE PROSTHESES

As treatment for CNS malformations, tumors, infections, injuries, and vascular disease has improved, congenital and acquired hydrocephalus has increasingly become a challenge for the neurosurgeon. Since their first application in the early 1960s, shunt devices have become an indispensible part of the neurosurgeon's armamentarium.[41,42] As with other prosthetic devices, however, infections occur in a significant number of patients. The management of these infections is difficult because of the need to maintain CSF diversion throughout the treatment period. This difficulty has prompted some neurosurgeons to devise a variety of clinical approaches for the management of this infection.

Etiology and Pathogenesis of Shunt Infections

Shunt infections are most common in infants and very elderly patients. The incidence varies from 3 to 40 percent in various series, but rates of 10 to 15 percent are most commonly reported.[43-45] Most shunt infections become apparent within 6 months of the operative procedure. The commonest causative organism is *Staphylococcus epidermidis,* with viridans streptococci, *Staphylococcus aureus,* and diphtheroids causing the majority of remaining cases. In newborns Enterobacteriaceae and the enterococcus are common etiologic agents. The fact that most infections occur soon after surgery and are caused by organisms which commonly reside in the epidermis suggests that the pathogenesis usually involves contamination of the prosthesis at the time of surgery.[46] A number of technical factors seem to influence the rate of infection, including the experience of the surgeon, duration of surgery, and host defenses of the patient. Venes advocates an operative regimen that includes prophylactic antibiotics, careful skin preparation, and isolation of incisional skin edges from the prosthesis, an approach which has reduced infections in her patients.[46]

The presence of shunt components appears to impair leukocytic function. Bayston and Penny describe the excessive production by *S. epidermidis* type SIIA of a mucoid substance, which enables it to remain adherent to the walls of colonized shunt valves.[47] Such glycocalyx-enclosing biofilms are commonly seen in prosthesis-related infections and probably are of primary significance in resistance to host defense mechanisms and antimicrobial therapy (see Chapter 2).

Like totally implantable ventriculoperitoneal or ventriculoatrial shunts, external ventricular drainage systems are susceptible to infection.[48] Narayan et al. reported a 6 to 7 percent infection rate in a large series of head-injured patients who had had ventriculostomies for intracranial pressure measurement.[49] The rate of infection may be lower for patients who undergo temporary (2- to 5-day) treatment for posterior fossa tumors or intraventricular hemorrhage. Prophylactic antibiotics do not seem to affect the incidence of external ventricular drainage system infections.[48] The incidence of infection with subarachnoid screws or bolts for the measurement of intracranial pressure is much lower than that for ventriculostomies.[50,21]

Clinical Features of CSF Shunt Infections

Patients with CSF shunt infections may present in a variety of ways.[51] Meningitis (or ventriculitis) usually becomes manifest with fever, changes in appetite or feeding behavior, irritability, or excessive somnolence. In children these symptoms may be difficult to distinguish from those of otitis media, viral gastroenteritis, or urinary tract infection. Children with such symptoms and

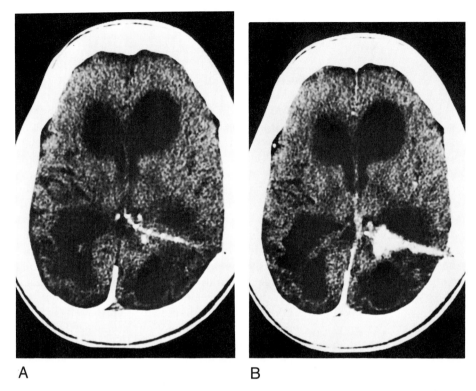

A   B

Fig. 6-12. Cerebritis surrounding the ventricular shunt catheter. This unusual complication of CSF shunts is apparent when the unenhanced CT (A) is compared with the enhanced CT (B). This ventricular catheter was removed during treatment of this shunt infection.

no readily identifiable source of infection should have a CSF culture and examination. Nuchal rigidity is not common in these patients.[51]

Although meningitis is the most common clinical indicator of shunt infection, a variety of other presentations has been reported. Shunt malfunction due to obstruction of the valve or distal tubing may result from infection. Patients may also present with an intra-abdominal mass due to loculation of CSF within the peritoneal cavity caused by an inflammatory exudate. Cysts such as this are diagnosed by ultrasonography or CT and may occur in the absence of infection. Findings such as fever or alteration in level of consciousness should point to the diagnosis of shunt infection in patients with these cysts.

Widespread peritonitis may also be the first indicator of shunt infection but must be distinguished from other intra-abdominal processes, such as appendicitis. Infections of ventriculoatrial shunts may be complicated by a circulating immune complex–mediated nephritis with fever, hematuria, and proteinemia; *Corynnebacterium bovis* and *S. epidermidis* have been associated with this complication. Wound infections are unusual forms of shunt-related infections.[53]

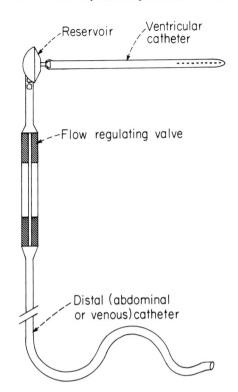

Fig. 6-13. Schematic diagram of ventriculoperitoneal or ventriculovenous shunt. The components of the shunt system are shown diagramatically. "Externalization" of a shunt may be performed at a level above (proximal to) or below (distal to) the flow regulating valve. The chest wall is frequently chosen as a convenient site for externalization of the distal catheter.

Management of Shunt Infection

The conventional approach to shunt infection management centered upon removal of the colonized prosthesis (Fig. 6-12). Recently some neurosurgeons have advocated medical management of some of these infections without surgical removal of shunt components[52] (Fig. 6-13). There are a number of alternative treatment schemata that rely to varying degrees on antibiotic therapy and shunt apparatus removal. However, the most difficult aspect of treating these patients is still the need for continuing CSF drainage or diversion during and after eradication of the infection by antibiotics.

Frame and McLaurin advocate primary antibiotic treatment of shunt infections, with resort to surgery reserved for obstructive malfunction or failure of antibiotic therapy.[52] Their approach depends upon daily CSF cultures, quantitative antibiotic susceptibilities and CSF inhibitory titer determinations. Intraventricular (IV) and parenteral or oral antibiotics are given for 2 weeks after the last positive CSF culture (or shunt replacement, if necessary). For *S. aureus* or *S. epidermidis* infections they administer nafcillin (or a cephalosporin) IV and intrathecally (IT) and gentamicin IT if the minimal inhibitory concentration (MIC) of the isolate is 1.0 μg/ml or less. For nafcillin-resistant staphylococci, a course of oral rifampin and trimethoprim plus parenteral and IT vancomycin is given. Enterobacteriaceae infections are treated with combination IT and IV β-lactam and aminoglycoside antibiotics. These investigators reported the

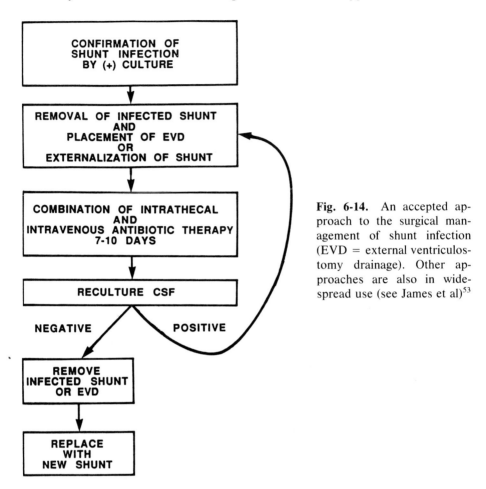

CONFIRMATION OF
SHUNT INFECTION
BY (+) CULTURE

REMOVAL OF INFECTED SHUNT
AND
PLACEMENT OF EVD
OR
EXTERNALIZATION OF SHUNT

COMBINATION OF INTRATHECAL
AND
INTRAVENOUS ANTIBIOTIC THERAPY
7-10 DAYS

RECULTURE CSF

NEGATIVE   POSITIVE

REMOVE
INFECTED SHUNT
OR EVD

REPLACE
WITH
NEW SHUNT

Fig. 6-14. An accepted approach to the surgical management of shunt infection (EVD = external ventriculostomy drainage). Other approaches are also in widespread use (see James et al)[53]

treatment of 12 shunt infections in children with a combination of oral rifampin and trimethoprim and IT vancomycin; long-term cures were achieved in 8 of these patients. They stressed the importance of antibiotic susceptibility testing and adequate shunt function if this mode of therapy is to be used. However, shunt revision, externalization, or removal was required in all but three of these cases.

James et al. reported the results of a randomized prospective study of shunt infections.[53] Patients were assigned to one of three groups: shunt removal plus systemic antibiotics with external ventricular drainage (A); immediate shunt removal and replacement with new components, plus intrashunt antibiotic therapy (B); IV and IT antibiotics alone without removal or replacement of the shunt (C). Most patients in groups A and B had prompt resolution of their infections with shorter hospital stays. Group C patients had longer hospital stays, and only 30 percent responded to treatment. James et al. concluded that removal of the infected shunt and either immediate or delayed replacement was the most effective approach to therapy.

Three alternative approaches for the treatment of shunt infection are currently in use: (1) immediate removal of the infected shunt, insertion of external ventricular drainage, administration of intrathecal and intravenous antibiotics, and replacement of shunt after CSF sterility is established; (2) immediate removal of the infected shunt and replacement with a new shunt, followed by intrashunt and intravenous antibiotics for 2 weeks; (3) externalization of the distal catheter at the chest wall, and administration of intrashunt and intravenous antibiotics followed by replacement of the infected shunt with a new prosthesis (see Fig. 6-14). If the infection is caused by *S. epidermidis* and there is no distal shunt obstruction, a 10-day course of therapy without externalization has been recommended.[52] This is followed by removal of the infected shunt and replacement with a new one.

Antibiotic Prophylaxis of Shunt Infection

Since intraoperative inoculation of the shunt with *S. epidermidis* is a common mode of shunt infection, there have been many attempts at perioperative antibiotic prophylaxis. Malis reports as part of an uncontrolled series 123 shunt procedures without a single infection.[54] The antibiotic regimen in this series consisted of a single parenteral dose of tobramycin and vancomycin, with streptomycin irrigation solution. Slight et al. report no difference in rate of infection when vancomycin was administered prophylactically.[55] Wang et al. report that the perioperative intravenous administration of sulfamethoxazole and trimethoprim did not reduce the incidence of shunt infection in a randomized, prospective, double-blind clinical trial.[56] There is no conclusive evidence that prophylactic antibiotics significantly decrease the rate of shunt infection.

REFERENCES

1. Hammon WM: Analysis of 2187 consecutive penetrating wounds of the brain from Vietnam. J Neurosurg 34:127, 1971
2. Hubschmann O, Shapiro K, Baden M, et al: Craniocerebral gunshot injuries in civilian practice—prognostic criteria and surgical management: experience with 82 cases. J Trauma 19:6, 1979
3. Hyslop NE Jr, Montgomery WW: Diagnosis and management of meningitis associated with cerebrospinal fluid leaks. p. 254. In Remington JS, Swartz MN (eds): Current Clinical Topics in Infectious Diseases. Vol. 3. McGraw-Hill, New York, 1982
4. Klastersky J, Sadeghi M, Brihaye J: Antimicrobial prophylaxis in patients with rhinorrhea or otorrhea: a double-blind study. Surg Neurol 6:111, 1986
5. Hand WL, Sanford JP: Posttraumatic bacterial meningitis. Ann Intern Med 72:869, 1970
6. Ignelzi RJ, VanderArk GD: Analysis of the treatment of basilar skull fractures with and without antibiotics. J Neurosurg 43:721, 1975
7. Hoff JT, Brewin A, U HS: Antibiotics for basilar skull fracture. J Neurosurg 44:649, 1976

8. Haines SJ: Systemic antibiotic prophylaxis in neurological surgery. Neurosurgery 6:355, 1980
9. Harsh GR: Infection complicating penetrating craniocerebral trauma. p. 135. In U.S. Army Medical Service: Neurological Surgery of Trauma. Office of the Surgeon General, Washington, 1965
10. Jennett B, Miller JD: Infection after depressed fracture of the skull. Implications for management of nonmissile injuries. J Neurosurg 36:333, 1972
11. Kriss FC, Taren JA, Kahn EA: Primary repairs of compound skull fractures by replacement of bone fragments. J Neurosurg 30:698, 1969
12. Nadell J, Cline DG: Primary reconstruction of depressed frontal sinus fractures including those involving the sinus, orbit and cribriform plate. J Neurosurg 41:200, 1974
13. Kaufmann DM, Miller MH, Steigbigel NH: Subdural empyema: analysis of 17 recent cases and review of the literature. Medicine 54:485, 1975
14. Dunker RO, Khakoo RA: Failure of computed tomographic scanning to demonstrate subdural empyema. JAMA 246:1116, 1981
15. Luken MG, Whelan MA: Recent diagnostic experience with subdural empyema, J Neurosurg 52:764, 1980
16. Stephanov S, Joubert MJ, Welchman JM: Combined convexity and parafalx subdural empyema. Surg Neurol 11:147, 1979
17. Morgan H, Wood M, Murphey F: Experience with 88 consecutive cases of brain abscess. J Neurosurg 38:689, 1973
18. Garfield J: Management of supratentorial intracranial abscess: a review of 200 cases. Br Med J 2:7, 1969
19. Garvey G: Current concepts of bacterial infections of the central nervous system, bacterial meningitis and bacterial brain abscess. J Neurosurg 59:735, 1983
20. Molinari GF: Septic cerebral embolism. Stroke 3:117, 1972
21. Winn HR, Mendes M, Moore P, et al: Production of experimental brain abscess in the rat. J Neurosurg 51:685, 1979
22. Mendes M, Moore P, Wheeler CB, et al: Susceptibility of brain and skin to bacterial challenge. J Neurosurg 52:772, 1980
23. Britt RH, Enzmann DR, Placone RC Jr, et al: Experimental anaerobic brain abscess. J Neurosurg 60:1148, 1984
24. Britt RH, Enzmann DR, Yeager AS: Neuropathological and computerized tomographic findings in experimental brain abscess. J Neurosurg 55:590 1981
25. Bohl I, Wallenfang T, Bothe H, Schurmann K: The effect of glucocorticoids in the combined treatment of experimental brain abscess in cats. Adv Neurosurg 9:125, 1981
26. Haley EC Jr, Costello GT, Rodeheaver GT, et al: Treatment of experimental brain abscess with penicillin and chloramphenicol. J Infect Dis 148:737, 1983
27. deLouvois J: Antimicrobial chemotherapy in the treatment of brain abscess. J Antimicrob Chemother 11:205, 1983
28. Dacey RG, Winn HR: Brain abscess and perimeningeal infections. p. 1503. In Stein JH, Cline MJ, Daly WJ et al (eds): Internal Medicine. 2nd ed. Little Brown, Boston, 1987
29. Britt RH, Enzmann DR: Clinical stages of human brain abscess on serial CT scans after contrast infusion. Computerized tomographic, neuropathological, and clinical correlations. J Neurosurg 59:972, 1983
30. Heineman HS, Braude AI: Anaerobic infection of the brain. Observations on eighteen consecutive cases of brain abscess. Am J Med 35:682, 1963

31. Heineman HS, Braude AI, Osterholm JL: Intracranial suppurative disease: early presumptive diagnosis and successful treatment without surgery. JAMA: 218:1542, 1971

32. Scheld WM, Winn HR: Brain abscess. p. 585. In Mandell GL, Douglas RG, Bennett JE (eds): Principles and Practices of Infectious Diseases. 2nd Ed. Wiley, New York, 1985

33. Ingham HR, Selkon JB, Roxby CM: Bacteriological study of otogenic cerebral abscesses: chemotherapeutic role of metronidazole. Br Med J 2:991, 1977

34. Rosenblum ML, Hoff JT, Norman D, et al: Non-operative treatment of brain abscesses in selected high risk patients. J Neurosurg 52:217, 1980

35. Jaffe HW, Bregman DJ, Selik RM: Acquired immune deficiency syndrome in the United States: the first 1000 cases. J Infect Dis 148:339, 1983

36. Levy RM, Bredesen DE, Rosenblum ML: Neurological manifestations of the acquired immunodeficiency syndrome (AIDS): experience at UCSF and review of the literature. J Neurosurg 62:475, 1985

37. Bredesen DE, Lipkin WI, Messing R, et al: Prolonged recurrent aseptic meningitis with prominent cranial nerve abnormalities: a new epidemic in gay men? Neurology 33: suppl 2, 85, 1983 (Abstract)

38. Snider WD, Simpson DM, Nielsen S, et al: Neurological complications of the acquired immune deficiency syndrome: analysis of 50 patients. Ann Neurol 14:403, 1983

39. Levy RM, Pons VG, Rosenblum ML: Central nervous system mass lesions in the acquired immune deficiency syndrome (AIDS). J Neurosurg 61:9, 1984

40. Centers for Disease Control: Prevention of acquired immune deficiency syndrome (AIDS): report of interagency recommendations. MMWR 32:101, 1983

41. Nulsen FE, Becker DP: Control of hydrocephalus by valve-regulated shunt. Infections and their prevention. Clin Neurosurg 14:256, 1966

42. Ames RH: Ventriculo-peritoneal shunts in the management of hydrocephalus. J Neurosurg 27:525, 1967

43. McLaurin RL: Infected cerebrospinal fluid shunts. Surg Neurol 1:191, 1973

44. Schoenbaum SC, Gardner P, Shillito J: Infections of cerebrospinal fluid shunts: Epidemiology, clinical manifestations and therapy. J Infect Dis 131:543, 1975

45. George R, Leibrock L, Epstein M: Long-term analysis of cerebrospinal fluid shunt infections: a 25 year experience. J Neurosurg 51:804, 1979

46. Venes JL: Control of shunt infection: report of 150 consecutive cases. J Neurosurg 45:311, 1976

47. Bayston R, Penny SR: Excessive production of mucoid substance in *Staphylococcus* SIIA: a possible factor in colonisation of Holter shunts. Dev Med Child Neurol 14: suppl. 27, 25, 1972

48. Mayhall CG, Archer NH, Lans A, et al: Ventriculostomy-related infections. N Engl J Med 310:553, 1984

49. Narayan RK, Kishore PR, Becker DP, et al: Intracranial pressure: to monitor or not to monitor? A review of our experience with severe head injury. J Neurosurg 56:650, 1982

50. Vries JK, Becker DP, Young HF: A subarachnoid screw for monitoring intracranial pressure. Technical note. J Neurosurg 39:416, 1973

51. James HE: Infections associated with cerebrospinal fluid prosthetic devices. p. 23. In Sugarman J, Young EJ (eds): Infections Associated with Prosthetic Devices. CRC Press, Boca Raton, 1984

52. Frame PT, McLaurin RL: Treatment of CSF shunt infections with intrashunt plus oral antibiotic therapy. J Neurosurg 60:354, 1984

53. James HE, Walsh JW, Wilson HD, et al: Prospective randomized study of therapy in cerebrospinal fluid shunt infection. Neurosurgery 7:459, 1980
54. Malis LI: Prevention of neurosurgical infection by intraoperative antibiotics. Neurosurgery 5:339, 1979
55. Slight PH, Gundling K, Plotkin SA, et al: A trial of vancomycin for prophylaxis of infections after neurosurgical shunts (Letter). N Engl J Med 312:921, 1985
56. Wang EE, Prober CG, Hendrick BE, et al: Prophylactic sulfamethoxazole and trimethoprim in ventriculoperitoneal shunt surgery. A double-blind, randomized, placebo-controlled trial. JAMA 251:1174, 1984

7 | Infection in Cardiac and Other Organ Transplant Recipients

Robert H. Rubin

One of the most remarkable success stories in modern medicine is that of organ transplantation. In just a few decades organ transplantation has evolved from an interesting experiment in human immunobiology to the treatment of choice for end-stage cardiac, renal, and liver disease. Today, recipients of cadaveric organ transplants can expect a 75 percent chance of surviving the critical first year post-transplant with a functioning allograft, as compared with a mortality rate, in the case of heart and liver recipients, that approaches 100 percent without such transplants. The successful transplant recipient has overcome the two major barriers to successful organ transplantation—rejection and infection—because of the great progress made in several areas (Table 7-1). The result of this progress is better control of rejection and better prevention and treatment of infection.[1,2]

It is important to emphasize that these two all-important processes are closely interrelated: any intervention that decreases the incidence or severity of rejection and thereby lowers the immunosuppressive requirement will decrease the incidence and severity of infection; any intervention that decreases the risk of infection will permit the safer utilization of more intense immunosuppressive therapy and thus decrease allograft rejection. Thus, any consideration of the infectious complications of organ transplantation must recognize the relative contributions of immunosuppressive therapy and the rejection process to the clinical picture. That infection remains an important part of organ transplantation is underlined by two observations: more than two-thirds of

95

Table 7-1. Major Areas of Progress in Organ Transplantation

1. Improved matching of the donor organ to potential recipient
2. Careful assessment, procurement, and preservation of the donor organ, and proper preparation of the recipient
3. Improved surgical technique, resulting in a minimum of tissue injury, secure anastamoses, and prevention of fluid collections
4. More precise management of the immunosuppressive regimen
5. Prompt diagnosis and specific therapy of those infections that do occur

(Modified from Rubin RH: Infection in the renal transplant patient. p. 553. In Rubin RH, Young LS (eds): Clinical Approach to Infection in the Compromised Host. Plenum, New York, 1981.)

transplant recipients have at least one infection in the first 6 months post-transplant and the majority of deaths are due to infection.[1-5]

Because of the life-long need for broadly acting immunosuppressive therapy to prevent allograft rejection, the infectious disease clinician responsible for the care of patients with organ transplants is challenged by several unique problems[6]:

(1)   The potential sources of infection for the transplant recipient are many—endogenous organisms, the environment, the allograft, even the patient's food and water supply.

(2)   Chronic immunosuppression complicated by invasion by certain microbes, particularly viruses, can result in a chronic progressive disease including a range of clinical syndromes not caused by these organisms in the normal host.

(3)   Prevention of infection in these patients is far preferable to therapy; in particular, the prevention of nosocomial infection is of critical importance.

(4)   The signs and symptoms of infection in these patients are often greatly reduced by the anti-inflammatory effects of the immunosuppressive therapy being administered. This may complicate early diagnosis and aggressive therapy.

It is the purpose of this review to provide a guideline to the infectious disease problems that complicate organ transplantation, concentrating particularly on the cardiac allograft recipient.

TIMETABLE OF INFECTION IN THE ORGAN TRANSPLANT RECIPIENT

Different infections are likely to occur at different points in the post-transplant course; that is, the risk for particular infections is variable depending on how much time has elapsed since the transplant. All three of the major forms of organ transplantation—cardiac, renal, and liver have similar timetables, according to which different infections are likely to occur, which are due to common forms of immunosuppression. This timetable is delineated in Figure

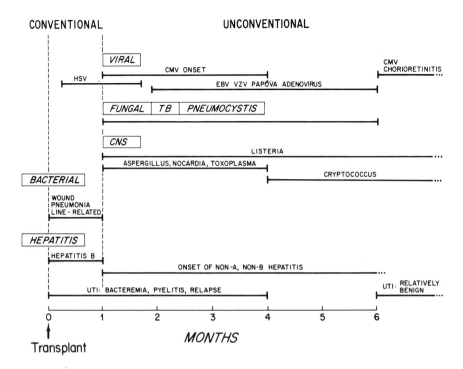

CONVENTIONAL   UNCONVENTIONAL

Fig. 7-1. Timetable for the occurrence of infection in the organ transplant patient. Abbreviations used: CMV, cytomegalovirus; HSV, herpes simplex virus; EBV, Epstein-Barr virus; VZV, varicella-zoster virus; CNS, central nervous system; UTI, urinary tract infection. (Modified from Rubin RH, Wolfson JS, Cosimi AB, Tolkoff-Rubin NE: Infection in the renal transplant patient. Am J Med 70:405, 1981.)

7-1, which divides the infectious disease problems in organ transplant recipients into three convenient time periods.[1,2,6]

1. *First month post-transplant:* The infections occurring in the first month post-transplant can be grouped into one of three categories: continuing infections that were present prior to the transplant procedure; infection acquired with the allograft; and routine postoperative bacterial infections related to the surgical wound, intravenous lines, bladder catheters, and the lungs.

2. *One to six months post-transplant:* This is the time period when the risk of infection is the greatest, corresponding to the development of significant immunosuppression by treatment to prevent rejection. This is also the period when major viral infections, such as cytomegalovirus (CMV), Epstein-Barr virus (EBV), and non-A non-B hepatitis, become apparent. Present evidence would suggest that these viral agents also contribute to the net state of immunosuppression.

3. *Late period, more than six months post-transplant:* Patients surviving into the late period with functioning allografts can be divided into three major

categories in terms of their infectious disease problems: those with chronic or progressive effects of infections acquired earlier in the post-transplant course; those with minimal rejection activity, not requiring alterations in immunosuppressive therapy, and those who have had chronic rejection activity and are receiving larger amounts of chronic and acute immunosuppressive therapy. This last group is at highest risk for a life-threatening opportunistic infection.

Knowledge of this timetable of infections in the post-transplant period can be utilized by the clinician in two ways: first, it can be helpful in generating a differential diagnosis when a patient presents with a particular infectious disease syndrome; for example, pneumonia occurring 2 weeks post-transplant is highly likely to have a very different etiology and differential diagnosis than pneumonia occurring 3 months post-transplant. Even more important, however, is the epidemiologic information that can be gained from the comparison of the timetable with the actual diagnosis in a given patient. As will be discussed subsequently, immunosuppressed patients are at high risk of being infected by organisms present in the environment in excessive numbers. An important clue to the presence of such an excess epidemiologic hazard is the occurrence of certain infections at unlikely times post-transplant. For example, nosocomial epidemics of *Aspergillus, Legionella, Pseudomonas,* or *Nocardia* infection often declare themselves by causing infection in the first month post-transplant. *A single case of infection with an opportunistic pathogen in the first month following renal transplantation constitutes significant evidence of a nosocomial epidemic.*

INFECTION IN THE FIRST MONTH POST-TRANSPLANT

In order to decrease morbidity and mortality post-transplant, it is important for the clinician to identify and eradicate, if possible, any active infectious process before immunosuppressive therapy is instituted. In addition to the usual bacterial infections (especially infections of the lung and those that could enter the bloodstream and threaten the transplant vascular anastamosis), particular concerns are mycobacterial and fungal infections and the parasitic infestation *Strongyloides stercoralis.* In the immunosuppressed host *S. stercoralis* can cause a devastating hyperinfection syndrome or disseminated disease, which is associated with an extremely high mortality.[7-9] Each of these problems is best identified and treated pretransplant.

The allograft itself can be a source of serious infection. This has been particularly well documented with renal transplantation, in which two general categories of allograft contamination have had important effects on the transplant recipient.[1,7] The first category is that of long-standing infection predating the terminal illness that leads to organ donation. This includes mycobacterial infection, fungal infection, hepatitis B, and CMV. A potential new worry in this category is human immunodeficiency virus (HIV), the causative agent of the acquired immunodeficiency syndrome (AIDS). Because of the epidemiologic similarities between hepatitis B and HIV, one must assume that this virus is potentially transmittable with the allograft. The risk of chronic infection transmission can be minimized by appropriate serologic testing and the acquisition of a thorough clinical history on the donor.

More difficult are the acute infections in cadaveric allograft donors that complicate their terminal care. Because of the nature of these individuals' terminal illness, most prospective cadaveric donors have had indwelling bladder catheters, endotracheal tubes, and a variety of intravascular lines. All these can lead to sepsis that could seed the allograft, so at present all potential donors with clear-cut systemic sepsis are eliminated from consideration. However, it has been clearly demonstrated that contamination of the allograft may occur without clinical signs in the donor. This can lead to disastrous complications due to disruption of vascular anastomoses.[1,7,10]

In order to prevent such catastrophic events, the following guidelines have been proposed for assessing the suitability of potential cadaveric donors: (1) Any potential donor with documented sepsis, systemic viral infection, viral encephalitis, etc. is eliminated from consideration. (2) Even in the absence of symptoms, careful preterminal culturing of the donor (including blood cultures) and of perfusates or fluids in which the allograft is placed following harvest is carried out. Systemic antimicrobial therapy is initiated for positive cultures, the duration of therapy being shorter (less than 7 days) for low-virulence organisms and longer (more than 14 days) if the cultures yield gram-negative bacilli, *Staphylococcus aureus,* or *Candida spp.* (3) Certain potential donors are at particularly high risk for occult sepsis and should not be utilized: these include victims of drowning (who may be infected with microorganisms found in water), burn victims, and patients who have been maintained on a respirator with indwelling lines and catheters for more than 7 days.[7,10]

The most common form of treatable infection found in the first month post-transplant is wound infection.[11] The incidence of wound infection in cardiac transplant patients ranges from 3.6 to 62.5 percent in different series and is particularly common in patients who have to undergo re-exploration for post-operative bleeding.[12,13] A second form of wound infection unique to cardiac transplantation is that due to the prolonged presence of chest tubes in the pleural spaces. This often leads to colonization and then invasion of the pleural space by a variety of pathogens but particularly by the gram-negative bacilli resident in the hospital environment.[12,13] Data from a variety of transplant populations indicates that the most important factor in the prevention of wound infection is the technical quality of the surgery performed. The incidence of wound sepsis is directly related to the occurrence of wound hematoma, lymph leakage, and tissue injury created by the surgery. Meticulous wound and catheter care and the early removal of all foreign devices will also contribute significantly to a decrease in the occurrence of wound infection in this patient population.[62,11]

It is particularly important to emphasize that the diagnosis of wound infection requires an extremely high index of suspicion, as the signs of such infection may be obscured by immunosuppressive therapy. Therefore any transplant patient with an unexplained fever in the first month post-transplant should be subjected to two procedures: sterile needle exploration of the wound and either ultrasonographic or computerized tomographic scanning of the deeper operative sites.[14]

Unless absolutely essential, plastic catheters for intravenous use are to be discouraged, particularly central venous pressure catheters or Swan-Ganz pulmonary artery catheters for hemodynamic monitoring. While avoidance of such devices in patients undergoing renal transplantation is relatively simple,[14] intravenous line–related sepsis is not uncommon in patients undergoing cardiac and liver transplantation. Bacteremia complicates the invasive hemodynamic monitoring equipment that is usually required. Meticulous attention to the care and changing of such lines at a minimum of every 72 hours can limit the incidence and severity of such problems.[5,12,13]

As in nonimmunosuppressed patients undergoing major surgery, urinary tract infections secondary to bladder catheterization and pneumonia can be important problems in the first month post-transplant. Pneumonia, in particular, has been a major problem in the cardiac transplant recipient because of the frequent presence of underlying lung disease and, probably more important, a prolonged period of intubation.[5,12,13,15] Studies carried out in renal transplant patients have suggested that the risk of life-threatening pneumonia increases significantly after 3 days of intubation.[16]

INFECTION ONE TO SIX MONTHS POST-TRANSPLANT

In the second through sixth months post-transplant period the bacterial infections resulting from technical complications of the transplant procedure have largely run their course. The most important infections occurring during this time period are those that are directly related to the immunosuppressed state of the patient. This is the critical time period for most transplant patients in terms of greatest risk for life-threatening infection. The reasons for this are twofold: first, the duration of immunosuppressive therapy has been sufficient to generate a major depression of host defenses; second, largely because of such immunosuppressive therapy, infection with a variety of viruses becomes manifest during this time period. These viruses include CMV, EBV and the hepatitis viruses. In addition to their direct clinical manifestations, these viruses have broad-reaching effects on host defenses, contributing to the net state of immunosuppression, and they play a significant role in pathogenesis of the relatively high incidence of opportunistic infection during this period. The clinical illnesses produced by these viruses are greatly modulated by the two phenomena that are unique to transplantation—allograft rejection and the chronic state of immunosuppression. Indeed, the intensity and kind of immunosuppressive therapy administered is probably the major determinant of the clinical course these viruses take. Two effects are noted: those viruses that latently infect most of the normal population will be reactivated, and the ability of the host to eliminate active infection will be impaired. This leads to a state of chronic viral infection, with a much broader range of clinical effects.[1,2,17,18]

Although there is no documentation for this phenomenon at the present time, it is highly likely that the causative agent of AIDS, HIV will have to be added to this list of important viral infections. Transfusion-associated HIV infection of the dialysis population has already been documented (Rubin RH, unpublished observations), and it seems only a matter of time until this virus begins to appear in transplant recipients because of the large number of transfusions that such patients receive. However, the nation-wide use of the ELISA test to detect antibodies to HIV should keep transfusion-related HIV infection in the dialysis population at a very low frequency.

Herpes Virus Group

There are four human herpes viruses: CMV, EBV, herpes simplex virus (HSV), and varicella-zoster virus (VZV). These are the most common infections found in the transplant recipient.

Cytomegalovirus

The most important single infectious agent affecting transplant recipients is CMV, with more than two-thirds of cardiac, renal, and liver transplant recipients showing evidence of active CMV infection post-transplant.[17–19] There are two major patterns of transmission of CMV infection in transplant recipients.[17–21] The first, *primary infection,* occurs when a seronegative transplant recipient acquires infection transmitted in latent fashion from a seropositive donor. In the kidney transplant recipient it is quite clear that the allograft is the source of such latent virus in some 80 to 95 percent of instances,[20,21] with leukocyte-containing blood transfusions accounting for virtually all the remaining cases.[22] Epidemiologic studies in human cardiac transplant recipients similarly implicate the heart allograft as a source of primary infection,[23] and direct studies of CMV in a murine model have clearly established that this can occur.[24–26] The source of primary CMV infection in liver transplant recipients has not yet been established but is probably similar. The second major pattern of transmission of CMV infection is so-called *reactivation.* In this instance the transplant recipient has had his primary infection previously, remains latently infected with the virus (and is seropositive for CMV prior to transplant), and reactivates endogenous latent virus post-transplant. Virtually every seropositive individual will reactivate virus post-transplant.[17,21]

With both primary and reactivation CMV disease clinically apparent infection begins 1 to 6 months post-transplant, with a peak occurrence approximately 6 to 8 weeks after the onset of immunosuppression. There is a major difference in the clinical significance of primary and reactivation CMV infection. Whereas approximately 60 percent of individuals with primary CMV infection become symptomatic, only about 20 percent of individuals with reactivation disease become symptomatic.[17–19] As previously noted, the major

Table 7-2. Clinical Effects of Cytomegalovirus in the Organ Transplant Patient

1. Production of a variety of infectious disease syndromes by the virus itself:
   "Early" syndromes: Mononucleosis, pneumonia, leukopenia, thrombocytopenia, hepatitis, gastrointestinal ulcerations
   "Late" syndrome: Progressive chorioretinitis
2. Production of a major depression in host defenses by the virus, leading to the occurrence of potentially lethal superinfection with a variety of opportunistic pathogens
3. Possible production of allograft injury
4. Possible role in the pathogenesis of Kaposi's sarcoma

factor influencing the severity and clinical significance of CMV infection is the intensity and type of immunosuppression administered.[17-19] In the early days of renal transplantation, when steroids alone were used for immunosuppression, CMV was essentially unknown. The addition of such cytotoxic drugs as azathioprine and cyclophosphamide to the regimen resulted in the widespread occurrence of CMV infection.[17-19] A similar risk of clinically apparent infection exists in patients receiving cyclosporine and prednisone.[27] However, of all the immunosuppressive regimens, those which include antilymphocyte therapies (antithymocyte globulin, antilymphocyte serum, or the more recently available anti-T-cell monoclonal antibodies such as OKT 3) have the most dramatic CMV-promoting effect.[17-19,23,27,28] For example, in studies of renal transplant recipients, Cheeseman et al.[28] have noted that the addition of antithymocyte globulin to conventional azathioprine and prednisone regimens (as has been traditionally prescribed) promoted a higher rate of viremia and symptomatic disease. Furthermore, the beneficial effects of a prophylactic course of interferon-alpha were abrogated. Reductions in the dosages of azathioprine, prednisone, and perhaps cyclosporine therapy at the time of the antilymphocyte treatment may reduce clinically apparent CMV infection.[29]

The clinical manifestations of CMV infection in the transplant patient are outlined in Table 7-2 and can be grouped into an early category and a late category. The most common early manifestation is a clinical syndrome that closely resembles mononucleosis in the nonimmunosuppressed individual and entails anorexia, fever, malaise, myalgias, and arthralgias. Indeed, small numbers of atypical lymphocytes can be observed in the peripheral blood of patients with this syndrome. In approximately one-third of patients who develop a febrile illness due to CMV, signs of pneumonitis may develop, usually with a dry, nonproductive cough. The x-ray picture associated with CMV pneumonia may take a variety of forms: most commonly a bilateral, symmetrical predominantly lowerlobe peribronchovascular (interstitial) process; less commonly, a focal consolidation or even a solitary nodule may be observed.[17-19]

The important question for the clinician to answer when dealing with a transplant patient with an interstitial pneumonia 1 to 6 months post-transplant is not so much whether or not CMV is present but is almost invariably: Is there present some treatable form of superinfection, particularly that due to *Pneumocystis carinii?* CMV and *P. carinii* cause similar clinical syndromes, and moreover both are often found together. A particular association between primary CMV infection and *P. carinii* pneumonia has been noted in the cardiac transplant patient.[30-32]

Other major effects of CMV are on the hematologic and gastrointestinal systems. Leukopenia, thrombocytopenia, and atypical lymphocytes are observed commonly,[17-19] and approximately one-third of patients will have some mild evidence of hepatocellular dysfunction.[33] Much more dramatic is the occurrence of gastrointestinal hemorrhage, apparently due to ulcerations caused by local CMV invasion of the gastrointestinal tract. Such CMV lesions are particularly common in the right colon.[17-19,34]

The most important effect of CMV infection is a further depression of host defenses. Patients will rarely die from CMV alone; rather, death is caused by superinfection with a variety of opportunistic agents. The adverse effects of CMV infection on host defenses are numerous,[36-38] the most obvious being the severe leukopenia which may be observed. More important is the further suppression of cell-mediated immunity. One laboratory marker of CMV- (and EBV-) induced depression of cell-mediated immunity is provided by measurement of T cell subsets. Both in normals and in renal transplant patients, these viruses cause some decrease in the T helper cells and a marked increase in the T cytotoxic-suppressor cells. Studies in transplant patients have shown that the great majority of opportunistic infections occur in the subgroup of renal transplant patients with viral-induced inverted helper to suppressor T cell ratios.[39] Thus, any patient with an inverted ratio should be treated rather gingerly in terms of the intensity of immunosuppressive therapy. The few occurrences of opportunistic infection in the setting of normal T cell subsets have in our experience been almost invariably in the circumstance of an excessive environmental nosocomial hazard.

A major late manifestation of CMV infection is a progressive chorioretinitis. This usually begins 4 to 8 months post-transplant and then is usually relentlessly progressive—causing blindness either directly or via secondary retinal detachment, anterior uveitis, or glaucoma.[17-19,40]

The other possible late manifestation of CMV infection is Kaposi's sarcoma. There is an increasing body of circumstantial evidence in African populations, among transplant recipients, and among AIDS patients that CMV may be involved in the pathogenesis of this tumor.[17-19]

Epstein-Barr Virus Infection

Evidence of reactivation of EBV infection may be seen in as many as two-thirds of transplant recipients. What is less clear is the exact clinical consequence of this viral reactivation. Because of the ubiquity of CMV infection, it has been difficult to sort out the relative contribution of EBV to the infectious disease morbidity observed in transplant recipients. It is not an unreasonable hypothesis, however, to assume that CMV disease syndromes can be caused also by EBV.[1,17,41,42]

Much more convincing, however, is the increasing evidence that EBV is an important factor in the development of a particular type of lymphoid malignancy observed in transplant patients. As many as 15 percent of the malignancies observed in these patients are a form of lymphoma called *immunoblastic sarcoma*. Many of these are due to B cell proliferation. EBV specific antibody titers, immunofluorescent staining of tumors for the presence of EBV nuclear antigen, and DNA hybridization studies all strongly implicate EBV as the probable etiologic agent in these disorders.[17,43-48] Of great interest is the report of a renal transplant patient with a polyclonal B cell lymphoproliferative disorder who responded clinically on two occasions to acyclovir, an antiviral agent with anti-EBV effects in vitro but no inherent antilymphoma properties.[49]

The mechanism by which EBV plays a role in the pathogenesis of these B cell lymphoproliferative syndromes in the immunosuppressed host is only partially understood. Like other herpes viruses, EBV has been shown to have oncogenic potential. In vitro EBV infection of B cell lines will cause the establishment of immortalized B cell lines (the in vitro correlate of malignant transformation). It is believed that EBV has a similar potential in the normal host. However, in such individuals specific memory T cells mount a vigorous cytotoxic response against EBV-infected B cells, thus preventing the establishment of B lymphoid malignancies. It is postulated that immunosuppression in transplant patients interferes with this T cell surveillance mechanism, leading to unopposed B cell proliferation. Immunosuppression with cyclosporine has been associated with an undue incidence of B cell lymphoproliferative disease, particularly in individuals receiving the earlier, high-dose regimens of this drug.[50-52]

Herpes Simplex Virus

Approximately one-third to one-half of all transplant recipients will develop mucocutaneous lesions due to herpes simplex virus, usually beginning approximately one month post-transplant. These mucocutaneous lesions may be due to either HSV type 1, in which case they are usually around the nose and mouth, or HSV type 2, in which case anogenital involvement is the rule. The severity of HSV type 1 infections may be greatly exacerbated if the nasal or oral mucosa is traumatized by the presence of an endotracheal or nasogastric tube. The intensity and severity of HSV infection is likewise influenced by the immunosuppressive therapy administered. In particular, antilymphocyte therapies appear to be the major promoters of HSV infection. Fortunately, in the case of this virus acyclovir is quite effective in the treatment of mucocutaneous HSV infection. It must be pointed out, however, that if a course of antilymphocyte therapy or other high-dose immunosuppression is being maintained, the HSV infection will recur quite promptly following the completion of a course of acyclovir.[1,17,53]

Less common forms of HSV infection include zosteriform lesions on the buttocks and eczema herpeticum in patients with preceding eczema. Unlike bone marrow transplant recipients, organ transplant recipients experience disseminated visceral HSV infection or primary HSV pneumonia only exceedingly rarely.[1,17,53]

Varicella-Zoster Virus

Reactivation VZV infection is quite common in organ transplant recipients, occurring in approximately 10 percent of these patients in the post-transplant period. It should be emphasized that, unlike the situation with lymphoma patients, reactivation VZV infection rarely disseminates in organ transplant patients, and the routine use of antiviral chemotherapy has therefore not been recommended in such patients.[1,17]

In direct contrast to the relative benignity of reactivation VZV infection is the malignant course that primary VZV (chickenpox) can take in this group of patients, as in any immunosuppressed patient population. Chickenpox in these patients is a devastating illness characterized by severe pneumonia, gastrointestinal lesions with hemorrhage, central nervous system involvement, and disseminated intravascular coagulation. Therefore, a careful check of past chickenpox experience and current exposure is essential, with immediate zoster immune globulin prophylaxis for any significant exposures and institution of antiviral therapy with acyclovir at the earliest stage of clinical disease.[1,17]

Hepatitis Viruses

Because of the large number of transfusions that are administered to organ transplant recipients, it is not surprising that approximately 10 to 15 percent of transplant recipients develop evidence of hepatitis post-transplant. With the advent of universal blood bank screening for hepatitis B, the incidence of hepatitis B infection has fallen dramatically at all transplant centers. However, the incidence of hepatitis has been largely unchanged because of our inability to adequately protect against transfusion-related non-A, non-B hepatitis. The impact of such infections is potentially great if the experience garnered in renal transplant patients is any guide.

Approximately 80 percent of individuals who develop non-A, non-B hepatitis post-transplant will develop chronic infection. Non-A, non-B hepatitis appears to contribute to further immunosuppression, as manifested by an increased incidence of life-threatening and life-taking nonhepatic infectious processes as well as an increased rate of kidney allograft survival in these patients. In addition, the chronicity of the infection will result in occult development of cirrhosis, a number of patients presenting 3 to 10 years post-transplant with ascites, bleeding esophageal varices, spontaneous bacterial peritonitis, etc., as a result of their smoldering chronic non-A, non-B hepatitis. We currently do not have an adequate means to either prevent or treat this complication of transplantation.[1,17,54]

LATE PERIOD, MORE THAN SIX MONTHS POST-TRANSPLANT

As previously noted, patients surviving with functioning organ transplants in place and continuing immunosuppression can be divided into three general categories in terms of infectious disease risk[1,2,17]:

1. The majority of individuals with good allograft function, minimal chronic immunosuppressive therapy, no recent acute antirejection therapy, and no evidence of chronic viral infection are at minimal risk for opportunistic infection. Those infections that do develop closely resemble those seen in the general community.

2. There is a small group of patients who have had chronic rejection, such that both their chronic level of immunosuppressive therapy and the intensity and duration of acute high-dose antirejection therapy have been unduly great. These have also been associated with a high incidence of chronic infection with such immunosuppressing viruses as CMV and non-A, non-B hepatitis. This is the subgroup of patients who are at highest risk for life-threatening opportunistic infection, particularly by *Cryptococcus neoformans*. In kidney transplantation it is clear that these patients are best served by giving up on the allograft, returning the patient to dialysis, and perhaps retransplanting at a later date. Unfortunately, in cardiac and liver transplantation this is not a feasible choice.

3. The third group consists of patients with lingering effects of infection acquired earlier; the prime examples of this are chronic hepatitis and progressive chorioretinitis due to CMV.

INFECTIOUS DISEASE SYNDROMES OF PARTICULAR IMPORTANCE IN THE TRANSPLANT RECIPIENT

Central Nervous System Infection

Infection involving the central nervous system occurs in some 5 to 10 percent of transplant recipients. As delineated in Table 7-3, there are four distinct clinical syndromes observed in the transplant patient—acute meningitis, subacute-chronic meningitis, meningoencephalitis, and localized mass lesions of the brain. It is not so much that these clinical syndromes are different from those observed in the normal hosts but rather that the etiologies of these clinical syndromes are very different. Furthermore, the clinical manifestations are often greatly muted as a result of the anti-inflammatory effects of the immunosuppressive therapy. Thus, many transplant patients with acute meningitis will have little or no evidence of meningeal irritation. Similarly, only mild changes in the state of consciousness may be present in the face of florid central nervous system infection. Because of this the clinician must be extremely alert to the possibility of central nervous system involvement and, indeed, the most reliable indication for a neurologic evaluation is the presence of an unexplained

Table 7-3. Clinical Syndromes Due to Central Nervous System Infection and their Etiologies in the Transplant Patient

Clinical Syndromes	Microbial Etiology
Acute meningitis	*Listeria monocytogenes*
Subacute-chronic meningitis	*Cryptococcus neoformans* (*Candida* spp, *Mycobacterium tuberculosis, Listeria monocytogenes, Coccidioides immitis, Histoplasma capsulatum, Strongyloides stercoralis*)
Encephalitis or meningoencephalitis	*Listeria monocytogenes, Toxoplasma gondii*, JC papovavirus
Localized mass lesion	*Aspergillus* spp, *Nocardia asteroides, Toxoplasma gondii, Listeria monocytogenes*

(Modified from Rubin RH, Hooper DC: Central nervous system infection in the compromised host. Med Clin North Am 69:281, 1985.)

headache or behavioral change, particularly when accompanied by fever. Such neurologic evaluation should include both CT scan and lumbar puncture.[55,56]

Dermatologic Manifestations of Infection

For the clinician caring for the transplant recipient, careful attention to the skin and subcutaneous tissues is extremely important. First, the skin and the mucosal surfaces of the body are the primary barriers against infection, with such primary barriers being of particular importance in immunocompromised patients whose secondary host defenses are impaired by the immunosuppressive therapy. Secondly, the skin's rich blood supply provides an opportunity for metastatic spread of infection both from this site as the initial portal of entry and to this site from other sources (Fig. 7-2). Finally, the anti-inflammatory effects of immunosuppressive therapy greatly modify the appearance of infection in the skin, necessitating biopsy for diagnosis.[57,58]

Important aspects of skin infection in transplant patients that merit particular emphasis are the following:

1. Typical cellulitis-appearing lesions commonly due to gram-positive organisms may be due to such unusual etiologies as *C. neoformans, Candida* spp, or gram-negative organisms in the transplant recipient. Hence the need for biopsy in any patient who does not rapidly respond to antibacterial therapy aimed at gram-positive organisms.

2. Injury to the skin, as with occlusive dressings, has been associated with invasion by a variety of opportunistic organisms but most particularly *Aspergillus, Candida,* and *Rhizopus* spp. Such invasion has not uncommonly resulted in systemic dissemination.

3. The skin may provide the first clinically assessable manifestation of disseminated opportunistic infection. In particular, some 20 to 30 percent of patients with cryptococcal infection will develop skin lesions weeks to months

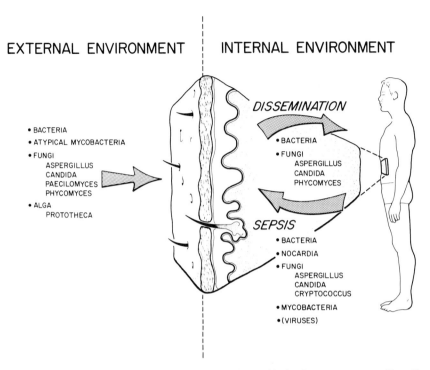

EXTERNAL ENVIRONMENT | INTERNAL ENVIRONMENT

DISSEMINATION

- BACTERIA
- ATYPICAL MYCOBACTERIA
- FUNGI
  ASPERGILLUS
  CANDIDA
  PAECILOMYCES
  PHYCOMYCES
- ALGA
  PROTOTHECA

- BACTERIA
- FUNGI
  ASPERGILLUS
  CANDIDA
  PHYCOMYCES

SEPSIS

- BACTERIA
- NOCARDIA
- FUNGI
  ASPERGILLUS
  CANDIDA
  CRYPTOCOCCUS
- MYCOBACTERIA
- (VIRUSES)

Fig. 7-2.   Schematic representation of the role of the skin in the occurrence of localized and disseminated infection in the organ transplant patient. (Reproduced with permission from Wolfson JS, Sober AJ, Rubin RH: Dermatologic manifestations of infections in the compromised host. Ann Rev Med 34:205, 1983. © 1983 by Annual Reviews Inc.)

prior to the development of central nervous system disease. Some 10 to 15 percent of patients with disseminated candidal infection will similarly have early development of skin lesions. Clinical experience has demonstrated that it is far easier to treat fungal infection metastatic to the skin than to treat such infection once it has reached the brain. Thus, close examination of the skin and aggressive attention to even the most innocuous of unexplained skin lesions can provide an early warning of life-threatening infection. The opportunity for early therapy increases the chances of cure.[57,58]

SUMMARY

Great progress has been made in the technical and immunologic manipulations of organ transplant recipients, resulting in the rehabilitation of increasing numbers of individuals previously condemned to an early demise. Rejection and infection remain, however, as the twin barriers to successful transplantation, with infection still accounting for the majority of deaths. Although the need for chronic immunosuppressive therapy influences the incidence and severity of all forms of infection in these patients, certain types of infection appear to be preventable: those present in the recipient pretransplant or conveyed with the allograft; those due to technical errors (these include operative errors resulting in undue tissue trauma, hematomas, lymph accumulations, etc. and the inappropriate management of intravenous lines and surgical drains); and those due to excessive environmental contamination (as with *Aspergillus* spp, *Legionella* spp, or *Pseudomonas aeruginosa*). In addition, there is a group of viral infections which are greatly modulated by the intensity and type of immunosuppressive therapy being administered; these are ubiquitous in transplant patients and have a broad range of clinical effects. The viral agents include CMV, the other herpes group viruses, and the hepatitis viruses. At present our techniques for preventing and treating such infections are less than ideal.

Despite those challenges the impact of infection in organ transplant recipients can be minimized if one important tenet is kept in mind: the anti-inflammatory effects of the immunosuppressive therapy will greatly influence, attenuate, and modify the clinical manifestations of a particular infectious process. Therefore, clinical success in this field depends greatly on detecting the earliest signs of invasive infection. An unimpressive skin lesion, a mild but persistent headache, or a mild cough may be the only clue to life-threatening disease, and the clinician must act accordingly. If he does, the rewards for his patient will be many.

ACKNOWLEDGMENT

Supported in part by Grant HL 1864b from the U.S. Public Health Service.

REFERENCES

1. Rubin RH: Infection in the renal transplant patient. p. 553. In Rubin RH, Young LS (eds): Clinical Approach to Infection in the Compromised Host. Plenum, New York, 1981
2. Rubin RH, Wolfson JS, Cosimi AB, Tolkoff-Rubin NE: Infection in the renal transplant patient. Am J Med 70:405, 1981
3. Pennock JL, Oyer PE, Reitz BA, et al: Cardiac transplantation in perspective for the future: survival, complications, rehabilitation, and cost. J Thorac Cardiovasc Surg 83:6, 1982
4. Bieber CP, Hunt SA, Schwinn DA, et al: Complications in long term survivors of cardiac transplantation. Transplant Proc 13:207, 1982
5. Dummer JS, Bahnson HT, Griffith BP, et al: Infections in patients on cyclosporine and prednisone following cardiac transplantation. Transplant Proc 15:suppl 1–2, 2779, 1983
6. Auchincloss H Jr, Rubin RH: Clinical management of the critically ill renal transplant patient. In Parrillo JE, Masur H: The Critically Ill Immunosuppressed Patient: Diagnosis and Management. Aspen Press (in press)

7. Scowden EB, Shaffner W, Stone WJ: Overwhelming strongyloidosis: an unappreciated opportunistic infection. Medicine 57:527, 1978

8. Vishwannath S, Baker RA, Mansheim BJ: Strongyloides infection and meningitis in an immunocompromised host. Am J Trop Med Hyg 31:857, 1982

9. Ruskin J: Parasitic diseases in the compromised host. p. 269. In Rubin RH, Young LS (eds): Clinical Approach to Infection in the Compromised Host. Plenum, New York, 1981

10. Nelson PW, Delmonico FL, Tolkoff-Rubin NE, et al: Unsuspected donor *Pseudomonas* infection causing arterial disruption after renal transplantation. Transplantation 37:313, 1984

11. Kyriakides GK, Simmons RL, Najarian JS: Wound infection in renal transplant wounds: pathogenetic and prognostic factors. Ann Surg 186:770, 1975

12. Remington JS, Gaines JD, Gripp RB, et al: Further experience with infection after cardiac transplantation. Transplant Proc 4:699, 1972

13. Montgomery JR, Barrett FF, Williams TW: Infectious complications in cardiac transplant patients. Transplant Proc 5:1239, 1973

14. Cosimi AB: Surgical aspects of infection in the compromised host. p. 607. In Rubin RH, Young LS (eds): Clinical Approach to Infection in the Compromised Host. Plenum, New York, 1981

15. Copeland DJ, Stinson EB: Human heart transplantation. Curr Probl Cardiol 3:4, 1980

16. Ramsey PG, Rubin RH, Tolkoff-Rubin NE, et al: The renal transplant patient with fever and pulmonary infiltrates: etiology, clinical manifestations, and management. Medicine 59:206, 1980

17. Rubin RH, Tolkoff-Rubin NE: Viral infection in the renal transplant patient. Proc Eur Dial Transplant Assoc 19:513, 1982

18. Rubin RH, Tolkoff-Rubin NE: The problem of cytomegalovirus infection in transplantation. p. 89. In Morris PJ, Tilney NL (eds): Progress in Transplantation. Vol. 1. Churchill Livingstone, Edinburgh, 1984

19. Ho M: Cytomegalovirus, Biology and Infection. Plenum, New York, 1982

20. Betts RF, Freeman RB, Douglas RG Jr, et al: Transmission of cytomegalovirus infection with renal allograft. Kidney Int 8:385, 1975

21. Ho M, Suwansirikul S, Dowling JN, et al: The transplanted kidney as a source of cytomegalovirus infection. N Engl J Med 293:1109, 1975

22. Rubin RH, Tolkoff-Rubin NE, Oliver D, et al: Multicenter seroepidemiologic study of the impact of cytomegalovirus infection on renal transplantation. Transplantation 40:243, 1985

23. Preiksaitis JK, Rosno S, Grumet C, et al: Infections due to herpesviruses in cardiac transplant recipients: role of the donor heart and immunosuppressive therapy. J Infect Dis 147:974, 1983

24. Rubin RH, Wilson EJ, Barrett LV, Medearis DN: Primary cytomegalovirus infection following cardiac transplantation in a murine model. Transplantation 37:306, 1984

25. Shanley JD, Billingsley AM, Shelby J, Corry RJ: Transfer of murine cytomegalovirus by heart transplantation. Transplantation 36:584, 1983

26. Wilson EJ, Medearis DN Jr, Barrett LV, Rubin RH: Activation of latent murine cytomegalovirus in cardiac explant and cell cultures. J Infect Dis 152:625, 1985

27. Bia MJ, Andiman W, Gaudio K, et al: Effect of treatment with cyclosporine versus azathioprine on incidence and severity of cytomegalovirus (CMV) infection post transplantation. Transplantation, 40:610, 1985

28. Cheeseman SH, Rubin RH, Stewart JA, et al: Controlled clinical trial of prophylactic human leukocyte interferon on renal transplantation. Effects on cytomegalovirus and herpes simplex virus infections. N Engl J Med 300:1345, 1979

29. Rubin RH, Cosimi AB, Hirsch MS, et al: Effects of anti-thymocyte globulin on cytomegalovirus infection in renal transplant recipients. Transplantation 31:143, 1981

30. Pollard RB, Rand KB, Arvin AM, et al: Cell mediated immunity to cytomegalovirus infection in normal subjects and cardiac transplant patients. J Infect Dis 137:541, 1978

31. Rand KH, Pollard RB, Merigan TC: Increased pulmonary superinfections in cardiac transplant patients undergoing primary cytomegalovirus infection. N Engl J Med 298:951, 1978

32. Pollard RB, Arvin AM, Gamberg P: Specific cell-mediated immunity and infections with herpes viruses in cardiac transplant recipients. Am J Med 73:679, 1982

33. Luby JP, Brunett W, Hull AR, et al: Relationship between cytomegalovirus and hepatic function abnormalities in the period after renal transplant. J Infect Dis 129:511, 1974

34. Goodman MD, Porter DD: Cytomegalovirus vasculitis with fatal colonic hemorrhage. Arch Pathol 96:281, 1973

35. Sutherland DER, Chan FY, Foucar E, et al: The bleeding cecal ulcer in transplant patients. Surgery 86:368, 1979

36. Simmons RL, Motas AJ, Rattazzi LC, et al: Clinical characteristics of the lethal cytomegalovirus infection following renal transplantation. Surgery 82:537, 1977

37. Rubin RH, Cosimi AB, Tolkoff-Rubin NE, et al: Infectious disease syndromes attributable to cytomegalovirus and their significance among renal transplant recipients. Transplant 24:458, 1977

38. Rubin RH, Russell PS, Levin M, Cohen C: Summary of a workshop on cytomegalovirus infections during organ transplantation. J Infect Dis 139:728, 1979

39. Schooley RT, Hirsch MS, Colvin RB, et al: Association of herpesvirus infection with T-lymphocyte-subset alterations, glomerulopathy, and opportunistic infections after renal transplantation. N Engl J Med 308:307, 1983

40. Pollard RB, Egbert PR, Gallagher JG, et al: Cytomegalovirus retinitis in the immunosuppressed host. Ann Intern Med 93:655, 1980

41. Moiker SC, Ascher NL, Kalis JM, et al: Epstein-Barr virus antibody responses and clinical illness in renal transplant recipients. Surgery 85:433, 1979

42. Cheeseman SH, Henle W, Rubin RH, et al: Epstein-Barr virus infection in renal transplant recipients: effects of antithymocyte globulin and interferon. Ann Intern Med 193:39, 1980

43. Hanto DW, Frizzera G, Gajl-Peczalska J, et al: The Epstein-Barr virus (EBV) in the pathogenesis of post-transplant lymphoma. Transplant Proc 12:756, 1981

44. Hanto DW, Frizzera G, Purtilo DT, et al: Clinical spectrum of lymphoproliferative disorders in renal transplant recipients and evidence for the role of Epstein-Barr virus. Cancer Res 41:4235, 1981

45. Thiru S, Calne RY, Nagington J: Lymphoma in renal allograft patients treated with cyclosporin-A as one of the immunosuppressive agents. Transplant Proc 13:359, 1981

46. Crawford DH, Thomas JA, Janossy G, et al: Epstein-Barr virus nuclear antigen positive lymphoma after cyclosporine-A treatment in patients with renal allograft. Lancet 1:1355, 1980

47. Hanto DW, Sakamoto K, Purtilo DT, et al: The Epstein-Barr virus in the pathogenesis of post-transplant lymphoproliferative disorders. Surgery 90:204, 1981

48. Dummer JS, Bound LM, Singh G, et al: Epstein-Barr virus-induced lymphoma in a cardiac transplant recipient. Am J Med 77:179, 1984
49. Hanto DW, Frizzera G, Gajl-Peczalska KJ, et al: Epstein-Barr virus-induced B-cell lymphoma after renal transplantation. N Engl J Med 306:913, 1982
50. Crawford DH, Sweny P, Edwards JMB, et al: Long-term T-cell mediated immunity to Epstein-Barr virus in renal allograft recipients receiving cyclosporin-A. Lancet 1:10, 1981
51. Bird AG, McLachlan SM, Britton S: Cyclosporin-A promotes spontaneous out-growth in vitro of Epstein-Barr virus-induced B-cell lines. Nature 289:300, 1981
52. Starzl TE, Porter KA, Iwatsuki S, et al: Reversibility of lymphomas and lympho-proliferative lesions developing under cyclosporin-steroid therapy. Lancet 1:583, 1984
53. Ho M: Virus infections after transplantation in man; brief review. Arch Virol 55:1, 1977
54. Laquaglia MP, Tolkoff-Rubin NE, Dienstag JL, et al: Impact of hepatitis on renal transplantation. Transplantation 32:504, 1981
55. Hooper DC, Pruitt AA, Rubin RH: Central nervous system infection in the chronically immunosuppressed. Medicine 61:166, 1982
56. Rubin RH, Hooper DC: Central nervous system infection in the compromised host. Med Clin North Am 69:281, 1985
57. Wolfson JS, Sober AJ, Rubin RH: Dermatologic manifestations of infection in the compromised host. Annu Rev Med 34:205, 1983
58. Wolfson JS, Sober AJ, Rubin RH: Dermatologic manifestations of infection in immunocompromised patients. Medicine 64:115, 1985

8 Biliary Tract Sepsis

W. Scott Helton
E. Patchen Dellinger

Infection is an important cause of morbidity and mortality in patients undergoing biliary surgery. Since 20 million people in the United States have gallstones and biliary tract surgery is the second most common operation performed, biliary sepsis will be a significant component of every general surgeon's practice. The intent of this chapter is to review the current state of knowledge about biliary sepsis, its occurrence in a variety of patient populations, and the proper treatment of a patient with established sepsis. Prophylaxis for those who are at risk for developing biliary sepsis and treatment of established sepsis demands an understanding of the pathogenesis of biliary infection, the factors associated with bacterbilia, the microbiology and antibiotic therapy of bacterbilia, and familiarity with the therapeutic options for relieving biliary obstruction.

The initiating events in acute and chronic biliary tract disease usually occur independently of bacteria. The serious complications and the mortality associated with biliary tract disease, however, are almost entirely mediated through bacterial infection. Many patients with biliary disease, such as those with acute cholecystitis or primary cholangitis, are at high risk for developing postoperative infectious complications because they come to operation with established infection.[1] Other patients with asymptomatic bacterbilia and even initially sterile bile are at risk for developing biliary and systemic sepsis during or after operative or T-tube cholangiography and percutaneous and endoscopic investigations and manipulations of the biliary tree.

The term *biliary sepsis* in its strictest sense refers to infection occurring within any area of the hepatobiliary tree. The term *cholangitis* literally means inflammation of the bile ducts but clinically refers to the manifestation of infected bile under pressure within the bile ducts. Cholangitis is not a single disease with a distinct, well-defined clinical appearance but a spectrum of disease with a wide range of severity. The appearance and course of cholangitis ranges from mild, intermittent, recurrent episodes of abdominal pain, jaundice, fever, and chills described by Charcot in 1877[2] to a rapidly progressive systemic illness resulting in shock, coma, and death as described by Reynolds and Dargin in 1959.[3] Although the pathogenesis of cholangitis is not entirely clear, its development requires the presence of at least three, and probably four, factors: (1) obstruction to the flow of bile; (2) colonization of the bile with bacteria (bacterbilia); (3) elevation of intraductal biliary pressure; and (4) some element of biliary mucosal inflammation or injury.

Obstruction to the flow of bile can happen anywhere within the biliary tree from the papilla of Vater in intrahepatic biliary radicals. Charcot in 1877 was the first to recognize this and attributed the occurrence of what he termed "intermittent hepatic fever" to stagnant bile resulting from stones, benign blockages, and malignancies.[2] Today the most common form of obstruction associated with cholangitis is obstruction secondary to calculi; the next most common causes are benign stricture of the ducts and malignancy.[4]

The mechanisms of bacterial colonization in a previously unoperated patient are not known. Four routes of bacterial entrance to the biliary tree have been proposed: (1) an ascending route from the intestine through the papilla of Vater; (2) migration of bacteria across intestinal mucosa into the portal circulation and then secretion into the bile ducts (portal-hepatic-biliary route); (3) hematogenous bacteremic seeding of the liver; and (4) spread from intestinal lymphatics. Clinical and laboratory evidence appears to support the first two mechanisms.[5-9]

In 1959 Reynolds and Dargin recognized that in cholangitis shock and delirium were sometimes associated with Charcot's triad of abdominal pain, fever and chills, and jaundice, creating what is now referred to as Reynolds' pentad. They showed that in such patients pus under pressure—not simply infection—had often developed within the biliary ducts and that this critical condition often improved with early surgical decompression. Subsequent authors have shown, however, that the clinical correlation between purulent cholangitis, Reynolds' pentad, and subsequent response to therapy is not a straightforward one.[10-12] Some patients present with systemic sepsis and shock and die without pus in the biliary tree. Others who present without the signs and symptoms of Reynold's pentad are found to have purulence under pressure within the biliary tree at the time of operation and do quite well after surgery.

Bacterbilia in the presence of obstruction does not always lead to cholangitis.[13,14] Experimental studies have demonstrated that increases in intraductal pressure lead to cholangiovenous and cholangiolymphatic reflux of bacteria and are probably responsible for the septic complications of cholangitis.[15-17] In addition to an increase in biliary ductal pressure, ductal mucosal inflammation or injury appears to be highly associated with the onset of cholangitis. Patients with biliary calculi may develop inflammation of the common bile duct mucosa secondary to either the presence or passage of stones, which subsequently allows the bacteria present within the duct to traverse the mucosal barrier. Instrumentation of the biliary tree intraoperatively, percutaneously, or endoscopically may result in injury to the biliary mucosa, again allowing bacteria to cross the epithelial barrier and gain access to the bloodstream. It is likely that for cholangitis to exist all four of these factors need to be present. Flemma[13] in 1969 and Suzuki[14] more recently have demonstrated that patients can have significant obstruction to the biliary tree with bacterbilia and be asymptomatic. Symptomatic cholangitis in patients with asymptomatic bacterbilia was noted only after manipulation of the biliary tree (resulting in transient increases in intraductal pressure or mucosal injury) or the onset of an inflammatory process. Further evidence to support the significance of elevated intraductal presure has been reported by Wayne and Dellinger.[18,19]

BACTERBILIA

The incidence of bacterbilia and the spectrum of bacterial species isolated differs according to the underlying biliary tract pathology and the techniques utilized in culturing the biliary tree. Several investigators have found that culturing the gallbladder wall will yield a higher incidence of bacterial isolation than culturing just the bile. In one series Keighley demonstrated that when culture of the gallbladder bile was negative, a culture of the gallbladder wall was positive 30 percent of the time.[20] The clinical utility of this information is unclear, however, since postoperative infectious complications result from contamination of the subhepatic space or the abdominal incision from spilled bile. If bacteria are confined to the gallbladder wall alone, the likelihood of contamination during its removal will be very small. When the gallbladder bile Gram stain is positive, there is no need to culture other sites since the bacteria isolated will be the same.[20]

Human bile is thought to be sterile in the absence of biliary tract pathology although there is some evidence that this is not always true. Lykkegaard Nielson[22] and Csendes[23] both failed to isolate bacteria from bile in 58 patients undergoing nonbiliary tract upper abdominal surgery. In a similar group of patients, however, Dye found that 20 percent had bacterbilia and that 17 percent of liver biopsies grew bacteria.[24] Greg failed to isolate any bacteria from the common duct bile of 45 patients undergoing endoscopic retrograde cholangiopancreatography (ERCP) and sphincterotomy for papillary stenosis after cholecystectomy.[25] The fact that bacterbilia is associated with several pathologic conditions of the biliary tree suggests intermittent passage of organisms through the bile in normal subjects but with rapid clearance. Impediment to bile flow by stones or foreign bodies may allow such bacteria to proliferate within the bile ducts, resulting in bacterbilia.[8]

Bacterbilia is associated most commonly with calculus biliary tract disease but is also present in other diseases that involve obstruction of the choledochus. Table 8-1 illustrates the incidence of bacterbilia in various pathologic conditions of the biliary tree. Those in which bacterbilia is more prevalent include common bile duct stones, prior biliary tract surgery, foreign bodies in the biliary tree, and acute inflammation. Sphincteroplasty and other biliary-enteric anasto-

Table 8-1. Incidence of Bacterbilia

Diagnosis	Positive Bile Culture (%)	Reference
Cholelithiasis		
No CBD stones/normal GB	5.3–12	5, 8, 26, 27
Chronic cholecystitis	18–33	28, 29, 30, 33
Acute cholecystitis	47–100	8, 23, 31, 32, 33, 34
Choledocholithiasis		
First operation	56–93	14, 34, 35, 36, 37, 38, 39, 49
Prior biliary operation	80–100	9, 18, 28, 40, 41, 42, 37, 49
Hepatolithiasis	96–100	14, 43
Biliary tubes		
T Tubes after CBDE	84–100	19, 40, 44, 45, 46
Percutaneous biliary drain	67	64
Malignant obstruction		
Partial	45	14
Complete	0–15	14, 47, 13, 9, 22
Biliary-enteric anastomosis	80–100	13, 48
Postsphincteroplasty sphincterotomy	70–76	25

moses lead to bacterbilia in almost all situations. The incidence of bacterbilia increases with age as well. It occurs in more than 50 percent of patients who are over 60 years old and approaches 90 percent in those over 80 years old.[33,49,56] Patients who require emergency operations for biliary tract disease have a higher incidence of bacterbilia than those having elective procedures. Among patients having elective procedures, jaundiced patients have bacterbilia more than nonjaundiced individuals.[1,51] The incidence of bacterbilia associated with malignant obstruction of the biliary tree is less than that with obstruction secondary to calculi or benign stricture. Furthermore, incomplete malignant obstruction is associated with a greater incidence of bacterbilia than is complete obstruction.[14]

BACTERIOLOGY

The most commonly isolated bacterium from bile in patients with biliary tract disease is *Escherichia coli,* followed by other *Enterobacteriaceae, Enterococcus,* and anaerobes—predominantly *Bacteroides* spp and *Clostridium* spp (Table 5-2). Recent authors using modern anaerobic culture techniques have reported anaerobes in 39 to 45 percent patients, accounting for about 20 percent of all isolates (see Table 8-3). Anaerobes are seldom found alone, usually occurring with *Enterobacteriaceae* and seldom causing bacteremia. England and Rosenblatt[51] found aerobes alone in 60 percent of 286 biliary tract cultures, aerobic and anaerobic mixed infection in 39 percent, and anaerobes alone in 1 percent. In that patient group 27 percent of patients with anaerobic bacterbilia had bacteremia, but only 11 percent of the bacteremic patients had anaerobes recovered from their blood.[53] Bacterbilia is usually polymicrobial (average, 3.2 isolates per patient) and rarely due to single isolates.[42,57]

Table 8-2. Biliary Bacteria: Three Combined Studies

Bacteria spp.	No. Isolates	Percent of Total
Escherichia coli	225	21
Klebsiella-Enterobacter spp	205	19
Enterococcus	154	14
Other gram-negative rods	149	14
Bacteroides fragilis	104	10
Clostridium spp	74	7
Other	166	15

(Data from Lykkegaard, Nielsen, and Justesen[22] England and Rosenblatt,[51] and Shimada et al.[52])

The type of underlying biliary pathology, the presence of T tubes, stents, transhepatic tubes, or catheters, previous operation, and the use of antibiotics all will alter the biliary flora.[14,54,55] The incidence of anaerobic recovery is increased by biliary enteric anastomosis, pigmented intrahepatic stones, and older age. Patients receiving antibiotics either acutely or chronically, for prophylaxis or for recurrent cholangitis and those with a previous operation on the choledochal apparatus have an increased recovery of less common species of bacteria such as *Pseudomonas* and *Serratia*.[54]

INFECTIOUS COMPLICATIONS

The presence of bacterbilia at the time of operation significantly increases the risk of developing postoperative infectious complications[13,35,56,58] (Table 8-4). Hence patients with the greatest chance of having bacterbilia (those with jaundice, acute cholecystitis, age greater than 70, common bile duct stones, previous biliary tract operation, or emergent operation) are at the greatest risk for developing postoperative wound infection and sepsis. Postoperative infection rates in patients with bacterbilia are $2\frac{1}{2}$ to 40 times higher than in patients with sterile intraoperative bile cultures.[34] In a study by Keighley, 90 percent of septic episodes and 64 percent of wound infections were caused by organisms isolated from bile intraoperatively.[35] Chetlin and Elliott found that cultures of blood and abscesses in patients with postoperative sepsis yielded the same organisms that were identified at operation.[34] Other investigators have reported

Table 8-3. Anaerobes in Bile

Study	No. Patients	No. with Anaerobes (%)		Year
England & Rosenblatt[51]	253	100	(40)	1977
Shimada et al[52]	40	18	(45)	1977
Lykkegaard Nielsen & Justesen[22]	41	16	(39)	1976
All isolates	1077[a]	213[b]	(20)[c]	

[a] Number of isolates from 334 patients.
[b] Number of anaerobic isolates.
[c] Percent of all isolates which were anaerobes.

Table 8-4. Incidence of Postoperative Infection Related
To Bacterbilia

Study	Operative Bile Cultures (%)	
	Sterile	Positive
Keighley[58]	11	39
Mason[56]	6	23
Chetlin & Elliot[34]	1	30
Wacha & Helm[59]	0	11

similar correlations.[35,56] Conversely, of patients with wound infections, the majority (77 to 88 percent) have had bacterbilia.[54] The most common infectious complications in patients with bacterbilia are wound infection, sepsis, and intra-abdominal abscess. The report by Chetlin and Elliott is representative, with a wound infection rate of 23 percent, sepsis rate of 12.5 percent, and intra-abdominal abscess rate of 6 percent. Keighley reported that other infections, such as pneumonia and urinary tract infections, were often caused by organisms also found in the bile at the time of operation.[35]

Patients who have had cholangitis associated with either intrahepatic duct strictures, intrahepatic stones, sclerosing cholangitis, or oriental cholangiohepatitis are at risk for developing intrahepatic microabscesses. The treatment of such abscesses requires first the relief of obstruction and then prolonged use of antibiotics and sometimes resection of involved liver parenchyma.[43,60–62]

DEVICE INTERVENTION

In patients who have sterile bile at an initial operation, the probability of bacterbilia increases dramatically after operation, especially if any complications occur or if indwelling tubes or drains are used. In several series the incidence of bacterbilia at initial common duct exploration was 40 to 80 percent. Of those patients with sterile bile in the operating room 44 to 100 percent became colonized in the postoperative period, leading to a postoperative incidence of T-tube bacterbilia of 76 to 100 percent (Table 8-5). In the patient

Table 8-5. Bacteria in T-Tube Bile: Percent of Patients with
Positive Cultures

Study	OR	Neg to Pos[a]	Final Pos[b]
Silen et al[44]	40	76	86
Pitt et al[45]	70	45	84
Dellinger et al[19]	53	58	85
Keighley[20]	56	44	76
Jackaman et al[40]	80	100	100

[a] Percent of patients with negative cultures in the operating room who subsequently developed positive T-tube bile cultures.
[b] Percent of all patients with positive T-tube bile cultures in the postoperative period

with retained common bile duct stones the likelihood of bacterbilia is large (76 to 100 percent).[40]

Patients with bacterbilia are at risk for bacteremic sepsis during postoperative cholangiography[19,46] or percutaneous and endoscopic diagnostic and therapeutic manipulations of the biliary tree. Thus it is important to recognize the incidence of bacterbilia and the setting in which it occurs. In some patients cholangitis, sepsis, and shock will be precipitated by diagnostic maneuvers such as ERCP and transhepatic, operative, and T-tube cholangiography, all of which can increase the pressure within the biliary system. When it is looked for, bacteremia is found following percutaneous transhepatic cholangiography and drainage in 5 percent (4 to 28 percent) of patients[63-66,116]; after T-tube tract manipulations for stone removal in up to 15 percent of patients[18]; after T-tube cholangiograms in 9 percent (5 to 15 percent) of all patients[19,46]; after T-tube cholangiograms in patients with known bacterbilia in 21 percent (11 to 51 percent)[46,57]; and after ERCP in 5 percent (0 to 14 percent) of patients.[67,68] Fever or some other manifestation of infection occurs in a greater percent of patients undergoing cholangiography.[19,46,69] These febrile reactions or septic episodes following biliary tract manipulations may be secondary to the effects of some unrecognized factors other than bacteria. Endotoxemia, for example, has been found to occur in 50 to 81 percent of patients with obstructive jaundice.[70-73] Ingolby found that preoperative endotoxemia in patients with obstructive jaundice was statistically associated with death after surgery in the biliary tree.[73] The total blood bile acid pool is increased in cholestatic jaundice,[74] and certain bile acids have been shown to be pyrogenic under experimental conditions.[75]

The presumed etiology of these episodes of bacteremia and other reactions is the close anatomic relation of the terminal biliary radicals and the hepatic sinusoids. Observations in laboratory animals and in man have confirmed that passage of bacteria-sized particles from the bile ducts into the bloodstream occurs readily at pressures in the biliary tree of 15 to 30 cm water, which is only slightly above resting pressures prior to manipulation.[9] Lygidakis and others have revealed that routine cholangiographic procedures in either the operating room or the radiology suite commonly exceed 40 cm water and that under these circumstances bacteremia and sepsis are more common.[57] It appears, therefore, that febrile reactions and the signs and symptoms of cholangitis may result from a disturbance (such as increases in pressure) within the biliary ducts, resulting in the systemic release of a pyrogenic bacterium, endotoxins, bile acids, or other unidentified toxic substances.

Attempts to prevent bacteremia and sepsis or to ameliorate their consequences during cholangiography have often focused on the use of antibiotics. Unfortunately, antibiotics are probably of little use for this purpose. Three separate studies on the incidence of bacteremia following cholangiography have failed to show any positive influence of antibiotic administration.[7,19,46] Two of these studies have related the incidence of bacteremia or serious reaction after cholangiography to the control of pressure during the study.[19,57] In a patient who is at risk for endocarditis the use of antibiotics to prevent valve colonization is advisable, but there is no evidence that their use will prevent bacteremia or reduce the incidence of febrile and hemodynamic reactions accompanying biliary tract manipulation. Dellinger reported no episodes of sepsis in patients undergoing postoperative T-tube cholangiography when a gravitational method was utilized.[19] The use of antibiotics did not prevent this complication when dye was injected. Similarly, Lygidakis[57] demonstrated a 51 percent incidence of bacteremia when the injection method of intraoperative cholangiography was utilized in patients with bacterbilia, compared with a 7 percent incidence of bacteremia when a gravitational method was used. In the latter study all patients received preoperative ampicillin and gentamicin.

PREVENTING POSTOPERATIVE INFECTIONS

Prophylactic administration of antibiotics preoperatively to patients with bacterbilia will lower the incidence of wound infection and intra-abdominal abscess (Table 8-6). Preoperative and preprocedural antibiotics do not, however, prevent the development of bacteremia and sepsis in patients with bacterbilia.[7,19,57] Holman reported a sepsis rate of 28 percent in patients undergoing operations for complex biliary problems despite the preoperative administration of antibiotics.[7] One reason for this is that patients with bacterbilia often have some element of obstruction, and while obstruction persists, antibiotics do not enter the bile in therapeutic concentrations. During operation manipulations of the common bile duct such as cholangiography result in transient elevations in intraductal biliary pressures, leading to cholangiovenous reflux of bacteria and endotoxin. While antibiotics may prevent colonization and metastatic infection resulting from transient bacteremia, they cannot affect the acute febrile and hemodynamic consequences of endotoxemia.[73]

The proper use of antibiotics for active biliary sepsis or for prevention of postoperative infection depends upon several factors. First, one must identify the patients at risk. Second, it is important to know which species of bacteria are likely to colonize the biliary tree under different pathologic circumstances and their likely sensitivities. Finally, the individual properties of the antibiotics, such as antibacterial spectrum, biliary excretion, tissue penetration, toxicity

Table 8-6. Antibiotic Effect on Wound Infection Rate

Study	Antibiotic	No Antibiotic (%)	With Antibiotic (%)	P Value
Cainzos et al[77]	Cefamandole	28	0	<.01[a]
Koufman et al[78]	Gentamicin	24.5	3.6	<.05
Lewis et al[76]	Cefazolin	19.6	2.2	<.005[a]
Keighley et al[80]	Gentamicin	21	6	<.05[a]
Strachan et al[82]	Cefazolin	17	4	<.025
Stone et al[81]	Cefazolin	11	2	<.01
Chetlin & Elliot[79]	Cephaloridine	11	4	NR[b]

[a] Randomized, prospective, controlled study
[b] Prospective
NR = Not reported

and cost, should be known. The presence of any of the risk factors listed in Table 8-1 are predictive of bacterbilia and of an increased chance of developing postoperative infection. Prophylactic preoperative use of antibiotics is therefore warranted in patients who have one or more of these risk factors.

The issue of tissue versus bile levels of antibiotics often arises in discussions of antibiotic use with biliary tract procedures. Several facts suggest that adequate tissue levels of antibiotics are more important than high excretion rates of antibiotics into the bile. First, antibiotics that have poor biliary excretion, such as the aminoglycosides, are effective both for prevention of postoperative infections and for treatment of established infections. Keighley treated two groups of patients with bacterbilia undergoing biliary surgery with preoperative antibiotics. One group received rifampin, which is highly secreted into the bile. The other group received gentamicin, which is poorly secreted into the bile but which has good tissue levels and a better sensitivity spectrum. Infection rate in the gentamicin group was 6 percent versus 22 percent in the group receiving rifampin.[80] Further evidence to support this concept is the fact that all serious infections in the biliary tree occur in the presence of bile duct obstruction. If the bile duct is obstructed, no antibiotic achieves therapeutic levels in the bile. No antibiotic administered preoperatively or preprocedure has reduced the incidence of positive bile culture at operation or percutaneous cholangiography.

The timing of antibiotic administration is quite important for prophylaxis. To be effective, preoperative antibiotics need to be administered 3 to 60 minutes before the operation commences so that tissue levels are high in the wound and around the area of dissection in the biliary tree.[21,81] Stone showed that if antibiotics were delivered 1 hour preoperatively, with two additional postoperative doses, wound infection rates were reduced fivefold.[81] Strachan showed that a single preoperative dose of cefazolin could decrease wound infection fourfold.[82] Depiro et al. determined that intraoperative serum and tissue concentrations of cefazolin and cefoxitin were higher if administered at induction of anesthesia as compared with on-call to the operating room.[21] On the other hand, Chetlin, Elliott, and Stone demonstrated that antibiotics started postoperatively did not lessen the infection rate.[79,81] Three prospective studies show no difference in the incidence of bacterbilia measured at the time of operation in groups of patients undergoing biliary surgery who did and did not receive antibiotics.[79,80,82] In one study of bacteria isolated following common duct exploration, the bacterial flora changed postoperatively; increases being found in resistant organisms, gram-negative anaerobic organisms, yeast, and the absolute number of different species being found. The use of antibiotics did not change this but instead resulted in an increase in the isolation of anerobes.[54]

Because gram-negative enteric bacteria are the most common species found in patients with bacterbilia and are the most frequent cause of postoperative wound infections and bacteremia, antibiotics effective against these organisms should be selected for prophylaxis. Cephalosporins, new-generation penicillins, and aminoglycosides all offer excellent broad-spectrum coverage in this setting and have good tissue penetration. Since the first-generation cephalosporin cefazolin is the least expensive, has the fewest side effects, and has established efficacy along with prolonged elevation of serum levels, it is an excellent first choice drug for prophylactic use in patients with bacterbilia. Cephalosporins do not cover for enterococcus, which, however, is rarely responsible for postoperative infections.

TREATING ESTABLISHED BILIARY INFECTION

The treatment of biliary sepsis differs from prophylaxis in the need for more specific antimicrobial therapy dictated by the particular patient's underlying pathology. For example, patients with previous biliary enteric anastomoses and patients with intrahepatic stones have a higher incidence of anaerobes. A patient with a stent or one recently operated on for cholangitis may have resistant flora, such as *Pseudomonas* and *Serratia* spp. Hence, until bacterial isolates are identified in these patients and sensitivities known, antibiotic coverage should be extended to cover virtually all potential biliary pathogens— aerobes and anaerobes, gram-negative and gram-positive enterics. Clindamycin or metronidazole and an aminoglycoside provide such broad-spectrum antimicrobial coverage. Some investigators believe that enterococcus should be covered as well, though this is controversial. Enterococci may be more likely to contribute to the clinical picture of cholangitis than to cause postoperative wound infections. Ampicillin can be added to cover for enterococus. The second- and third-generation cephalosporins (cefotaxime and ceftizoxime) and penicillins (mezlocillin and piperacillin) have been reported to be as effective in treating patients with biliary sepsis as clindamycin or metronidazole plus an aminoglycoside; however, the published literature is not adequate to draw definitive conclusions regarding relative efficacy.[107] Of the new agents, cefoxitin covers both anaerobes and aerobes but not enterococcus and is relatively cheap. Since the use of an aminoglycoside may be toxic in patients with cholangitis who are already at risk for renal failure because of sepsis, jaundice, and possible age-related renal disease, cefoxitin is a good second choice drug. Mezlocillin has been advocated by some[83] because it has, in addition to cefoxitin's spectrum, activity against enterococcus.

A patient with cholangitis from partial biliary obstruction may benefit from the use of an antibiotic that achieves high bile concentrations. Wacho[59] and Helm[84] have both treated separate groups of patients with nasobiliary decompression of obstructed common bile ducts with mezlocillin and ceftizoxime, respectively, and were able to completely eradicate the bacterbilia in most of their patients. However, if obstruction is not completely relieved and indwelling tubes and catheters remain in place, the chance of early recolonization is great and the next organism may be a resistant one.

Bacteria which persist in the biliary tract after invasive procedures such as common bile duct exploration with T-tube placement, percutaneous stone extraction, or stone dissolution are of some theoretical concern. Certainly the

Table 8-7. Mortality in Acute Cholangitis

Study	Year	Mortality (%)	Response to Initial Medical Management (%)
UCLA/Thompson et al[55]	1981	9	70
UCSF/Boey & Way[12]	1980	16	85
JHH/Saharia & Cameron[87]	1976	14	80
MGH/Welch & Donaldson[86]	1976	40	NR
UCSD/Saik et al[88]	1975	22	NR

NR = Not reported
UCLA = University of California, Los Angeles
UCSF = University of California, San Francisco
JHH = Johns Hopkins Hospital
MGH = Massachusetts General Hospital
UCSD = University of California, San Diego

overwhelming majority of patients who have had any indwelling biliary prosthesis, stent, or irrigation catheter will have bacterbilia. Little information exists concerning the fate of bacterbilia in this patient population because once the tubes and stents are out, access to bile for culture is gone without additional invasive procedures. We do know, however, that if these patients return with retained or recurrent stones or with a stricture, they are essentially 100 percent colonized with bacteria.

The persistence of these common duct bacteria may be important since there is evidence that long-term bacterial colonization of the bile ducts may predispose to formation of calcium bilirubinate stones through the deconjugation of bilirubin by bacterial beta-glucuronidase.[115] Bacteria commonly found in bile and possessing this enzyme include *Escherichia coli, Klebsiella* spp, *Bacteroides* spp, and *Clostridium* spp. It is an attractive concept that treatment of a patient with an antibiotic that is effective against the bacteria in his bile ducts and achieves high bile levels (such as mezlocillin or ceftizoxime) might succeed in clearing the ducts of bacterial colonization. If effective, this practice could in theory avoid some cases of recurrent common bile duct stone formation. This practice can only be effective, however, if done after all foreign bodies are out of the duct and anatomic abnormalities have been corrected to allow for unimpeded flow of bile.

As discussed above, biliary sepsis (cholangitis) is always associated with obstruction and bacterbilia although obstruction and bacterbilia can exist together without cholangitis. Since antibiotics will not change bacterbilia in the face of obstruction, the prime force of treatment for cholangitis must be directed at relieving obstruction. This is illustrated by the fact that the mortality rate due to severe suppurative cholangitis is close to 100 percent without operation[92,93] and approximately 40[12] to 54 percent[85] when operative treatment is undertaken.[12,85,86]

A review of the treatment of acute cholangitis from five major surgical centers in the United States shows that mortality varies from 9 to 40 percent (Table 8-7). Treatment strategies were similar and consisted of vigorous fluid and electrolyte replacement to achieve hemodynamic stability, nasogastric suction to reduce stimuli for pancreatic and biliary secretions, and the use of broad-spectrum I.V. antibiotics. On this regimen, 70 to 85 percent of patients with acute cholangitis improved and were able to undergo diagnostic studies prior to later operative decompression of the biliary tree and correction of the underlying pathology. The patients who failed to respond to medical therapy underwent emergent operation, and in this group mortality was high. In the patients from Hopkins, 50 percent of the deaths occurred because of recurrent or persistent biliary sepsis due to an inability to completely correct the underlying pathologic cause of obstruction. Saharia argues that if preoperative imaging of the biliary tree had been performed in these patients, it might have prevented some deaths. This is the argument for trying to stabilize a patient with antibiotics and resuscitation, thus providing the surgeon with the time to study the biliary tree radiologically.

In the 15 to 30 percent of patients in whom there is no dramatic reduction in fever and in whom abdominal tenderness and leukocytosis occur within 24 to 48 hours after the onset of nonoperative treatment for cholangitis, emergent operation to decompress the biliary tree should be performed. Death from cholangitis has been correlated with failure to respond to this early period of medical stabilization and antibiotic treatment ($P < .001$) irrespective of the time of operation.[55] In this group of refractory patients there was a high incidence of suppurative cholangitis and intrahepatic abscesses, which carried an operative mortality rate of 40 to 54 percent.[12,85] Thompson[55] reported that 86 percent of deaths in their patients occurred in those operated on after 72 hours. He did not believe, however, that adverse outcome was secondary to a delay in surgical decompression; rather, it was related to complex anatomic and pathologic abnormalities of the biliary tree. In contrast to Thompson's report, Welch and Donaldson[86] reported that operative mortality was 17 percent if patients were operated on within less than 24 hours and 50 percent if after 24 to 72 hours. It is hard to know from this latter study if mortality was truly related to time of operation alone because there was no analysis of deaths with respect to patient's underlying pathology, anatomy, and severity of cholangitis.

Thompson showed that the clinical course of acute cholangitis, predilection for fatal outcome, and recurrent attacks could be accurately predicted from the primary etiology of the first attack of acute cholangitis. For example, a high operative mortality occurred in patients with cholangitis secondary to malignant or congenital obstruction whereas mortality was rare in those with cholangitis secondary to calculi, primary sclerosing cholangitis, or benign strictures. Recurrent attacks of cholangitis were more frequent in obstruction secondary to stricture, biliary cancer, or sclerosing cholangitis. Reoperation for recurrent cholangitis was more common for stricture but was never required for cholangitis due to carcinoma or sclerosing cholangitis. In the latter two entities the cleansing and replacement of biliary tubes was generally effective in treating secondary attacks. Boey and Way also reported that benign duct stricture, sclerosing cholangitis, and 80 percent of choledocholithiasis cases were associated with less severe cholangitis, which usually responded to antibiotic treatment.[12]

The spectrum of acute cholangitis ranges from mild attacks, easily managed nonoperatively, to severe, unrelenting attacks, with sepsis, shock, and high mortality. It is the latter group of patients who are usually thought to have acute obstructive suppurative cholangitis and possibly miliary intrahepatic abscesses with complete bile duct obstruction needing emergent decompression. Boey,[12] O'Connor,[10] and Saharia[87] have all pointed out, however, that the correlation between suppuration in the bile duct and the clinical manifestations of cholangitis is inexact. Roughly half of patients with suppuration under pressure in the biliary tree will have shock and a deteriorating status. The other half of the patients can be medically stabilized and undergo radiologic diagnostic studies and elective operation.[10,87] Of all patients who have ascending cholangitis, only 50 to 70 percent will have all three components of Charcot's triad[10,12] The diagnosis of cholangitis must therefore often be made on a high index of suspicion, and the decision to operate must be based upon clinical judgment and evaluation of the patient's response to early aggressive non-operative therapy.

The traditional treatment for a first episode of acute cholangitis has been cholecystectomy, common bile duct exploration, and T-tube drainage.[89-93] In patients too ill to undergo cholecystectomy, cholecystostomy-tube drainage of the gallbladder is necessary because of the high incidence of cholecystitis in cholangitis.[92,93] Cholecystostomy drainage alone for acute cholangitis may provide inadequate decompression of the biliary tree and has a reported mortality of 80 percent, compared with 26 percent after common bile duct decompression.[88] These figures are, however, biased by case selection, with many surgeons performing cholecystostomy alone only on the most severely ill patients.

Choi and Wong have used operative sphincteroplasty and choledochojejunostomy for the initial treatment of cholangitis in over 400 patients with an operative mortality of 2.3 to 4.7 percent.[94,95] It should be noted that Choi's patients were all from Hong Kong and had benign disease, primarily oriental cholangiohepatitis. The majority of these patients respond to early medical management and are operated on semielectively. In those patients who required emergency operation, mortality was 12.9 percent.

Recently invasive radiologic and endoscopic techniques such as percutaneous transhepatic drainage and endoscopic drainage of the biliary tree have assumed a more prominent role in the initial treatment of cholangitis. Transhepatic catheter drainage of the biliary tree has been studied extensively for decompression of the uninfected, totally obstructed biliary tree.[63-66,96-103, 112,113,116] Its use as an emergent method of decompressing the infected obstructed duct has only recently been reported by several authors.[47,103-106] (Table 8-8). Fifty-one patients so treated for acute cholangitis have responded to such treatment, with a combined series mortality rate of 12 percent. In one study by Takata five patients had miliary intrahepatic abscesses secondary to calculus obstruction, all of which resolved after successful decompression of the biliary tree by percutaneous catheter.[104] These results appear at least comparable with those obtained by more traditional operative means.

Endoscopic sphincterotomy and nasal biliary drainage have been used to

Table 8-8. Transhepatic Percutaneous Drainage for Cholangitis

Study	No. Patients	No. with Purulence (Intrahepatic Abscess or Shock)	Deaths	Year
Nakayama et al[103]	9	4	1	1978
Kadir et al[105]	18	9	3	1982
Takada et al[104]	16	5	0	1976
Gould et al[106]	7	1	2	1985
O'Connor et al[47]	1	0	0	1981
Total	51	19 (37%)	6 (12%)	

treat acute cholangitis secondary to calculus biliary obstruction in elderly patients, with promising results in Europe and Japan.[110,114] Reiter has reported excellent results with endoscopic sphincterotomy as treatment of cholangitis in patients with the Sump syndrome secondary to choledochoduodenostomy.[110] His operative mortality was 1.5 percent, with a complication rate of 7 percent, compared with an operative mortality rate of 20 percent in patients over 70 years old from reoperative biliary tract disease.[111] Ikeda reported three patients with suppurative cholangitis secondary to calculus obstruction of the common bile duct, all of whom responded to emergent endoscopic cannulation of the common bile duct followed by endoscopic sphincterotomy.[112] The utility of these newer techniques may be greatest in the elderly, frail patient who has had previous biliary tract surgery. Evidence to date suggests that these procedures have a high rate of success in the desperately ill elderly patient.[66,109,110,114] The ultimate verdict regarding safety and therapeutic efficacy, however, will have to await prospective trials comparing them with traditional surgical means of treatment.

In summary, the surgeon's armamentarium for treating biliary tract disorders has been greatly expanded by the development of newly refined invasive radiologic, endoscopic, and operative techniques. Percutaneous and endoscopic manipulations of the biliary tree have opened a new arena for dealing with complicated severe biliary tract disorders, such as unresectable carcinoma complicated by purulent cholangitis. These techniques have the liability, however, of also introducing bacteria to the sterile obstructed biliary tree and of precipitating cholangitis. In a patient who already has bacterbilia, the risk of precipitating sepsis and bacteremia from such biliary tract manipulations is even higher. They should be used with caution and expertise, with special care to avoid sudden elevation of ductal pressures. It is clear that the surgical approach to decompression of the biliary tree for cholangitis will be guided by the nature of the underlying disease, its clinical severity, the extent and location of obstruction, the history of past surgical treatment, the operative techniques available, and the experience of the operator.

CONCLUSION

Prophylactic antibiotics in elective biliary tract surgery should be used in patients with a high probability of bacterbilia since they are at higher risk for developing wound complications and intra-abdominal abscess. Prophylactic antibiotics will not protect against bacteremia, which may be precipitated by cholangiography or manipulation of the biliary tree during operation. In patients at risk for endocarditis an antibiotic effective against bacteria found in the bile should be used prior to manipulations of the biliary tree. In other patients every effort should be made to avoid high pressures or undue trauma during procedures on the biliary tract. Bacteremia and other infectious complications following biliary tract surgery should be treated empirically when they occur. Antibiotics for this purpose should be chosen for their antimicrobial spectrum and effective serum levels and not for bile levels. Transient bacteremia without persistent symptoms occurring at the time of a procedure may not need specific treatment at all. Efforts to eliminate bacterbilia after correction of anatomic abnormalities and elimination of duct stones may be worthwhile. For this purpose, antibiotics which achieve high bile levels and are effective against the bacteria present in the bile are probably useful.

Treatment of biliary sepsis ideally involves a multidisciplinary approach, including hemodynamic stabilization, antibiotics, and a variety of methods for decompressing the obstructed biliary tree. Biliary sepsis is always associated with some element of underlying obstruction and bacterbilia. In addition, elevated intrabiliary pressures, with resulting cholangiovenous reflux and some element of mucosal damage or inflammation, are probably important. Roughly 80 percent of patients presenting with biliary sepsis can be controlled initially with rigorous medical resuscitation and systemic I.V. antibiotics. Selection of antibiotics should be based upon the patient's previous history of biliary tract disease and aimed at covering the potential pathogens that are known to exist with specific disease states. Roughly 15 to 20 percent of patients will not respond to such initial management, and in the majority of these patients failure is due to a totally obstructed biliary tree, resulting in persistent cholangiovenous reflux and the development of multiple intrahepatic abscesses. Mortality in this group of patients is extremely high even with early operative decompression. If stabilization of the patient does occur, radiologic imaging of the biliary tree should be performed in order to direct an accurately corrective operation.

Once operative decompression of the biliary tree is undertaken, a variety of methods may be used with equal efficacy. Currently there is no consensus regarding the optimal approach to patients with serious biliary sepsis—the operation used will be determined primarily by the type of obstructive biliary pathology, the history of previous biliary surgical treatment, and the preference of the surgeon. Nonoperative techniques such as endoscopic papillotomy, nasobiliary stents, and percutaneous catheters offer temporary means of stabilizing, and sometimes definitive treatment of, septic patients, particularly in the elderly population. Operative drainage of the common bile duct (by a variety of methods) is currently considered the most certain means of ensuring rapid and effective biliary drainage. When comparing results of methods used for the treatment of biliary sepsis, one must be aware of the patient populations under study and the nature of their underlying diseases.

Because of the diverse pathology, anatomic variabilities, range of severity at initial presentation, and relatively small number of cases in any one institution there have been no prospective trials comparing these different treatment plans in comparable groups of patients with cholangitis. In the absence of this type of information, dogmatic statements about optimal approaches for all patients with cholangitis cannot be made.

REFERENCES

1. Keighley MRB, Drysdale RB, Quoraishi AH, et al: Antibiotic treatment of biliary sepsis. Surg Clin North Am 55:1379, 1975
2. Charcot JM: Leçons sur les Maladies due Fore des Voies Bilares at des Veins. Paris, Faculte de Médecine de Paris, Recueillées et publiées par Bourneville et Sevestre, Paris, 1877
3. Reynolds BM, Dargan EL: Acute obstructive cholangitis. Ann Surg 150:299, 1959
4. Longmire WP: The diverse causes of biliary obstruction and their remedies. Curr Probl Surg 14:1, 1977
5. Lotveit T, Osnes M, Aune S: Bacteriological studies of common duct bile in patients with gallstone disease and juxta-papillary duodenal diverticula. Scand J Gastroenterol 13:93, 1977
6. Keighley MRB, Burdon DW: Identification of bacteria in the bile by duodenal aspiration. World J Surg 2:255, 1978
7. Holman JM Jr, Rikkers LF, Moody FG: Sepsis in the management of complicated biliary disorders. Am J Surg 138:809, 1979
8. Kune GA, Hibberd J, Morahan R: The development of biliary infection: an experimental study. Med J Aust 1:301, 1974
9. Scott AJ, Kahn GA: Origin of bacteria in the bile duct. Lancet 2:790, 1967
10. O'Connor MJ, Schwartz ML, McQuarrie DG, et al: Acute bacterial cholangitis: an analysis of clinical manifestation. Arch Surg 117:437, 1982
11. O'Connor MJ, Sumner HW, Schwartz ML: The clinical and pathologic correlations in mechanical biliary obstruction and acute cholangitis. Ann Surg 195:419, 1982
12. Boey JH, Way LW: Acute cholangitis. Ann Surg 191:264, 1980
13. Flemma RJ, Flint LM, Osterhout S, et al: Bacteriologic studies of biliary tract infection. Ann Surg 166:261, 1967
14. Suzuki Y, Kobayashi A, Ohto M, et al: Bacteriological study of transhepatically aspirated bile: relation to cholangiographic findings in 295 patients. Dig Dis Sci 29:109, 1984
15. Mixer HW, Rigler LG, Gonzales-Oddone MV: Experimental studies on biliary regurgitation during cholangiography. Gastroenterology 9:64, 1947
16. Jacobsson B, Kjellander J, Rosenbren B: Cholangiovenous reflux: an experimental study. Acta Chir Scand 123:316, 1962
17. Huang T, Bass JA, Williams RD: The significance of biliary pressure in cholangitis. Arch Surg 98:629, 1969
18. Wayne PH III, Whelan JG Jr: Susceptibility testing of biliary bacteria obtained before bile duct manipulation. AJR 140:1185, 1983
19. Dellinger EP, Kirshehbaum G, Weinstein M, et al: Determinants of adverse reaction following postoperative T-tube cholangiogram. Ann Surg 191:397, 1980
20. Keighley MRB: Microorganisms in the bile. A preventable cause of sepsis after biliary surgery. Ann R Coll Surg Engl 59:328, 1977
21. DiPiro JT, Vallner JJ, Bowden TA Jr, et al: Intraoperative serum and tissue activity of cefazolin and cefoxitin. Arch Surg 120:829, 1985

22. Lykkegaard Nielsen M, Justesen T: Anaerobic and aerobic bacteriological studies in biliary tract disease. Scand J Gastroenterol 11:437, 1976
23. Csendes A, Fernandez M, Uribe P: Bacteriology of the gallbladder bile in normal subjects. Am J Surg 129:629, 1975
24. Dye M, MacDonald A, Smith G: The bacterial flora of the biliary tract and liver in man. Br J Surg 65:285, 1978
25. Gregg JA, De Girolami P, Carr-Locke DL: Effects of sphincteroplasty and endoscopic sphincterotomy on the bacteriologic characteristics of common bile duct. Am J Surg 149:668, 1985
26. Goswitz JT: Bacteria and biliary tract disease. Am J Surg 128:644, 1974
27. Larmi TKI, Fock G, Vuopio P: Occurrence and antibiotical sensitivity of aerobic bacteria in bile and their role in postoperative inflammatory complications in biliary tract diseases. Acta Chir Scand 114:379, 1958
28. Engstrom J, Groth CG, Lundh G, Lonngrist B: Infectious complications after surgery for biliary calculus. Acta Chir Scand 138:357, 1972
29. Keighley MRB, Graham NG: Infective cholecystitis. J R Coll Surg Edinb 18:213, 1973
30. Robson MC, Bogart JN, Heggers JP: An endogenous source for wound infections based on quantitative bacteriology of the biliary tract. Surgery 68:471, 1970
31. Jarvinen HJ: Biliary bacteremia at various stages of acute cholecystitis. Acta Chir Scand 146:427, 1980
33. Funkunaga FH: Gallbladder bacteriology, histology, and gallstones: Study of unselected cholecystectomy specimens in Honolulu. Arch Surg 106:169, 1973
34. Chetlin SH, Elliott DW: Biliary bacteremia. Arch Surg 102:303, 1971
35. Keighley MRB, Lister DM, Jacobs SI, et al: Hazards of surgical treatment due to microorganisms in the bile. Surgery 75:578, 1974
36. Edlund Y, Mollstedt BO, Ouchterlony O: Bacteriological investigations of the biliary system and liver in biliary tract disease correlated to clinical data and microstructure of the gall bladder and liver. Acta Chir Scand 116:461, 1958
37. Maddocks AC, Hilson GRF, Taylor R: The bacteriology of the obstructed biliary tree. Ann R Coll Surg Engl 52:316, 1973
38. Cox JL, Helfrich LR, Pass HI, et al: The relationship between biliary tract infections and postoperative complications. Surg Gynecol Obstet 146:233, 1978
39. Wolloch Y, Feizeneberg Z, Zer M, et al: The influence of biliary infection on the postoperative course after biliary tract surgery. Am J Gastroenterol 67:456, 1977
40. Jackaman FR, Hilson RF, Lord Smith: Bile bacteria in patients with benign bile duct stricture. Br J Surg 67:329, 1980
41. Lygidakis NJ: Surgical approaches to postcholecystectomy choledocholithiasis. Arch Surg 117:481, 1982
42. Lygidakis NJ: Incidence of bile infection in patients with choledocholithiasis. Am J Gastroenterol 77:12, 1982
43. Tabata M, Nakayama F: Bacteriology of hepatolithiasis. Prog Clin Biol Res 152:163, 1984
44. Silen W, Wertheimer M, Kirshenbaum G: Bacterial contamination of the biliary tree after choledochostomy. Am J Surg 135:325, 1978
45. Pitt HA, Postier RG, Cameron JL: Biliary bacteria: significance and alterations after antibiotic therapy. Arch Surg 117:445, 1982
46. Pitt HA, Postier RG, Cameron JL: Postoperative T-tube cholangiography: Is antibiotic coverage necessary? Ann Surg 191:30, 1980
47. O'Connor MJ, Schwartz ML, McQuarrie DG, et al: Cholangitis due to malignant obstruction of biliary outflow. Ann Surg 193:341, 1981

48. Hitch DC, Lilly JR: Identification, quantification and significance of bacterial growth within the biliary tract after Kasai's operation. J Pediatr Surg 13:563, 1978
49. Lygidakis NJ: Incidence and significance of primary stones of the common bile duct in choledocholithiasis. Surg Gynecol Obstet 157:434, 1983
50. Soon-Shiong P, Debas HT: Prevention of infection in gastroduodenal and biliary surgery, p. 258. In Wilson SE, Finegold SM, Williams RA (eds): Intraabdominal Infection, McGraw-Hill, New York, 1982
51. England DM, Rosenblatt JE: Anaerobes in human biliary tracts. J Clin Microbiol 6:494, 1977
52. Shimada K, Inamatsu T, Yamashiro M: Anaerobic bacteria in biliary disease in elderly patients. J Infect Dis 135:850, 1977
53. Bourgault AM, England DM, Rosenblatt JE, et al: Clinical characteristics of anaerobic bactibilia. Arch Intern Med 139:1346, 1979
54. Pitt HA, Postier RG, Cameron JL: Biliary bacteria: significance and alterations after antibiotic therapy. Arch Surg 117:445, 1982
55. Thompson JE, Tompkins RK, Longmire WP: Factors in management of acute cholangitis. Ann Surg 195:137, 1982
56. Mason GR: Bacteriology and antibiotic selection in biliary tract surgery. Arch Surg 97:533, 1968
57. Lygidakis NJ: Potential hazards of intraoperative cholangiography in patients with infected bile. Gut 23:1015, 1982
58. Keighley MRB: Infection in biliary tract surgery. In Watts, McDonald, O'Brien, et al (eds): Infection in Surgery. Churchill Livingstone, Edinburgh, 1981
59. Wacha H, Helm EB: Efficacy of antibiotics and bacteriobilia. J Antimicrob Chemother suppl. A, 131, 1982
60. Choi TK, Wong J, Ong GB: The surgical management of primary intrahepatic stones. Br J Surg 69:86, 1982
61. Sato T, Suzuki N, Takahashi W, et al: Surgical management of intrahepatic gallstones. Ann Surg 192:28, 1980
62. Yamakawa T: Percutaneous transhepatic stone extraction technique for management of retained biliary tract stones. p. 253. In Okuna K, Nakayama F, Wong J (eds): Intrahepatic Calculi. Alan R. Liss, New York, 1984
63. Stambuk EC, Pitt HA, Pai OS, et al: Percutaneous transhepatic drainage: Risks and benefits. Arch Surg 118:1388, 1983
64. McPherson GAD, Benjamin IS, Habib NA, et al: Percutaneous transhepatic drainage in obstructive jaundice: advantages and problems. Br J Surg 69:261, 1982
65. Pollock TW, Ring ER, Oleaga JA, et al: Percutaneous decompression of benign and malignant biliary obstruction. Arch Surg 114:148, 1979
66. Ferrucci JT Jr, Mueller PR, Harbin WP: Percutaneous transhepatic biliary drainage. Radiology 135:1, 1980
67. Parker HW, Geenen JE, Bjork JT, et al: A prospective analysis of fever and bacteremia following ERCP. Gastrointest Endosc 25:102, 1979
68. Siegel JH, Berger SA, Sable RA, et al: Low incidence of bacteremia following endoscopic retrograde cholangiopancreatography (ERCP). Am J Gastroenterol 71:465, 1979
69. Bilbao MK, Dotter CT, Lee TG, et al: Complications of endoscopic retrograde cholangiopancreatography (ERCP). Gastroenterology 70:314, 1976
70. Wilkinson SP, Moodie H, Stamatakis JD, et al: Endotoxemia and renal failure in cirrhosis and obstructive jaundice. Br Med J 2:1415, 1976
71. Bailey ME: Endotoxin, bile salts and renal function in obstructive jaundice Br J Surg 63:774, 1976

72. Wardle EN: Renal failure in obstructive jaundice—pathogenic factors. Postgrad Med J 51:512, 1975
73. Ingoldby CJ, McPherson GAD, Blumgart LH: Endotoxemia in human obstructive jaundice. Am J Surg 147:766, 1984
74. Stiehl A: Disturbance of bile acid metabolism in cholestasis. Clin Gastroenterol 6:45, 1977
75. Bundy PK, Bodel P: Mechanism of action of pyrogenic antipyretic steroids in vitro. p. 101. In Wholstenholme GEW, Birch J (eds): Ciba Foundation Symposium. Churchill Livingstone, Edinburgh, 1971.
76. Lewis RT, Allan CM, Goodall RG, et al: A single preoperative dose of cefazolin prevents postoperative sepsis in high-risk biliary surgery. Can J Surg 27:44, 1984
77. Cainzos M, Potel J, Puente JL: Prospective randomized controlled study of prophylaxis with cefamandole in high risk patients undergoing operations upon the biliary tract. Surg Gynecol Obstet 160:27, 1985
78. Kaufman Z, Engelberg M, Eliashiv A, et al: Systemic prophylactic antibiotics in elective biliary surgery. Arch Surg 119:1002, 1984
79. Cletlin SH, Elliott DW: Preoperative antibiotics in biliary surgery. Arch Surg 107:319, 1973
80. Keighley MRB, Drysdale RB, Quoraishi AH, et al: Antibiotics in biliary disease: the relative importance of antibiotic concentrations in the bile and serum. Gut 17:495, 1976
81. Stone HH, Hooper CA, Kolb LD, et al: Antibiotic prophylaxis in gastric, biliary, and colonic surgery. Ann Surg 184:443, 1976
82. Strachan CJL, Black J, Powis SJA, et al: Prophylactic use of cephazolin against wound sepsis after cholecystectomy. Br Med J 1:1254, 1977
83. Pitt HA: Selective Antibiotic therapy in surgery. Part 3: The use of antibiotics in biliary tract surgery. Surgical Practice News, McMahon Publishing Co., June 1983
84. Helm EB, Wurbs D, Haag R, et al: Elimination of bacteria in biliary tract infections during ceftizoxime therapy. Infection 10:67, 1982
85. Pitt HA, Longmire WP: Suppurative cholangitis. In Hardy JD (ed): Critical Surgical Illness. 2nd Ed. WB Saunders, Philadelphia, 1980
86. Welch JP and Donaldson GA: The urgency of diagnosis and surgical treatment of acute suppurative cholangitis. Am J Surg 131:527, 1976
87. Saharia PC, Cameron JL: Clinical management of acute cholangitis. Surg Gynecol Obstet 142:369, 1976
88. Saik RP, Greenburg AG, Farris JM, et al: Spectrum of cholangitis. Am J Surg 130:143, 1975
89. Way LW, Dunphy JE: Management of choledocholithiasis. Ann Surg 176:347, 1972
90. DenBesten L, Doty JE: Pathogenesis and management of choledocholithiasis. Surg Clin North Am 61:893, 1981
91. Jordan GL Jr: Choledocholithiasis. Curr Probl Surg 19:722, 1982
92. Hinchey EJ, Couper CE: Acute obstructive suppurative cholangitis. Am J Surg 117:62, 1969
93. Dow RW, Lindenauer SM: Acute obstructive suppurative cholangitis. Ann Surg 169:272, 1969
94. Choi TK, Wong J, Lam KH, et al: Late result of sphincteroplasty in the treatment of primary cholangitis. Arch Surg 116:1173, 1981
95. Choi TK, Wong J, Ong GB: Choledochojejunostomy in the treatment of primary cholangitis. Surg Gynecol Obstet 155:43, 1982

96. Tylen U, Hoevels J, Vang J: Percutaneous transhepatic cholangiography with external drainage of obstructive biliary lesions. Surg Gynecol Obstet 144:13, 1977

97. Schwartz W, Rosen RJ, Fitts WT, et al: Percutaneous transhepatic drainage preoperatively for benign biliary strictures. Surg Gynecol Obstet 152:466, 1981

98. Ring EJ, Kerlan RK Jr: Interventional biliary radiology. AJR 142:31, 1984

99. Denning DA, Elison EC, Carey LC: Preoperative percutaneous transhepatic biliary decompression lowers operative morbidity in patients with obstructive jaundice. Am J Surg 141:61, 1981

100. Norlander A, Kalin B, Sundblad R: Effect of percutaneous transhepatic drainage upon liver function and postoperative mortality. Surg Gynecol Obstet 155:161, 1982

101. Gouma DJ, Wesdorp RIC, Oostenbroek RJ, et al: Percutaneous transhepatic drainage and insertion of an endoprosthesis for obstructive jaundice. Am J Surg 145:763, 1983

102. Hansson JA, Hoevels J, Simert G, et al: Clinical aspects of nonsurgical percutaneous transhepatic bile drainage in obstructive lesions of the extrahepatic bile ducts. Ann Surg 189:58, 1979

103. Nakayama T, Ikeda A, Okuda K: Percutaneous transhepatic drainage of the biliary tract. Gastroenterology 74:544, 1978

104. Takada T, Hanyu F, Kobayashi S, et al: Percutaneous transhepatic cholangial drainage: direct approach under fluoroscopic control. J Surg Oncol 8:83, 1976

105. Kadir S, Baassiri A, Barth KH, et al: Percutaneous biliary drainage in the management of biliary sepsis. AJR 138:25, 1982

106. Gould RJ, Vogelzang RL, Neiman HL, et al: Percutaneous biliary drainage as an initial therapy in sepsis of the biliary tract. Surg Gynecol Obstet 160:523, 1985

107. Solomkin JS, Meakins JL Jr, Allo MD, et al: Antibiotic trials in intra-abdominal infections: a critical evaluation of study design and outcome reporting. Ann Surg 200:29, 1984

108. Viceconte G, Viceconte GW, Pietropaolo V, et al: Endoscopic sphincterotomy: indications and results. Br J Surg 68:376, 1981

109. Cotton PB, Vallon AG: Duodenoscopic sphincterotomy for removal of bile duct stones in patients with gallbladders. Surgery 91:628, 1982

110. Reiter JJ, Bayer HP, Mennicken C, et al: Results of endoscopic papillotomy: a collective experience from nine endoscopic centers in West Germany. World J Surg 2:505, 1978

111. Vellacott KD, Powell PH: Exploration of the common bile duct: a comparative study. Br J Surg 66:389, 1979

112. Ikeda S, Tanaka M, Itoh H, et al: Emergency decompression of bile duct in acute obstructive suppurative cholangitis by duodenoscopic cannulation: a lifesaving procedure. World J Surg 5:587, 1981

113. Hatfield ARW, Terblanche J, Fataar S, et al: Preoperative external biliary drainage in obstructive jaundice. Lancet 2:896, 1982

114. Cotton PB, Vallon AG: British experience with duodenoscopic sphincterotomy for removal of bile duct stones. Br J Surg 68:373, 1981

115. Feretis CB, Contou CT, Manouras AJ, et al: Long term consequences of bacterial colonization of the biliary tract after choledochostomy. Surg Gynecol Obstet 159:363, 1984

116. Voegeli DR, Crummy AB, Weese JL: Percutaneous transhepatic cholangiography, drainage, and biopsy in patients with malignant biliary obstruction. Am J Surg 150:243, 1985

9 | Percutaneous Drainage of Abdominal Abscesses: The Role of the Radiologist

R. Brooke Jeffrey, Jr.

Newer radiologic imaging techniques have made a major impact on the management of patients with severe intra-abdominal infections. High-resolution computed tomography (CT) and ultrasound have greatly enhanced our ability to noninvasively diagnose and localize intra-abdominal abscesses.[1-10] When combined with modified angiographic techniques these modalities are often highly successful in guiding percutaneous abscess drainage.[11-18] In approximately 85 percent of patients this results in definitive therapy for the abscess, and thus surgery can be avoided with a minimum of patient discomfort, morbidity and cost.[11-16] This chapter will focus on current concepts in percutaneous abscess drainage and its role in managing patients with intra-abdominal sepsis.

DIAGNOSIS AND LOCALIZATION OF ABDOMINAL ABSCESSES

A variety of imaging techniques may be utilized to diagnose intra-abdominal abscesses. These include plain abdominal radiographs and radioisotope scans with ^{67}Ga and ^{111}In labeled white cells, as well as CT and ultrasound.[4,8] CT and ultrasound provide superior detail for defining complex anatomic re-

133

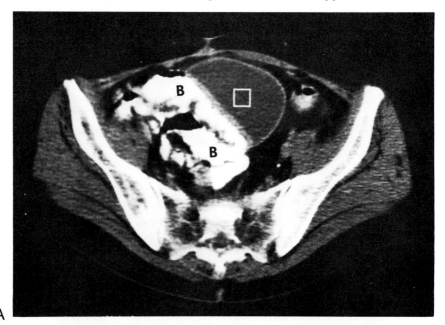

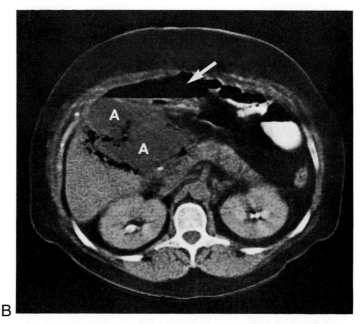

Fig. 9-1.   Spectrum of CT and ultrasound findings in abdominal abscesses. (Fig. A) Typical appearance of abdominal abscess with loculated fluid collection (cursor box), exhibiting mass effect and displacing bowel (B) adjacent to it. (Jeffrey RB Jr: Pelvic abscess. p. 55. In Walsh JR (ed): Computed Tomography of the pelvis. Churchill Livingstone, New York, 1985.) (Fig. B) Postoperative subhepatic abscess (A) containing multiple gas bubbles. Note pneumoperitoneum (arrow) from recent laparotomy. (*Figure continues.*)

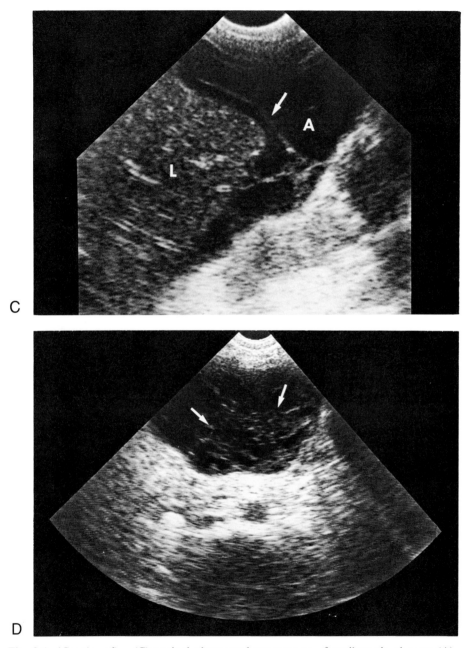

C

D

Fig. 9-1. (*Continued*).   (C) typical ultrasound appearance of perihepatic abscess (A). Longitudinal sonogram shows complex fluid collection with low-level echoes representing debris and septations (arrow) inferior to liver edge (L). (D) Infected pseudocyst in lesser sac. Sonogram demonstrates complex internal echoes within infected pseudocyst with multiple membranes and debris (arrows).

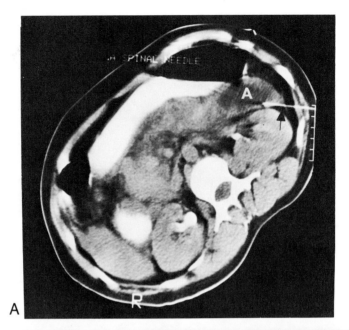

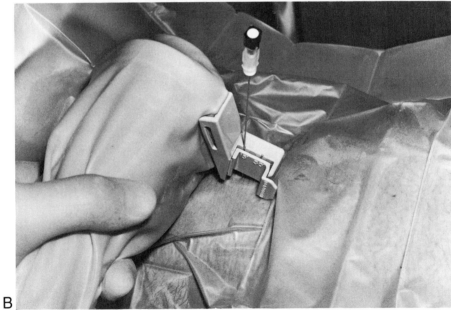

Fig. 9-2. CT and ultrasound guided-needle aspiration techniques. (A) Needle inserted into pancreatic abscess near the tail of the pancreas (arrow). (A = abscess.) Patient is in slight RPO decubitus position. (B) Ultrasound-guided needle aspiration. By using a special biopsy attachment with a slotted needle, the abscess can be punctured directly by a sterile technique under direct ultrasound monitoring.

lationships between abscess and surrounding structures. In addition they can readily guide diagnostic needle aspiration and catheter insertion for abscess drainage. The overall accuracy for CT and sonography in detecting abdominal abscesses is quite high, on the order of 90 to 95 percent.[8]

Ultrasound is particularly useful for diagnosing suspected right upper quadrant and pelvic abscesses.[4,13] This is because there is no intervening bowel gas to impede sonographic visualization. In patients with poorly localized abscesses and in postoperative patients with open surgical wounds and drains, CT is the imaging method of choice for abscess localization.[3]

On CT and ultrasound abscesses typically appear as complex fluid collections (Fig. 9-1A through D). Often, however, the imaging findings are nonspecific and can be mimicked by such abnormalities as hematomas, seromas, bilomas, lymphoceles, etc. This makes guided-needle aspiration essential for precise diagnosis of an infected intra-abdominal fluid collection. The presence of gas bubbles within a fluid collection is the most suggestive feature of an abscess (Fig. 9-1B). However, it is important to emphasize that only one-third of abdominal abscesses will demonstrate this finding.[1] On CT abscesses are often well-defined or encapsulated areas of decreased attenuation (CT numbers on the order of 0 to 20 Hounsfield units), exhibiting mass effect and often displacing bowel loops and adjacent structures (Fig. 9-1A). The sonographic features of an abscess are quite variable and range from complex fluid collections with fluid debris levels to sonolucent or echogenic masses (Fig. 9-1C and D). Because of this variability a high index of suspicion is essential for accurate diagnosis.

While most patients with intra-abdominal abscesses characteristically present with fever, localized pain, and leukocytosis, this is not invariably the case.[14] These clinical symptoms may be masked in patients with chronic, walled-off abscesses and modified in the presence of immunosuppression or prolonged antibiotic therapy. We have recently encountered nine patients with CT and surgical evidence of pyogenic abscesses without fever or leukocytosis.[14] Therefore, an abscess must be considered in the differential diagnosis of any abnormal abdominal fluid collection on CT or ultrasound.

In general, CT- or ultrasound-guided needle aspiration is initially performed with a 22-gauge needle (Fig. 9-2A and B). If no free-flowing fluid is obtained, then a larger, 18-gauge needle is inserted into the collection. Unless fluid can be aspirated from an 18-gauge needle, it is unlikely that the abscess is sufficiently liquefied to be successfully drained percutaneously. If the needle is confirmed to be in the area of abnormalitiy on repeat scanning, then cytologic material is sent as well as culture specimens. If there is any question regarding the nature of the aspirate, immediate Gram stain is mandatory for verification of an abscess.

PATIENT SELECTION FOR PERCUTANEOUS ABSCESS DRAINAGE

There are three important criteria in selecting patients for percutaneous drainage of abdominal abscesses.[15,16] First, there must be liquefied pus that

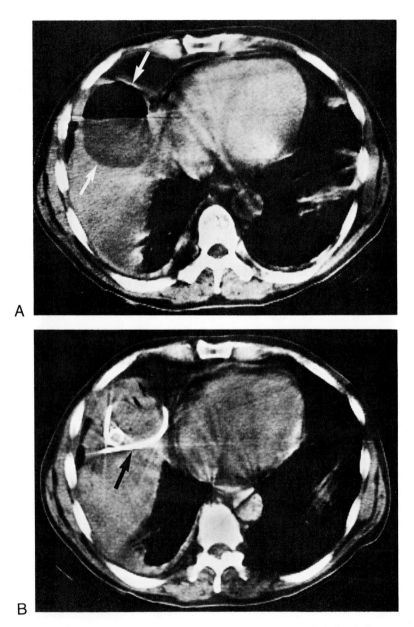

Fig. 9-3. Suitable abscess for percutaneous drainage. (A) A well-defined abscess cavity near the dome of the liver (arrows) with an air fluid level is shown. (B) Complete evacuation of the abscess cavity following insertion of percutaneous pigtail catheter (arrows). (*Figure continues.*)

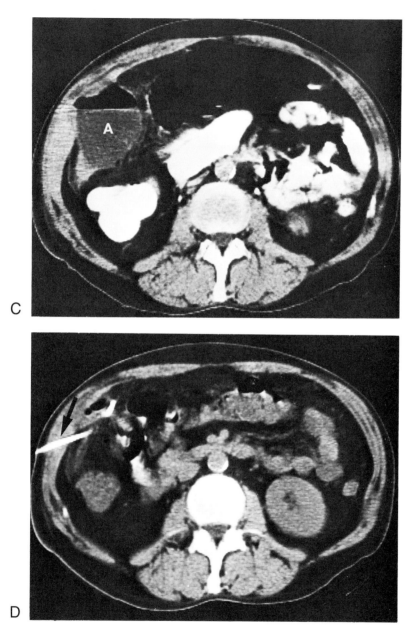

Fig. 9-3 (*Continued*).   (C) well-defined right paracolonic abscess cavity with air fluid level. This followed perforated duodenal ulcer treated medically. The patient had myocardial infarction and was not a good surgical candidate. (A = abscess. Note thickening of abdominal wall adjacent to the abscess.) (D) Complete abscess evacuation following percutaneous insertion of drainage catheter (arrow).

can be evacuated through a drainage catheter; second, the abscess must be well localized (either encapsulated or contained within a discrete anatomic compartment); and finally, there must be safe access for catheter insertion that avoids intervening bowel, pleura, and vascular structures (Figs. 9-3, 9-4).

In reviewing percutaneous abscess drainage in 250 patients Mueller[15] compared the similarities and differences between radiologic and surgical drainage. The major similarity is that complete abscess evacuation is the primary therapeutic effect. Generally, this is accomplished with large-bore sumps in surgically drained abscesses. However, small-bore catheters (including angiographic catheters and smaller sump catheters) have proved quite effective when inserted by radiologically guided techniques.[12] Mueller also noted that older surgical precepts regarding dependent drainage and preference for retroperitoneal versus intraperitoneal approach have not been critical to the success of percutaneous drainage.[15] This is likely due to the ability of CT to image the entire abdomen and provide precise anatomic detail for staging the extent of the abscess and following its subsequent drainage (Fig. 9-5). Finally, a key difference is that radiologically guided percutaneous techniques avoid general anesthesia in critically ill patients and can be accomplished with minimal morbidity, patient discomfort, and medical cost.

Once an abdominal abscess has been localized with CT or ultrasound and confirmed by guided-needle aspiration, a joint decision must be reached by referring clinicians, the interventional radiologist, and the surgeon regarding the feasibility of attempted percutaneous drainage. In general, CT has been the imaging method of choice to stage the extent of the abscess and to determine the safety of percutaneous drainage based on imaging criteria. CT affords more precise visualization of anatomic compartments and intervening bowel loops than sonography and is not hampered by overlying bowel gas, surgical drains, or dressings.

The CT criteria for attempted percutaneous drainage have evolved over several years. Initially it was felt that multilocular abscesses were not suitable for percutaneous drainage.[17] It has been shown that this is not the case and that in general many abscesses that appear multiseptated or multilocular in fact intercommunicate with a single dominant cavity and can often be drained via a single catheter.[17] More than one catheter can also be inserted into the abscess cavity if a true multilocular abscess exists. At present the major contraindications for abscess drainage are related primarily to lack of safe access because of intervening bowel, pleural, or major vascular structures.[15] Surgeons have stressed that prompt surgical debridement is necessary in patients with diffuse pancreatic abscesses because of the extensive associated pancreatic necrosis. While percutaneous drainage of infected pancreatic fluid collections may be useful as a temporizing maneuver to improve the patient's overall condition prior to laparotomy,[18] in general our approach has been to opt for early surgical debridement in widespread and multicompartmental pancreatic abscesses. Known or suspected echinococcal cysts or amebic abscesses are generally not referred for percutaneous abscess drainage.

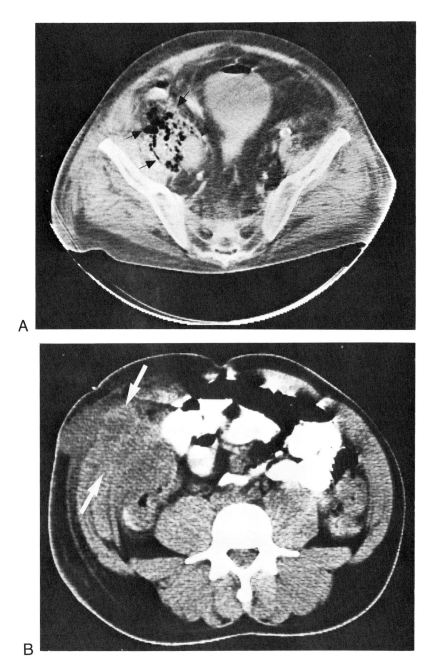

Fig. 9-4. Abscesses not suitable for percutaneous drainage. (A) Diffuse, poorly defined gas-forming abscess extending from the psoas muscle into the lower pelvis and abdomen (arrows). (B) Diffuse, periappendiceal and abdominal wall abscess following ruptured appendix. Because both these abscesses are so poorly defined, they are better treated surgically. (Arrows = abscess.)

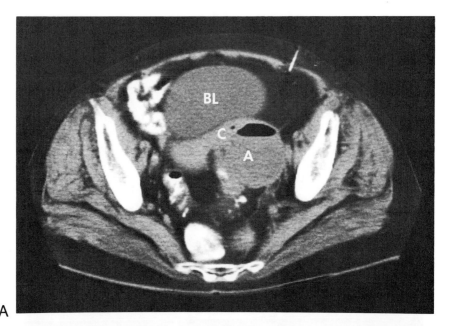

A

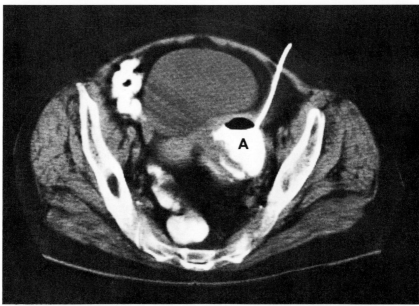

B

Fig. 9-5. CT-guided aspiration of paracolonic abscess from acute diverticulitis. (A) Abscess with air fluid level (A) adjacent to sigmoid colon (C). Urine-filled bladder (BL). Because there is no intervening bowel, a guided-needle aspiration was performed. Note needle in the subcutaneous tissues of the abdominal wall to guide subsequent catheter insertion. (B) Dilute contrast injected through abscess drainage catheter outlining the abscess cavity (A). (Jeffrey RB Jr. Pelvic abscess. p. 55. In Walsh JW (ed): Computed Tomography of the Pelvis. Churchill Livingstone, New York, 1985.) (Case courtesy of Henry I. Goldberg, M.D., San Francisco, California.)

TECHNIQUE OF ABSCESS DRAINAGE

There are several important technical points that need to be emphasized in using CT to guide abdominal abscess drainage. First, it is becoming increasingly clear that an intercostal approach to hepatic, splenic, and subphrenic abscesses runs the risk of traversing the pleura and converting an abdominal abscess into an empyema.[19] Radiologists performing percutaneous abscess drainage should be acutely aware of this problem and should puncture below the tenth intercostal space for all guided drainage procedures. Often this may require a "triangulation" approach, in which the needle is angled craniad from a more caudal entry site either below the twelfth rib posteriorly or by using an anterior subcostal approach.

Generally a combination of CT and fluoroscopy is utilized in performing abdominal abscess drainage. With use of sterile technique and local anesthesia, an abscess is initially localized and confirmed via percutaneous aspiration under CT guidance; then one of two methods may be employed for actual catheter insertion. For superficial abscess directly beneath the abdominal wall a trocar method under fluoroscopic control may be utilized. A second technique is a modified Seldinger approach using a guide wire and angiographic dilators. Once the abscess has been punctured, the guide wire is coiled within the abscess in the CT scanning area. The patient is then transported to the fluoroscopic interventional radiology suite, where subsequent catheter and guide wire manipulation are directly visualized under fluoroscopic control.

Prior to any catheter insertion it is important that the patient received an intravenous bolus of appropriate broad-spectrum antibiotics. In the interventional suite the patient is draped and given mild intravenous sedation and analgesia. Vital signs are closely monitored by nursing personnel. With the patient under a local anesthetic injected around the site of catheter insertion, a small skin incision appropriate for the catheter size is made. Generally, curved-end guide wires are coiled within the abscess cavity to prevent perforation of the cavity and leakage of its contents. Angiographic dilators are then passed over the guide wire to enlarge the percutaneous tract for subsequent catheter insertion.

The catheters utilized for percutaneous abscess drainage are generally of two types: 7 to 10 Fr angiographic pigtail catheters and larger, double-lumen 12 to 16 Fr sump catheters.[15,16] There are no controlled studies evaluating the efficacy of one catheter versus another, and many personal preferences dictate the use of drainage catheters. At our institution smaller abscess cavities (less than 100 cm^3), containing thin, free-flowing pus, are drained with 8 to 9 Fr angiographic pigtail catheters. Larger abscesses, containing more viscous fluid, require larger sump catheters (12 to 16 Fr) for complete evacuation of their contents. It is important to position the side holes of the drainage catheter in the most dependent position of the abscess cavity. Following the complete evacuation of the contents of the abscess, a small amount of dilute contrast is injected through the drainage catheter to determine the volume of the abscess and assess side hole position.

We have found real-time sonography to be quite helpful in determining the completeness of abscess drainage.[20] A portable real-time ultrasound unit can be brought directly into the interventional suite and a sterile glove placed over the transducer. Scans are obtained immediately before and after evacuation of the abscess, and a direct assessment can be made of how complete the abscess cavity, has been drained. Undrained locules of abscess can be identified which may require a second drainage catheter that can be placed directly under ultrasound guidance. In a series of 50 patients at our institution, ultrasound was successful in monitoring the abscess drainage in 45 (90 percent)[20] and in inserting a second catheter in 6 patients.

After the successful evacuation of the abscess the drainage catheter is securely fixed to the patient's skin. At this juncture several physicians advocate vigorous irrigation of the abscess cavity with large volumes of sterile saline to remove all debris and pus from the cavity.[15] Others, however, do not immediately irrigate the abscess out of concern for inducing bacteremia.[13,16] It should be noted that equal success rates have been reported in large series of patients both with and without vigorous irrigation of the abscess cavity, and its role is unclear at this time.[13,15] At our institution we prefer not to perform vigorous irrigation of the abscess cavity following the initial drainage. Catheter irrigation is performed only in patients with very viscous pus. This is generally done several days after appropriate intravenous antibiotics to ensure the sterility of the abscess cavity rather than after the initial drainage.[21]

CATHETER MANAGEMENT FOLLOWING PERCUTANEOUS ABSCESS DRAINAGE

Once the abscess has been completely evacuated, further management of the abscess catheter is directed by the radiology service in conjunction with the patient's physician. In order to ensure catheter patency small amounts of sterile saline (10 to 20 ml) are injected through the catheter several times a day at the patient's bedside. The volume of catheter drainage is measured daily. Major determinants of success in percutaneous abscess drainage include both objective clinical response (decreased fever and leukocytosis) and a significant decrease in the catheter drainage. Patients are maintained on intravenous antibiotics for a full course of therapy during the period of abscess catheter management. In successful cases patients show definite objective signs of clinical response 48 to 72 hours after initial catheter evacuation of the abscess. Patients show a decrease in fever and leukocytosis and an improved sense of well-being with decreasing pain in the region of the abscess cavity. In unilocular abscesses once the volume of the drainage decreases to 10 to 30 ml/day, the catheter can slowly be advanced over several days and can ultimately be removed. The exact length of time of catheter drainage is variable but is on the order of 5 to 10 days in the majority of patients with uncomplicated abscess.

In patients who do not respond clinically within the first 72 hours it is important to reevaluate the adequacy of initial drainage by abscess sinography

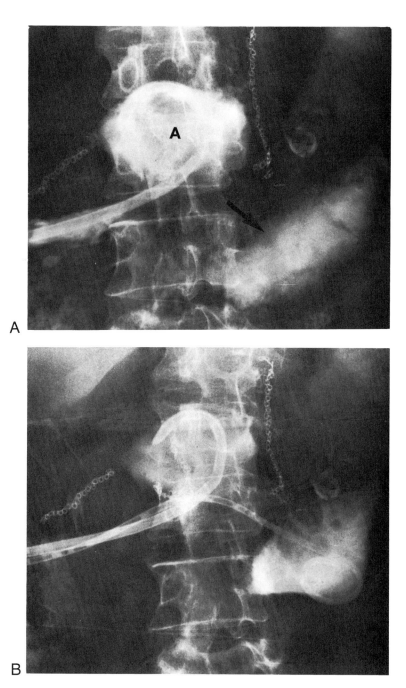

Fig. 9-6. Infected pancreatic pseudocyst with pancreatic fistula. (A) Abscess sinogram with filling of initial cavity drained percutaneously. (A = abscess. Arrow outlines second undrained infected pancreatic pseudocyst.) (B) Catheterization through initial drainage tract of second pseudocyst with placement of pigtail catheter within it. (*Figure continues.*)

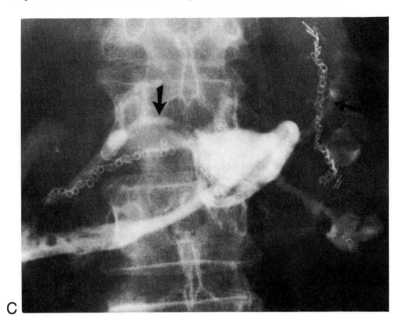

C

Fig. 9-6. (*Continued*).   Two weeks later there is a marked reduction in size of the abscess cavities but also a now well demonstrated fistula to pancreatic duct on contrast injection (arrow).

and CT. Abscess sinography is performed by fluoroscopically controlled injections of dilute contrast into the abscess cavity to define the volume of the residual abscess and detect unsuspected fistulas. After 3 days of intravenous antibiotics contrast can be injected into the cavity with minimal chances of inducing septicemia. Thus the abscess cavity can be directly studied radiographically. Abscess sinography is useful to document the presence of any fistulas to bowel, pancreas, or biliary tree and to ensure appropriate side hole positioning of the drainage catheter within the most dependent portion of the abscess (Fig. 9-6). It is important to note, however, that undrained locules of pus not in communication with the catheter will not be detected by abscess sinography. Repeat CT is necessary to evaluate whether there are additional areas of undrained pus. If a second undrained collection is identified, an additional catheter can be inserted at this juncture. The presence of abdominal fistulas (either high- or low-output) definitely affects the length of drainage and subsequent catheter management (see below).

COMPLICATIONS OF PERCUTANEOUS ABSCESS DRAINAGE

In reviewing percutaneous drainage of abdominal abscesses and fluid collections in 250 patients, van Sonnenberg noted minor complications in 6.6 percent of patients and major complications in 2.8 percent.[11] Minor complications

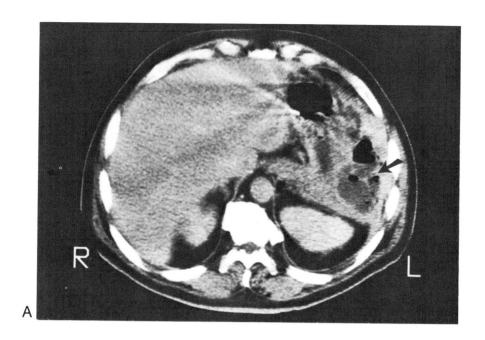

Fig. 9-7. Pancreatic abscess with colonic fistulas. (A) Fluid collection with gas bubbles and air-fluid level representing abscess (arrow). (B) Abscess sinogram demonstrates numerous colonic fistulas (arrows). All fistulas healed with a combination of hyperalimentation, abscess drainage, and antibiotic therapy.

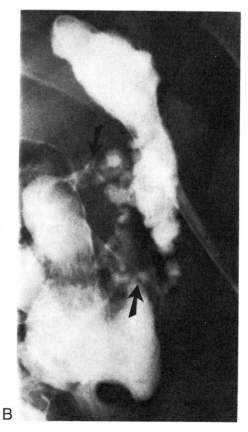

147

include transient septicemia without hypotension (five patients) and minor catheter back bleeding (five patients). In two patients incorrect triangulation methods were used to drain subphrenic abscess, which resulted in a pneumothorax or pleural effusion. In one patient accidental puncture of the hepatic flexure occurred during the trocar method. This was recognized at catheter sinography and the abscess catheter was repositioned without sequelae. Minor infection was noted adjacent to the site of catheter insertion in six patients and was treated with local wound care.

There were seven major complications, including one death.[11] The death resulted from laceration of a mesenteric vessel by a 16-gauge needle during an attempted drainage of a mesenteric abscess. Profound sepsis and disseminated intravascular coagulation were noted in two patients, two patients had septicemia with hypotension occurring after abscess drainage, and two other patients had superinfection of lymphoceles. In the remaining patient jejunal laceration with subsequent fistula formation occurred after drainage of an interloop abscess. The jejunal fistula was managed conservatively without development of peritonitis.

In reviewing the above complications it is clear that they fall in one of two categories, either septic complications or complications related to faulty access with transgression of either pleural, bowel, or major vascular structures. Nevertheless when compared with surgical series, the overall complication rate (10.4 percent with only 2.8 percent of major complications) is quite favorable.

SUCCESS RATE OF PERCUTANEOUS ABSCESS DRAINAGE

The overall success rates for percutaneous drainage of abdominal abscesses is on the order of 85 percent.[11-13] Recurrence rates have been noted to be on the order of 8 percent and are most frequently related to abscesses with underlying fistulas from either the bowel, kidney, pancreas, or biliary tree.[11] In some patients who ultimately require surgery, percutaneous drainage may be a useful temporizing maneuver prior to laparotomy.[18] Often surgery is undertaken to repair anastomoses or to resect fistulas following successful abscess drainage. In van Sonnenberg's series of 250 abscesses, 83.6 percent of patients were managed successfully without need for operation.[11]

In analyzing the causes of failure of percutaneous abscess drainage a number of important points need to be emphasized. Patients with infected phlegmons without significant liquefaction of the abscess are prone to fail percutaneous drainage. Similarly, patients with pancreatic abscesses often require extensive debridement of necrotic debris rather than catheter drainage. The pus in some intra-abdominal abscesses may be too viscous to drain through percutaneously placed catheters. Another cause of failed percutaneous drainage is the presence of fistulas associated with the abscess. In our own series of 72 patients with abdominal abscesses a surprisingly high percentage of low-output fistulas was documented by careful abscess sinograms in 32 patients (44 percent).[22] Although patients with fistulas required longer periods of catheter drainage, the fistulas closed in 27 of 37 patients with abscess drainage alone and without surgery.[22] Treatment failures were related to high-output fistulas and fistulas to the pancreatic duct.

SUMMARY

Percutaneous catheter drainage is a proven technique for management of patients with intra-abdominal abscess. This method can achieve a high rate of success in well selected patients. Complex abscesses and fistulas are frequently encountered in this procedure, and thus considerable experience is required for proper catheter management. Close communication among medical, surgical, and radiologic colleagues is essential to ensure the overall success of this technique.

REFERENCES

1. Callen PW: Computed tomographic evaluation of abdominal and pelvic infections. Radiology 131:171, 1982
2. Koehler PR, Moss AA: Diagnosis of intra-abdominal and pelvic abscesses by computerized tomography. JAMA 244:49, 1980
3. Wolverson MK, Jagannadharao B, Sundaram M, et al: CT as a primary diagnostic method in evaluating intraabdominal abscess. AJR 133:1089, 1979
4. Korobkin M, Callen PW, Filly RA, et al: Comparison of computed tomography, ultrasonography and gallium-67 scanning in the evaluation of suspected abdominal abscesses. Radiology 129:89, 1978
5. Haaga JR, Alfidi RJ, Havrella TR, et al: CT detection and aspiration of abdominal abscesses. Am J Roentgenol 128:465, 1977
6. Aronberg DJ, Stanely RJ, Levitt RG, et al: Evaluation of abdominal abscess with computed tomography. J Comput Assist Tomogr 2:384, 1978
7. Chin LC, Shapiro RL, Yiu VS: Abdominal abscess. Computed tomographic appearance, differential diagnosis and pitfalls in diagnosis. J Comput Assist Tomogr 2:195, 1978
8. Knochel JQ, Koehler PR, Lee TG, Welch DM: Diagnosis of abdominal abscesses with computed tomography, ultrasound, and ^{111}In leukocyte scans. Radiology 137:425, 1980
9. Newlin N, Silver TM, Stuck KJ, Sandler MA: Ultrasonic features of pyogenic liver abscesses. Radiology 139:155, 1981
10. Kressel HY, Filly RA: Ultrasonographic appearance of gas-containing abscesses in the abdomen. AJR 130:71, 1978
11. Van Sonnenberg E, Mueller PR, Ferrucci JT Jr: Percutaneous drainage of 250 abdominal abscesses and fluid collections. Radiology 151:337, 1984
12. Van Sonnenberg E, Ferrucci JT, Mueller PR, et al: Percutaneous drainage of abscess and fluid collections. Techniques, results and applications. Radiology 142:1, 1982
13. Kuligowska E, Conners SK, Shapiro JH: Liver abscess: sonography in diagnosis and treatment. AJR 138:253, 1982

14. Jeffrey RB Jr, Federle MP, Laing FC: Computed tomography of silent abdominal abscesses. J Comput Assist Tomogr 8:67, 1984
15. Mueller PR, van Sonnenberg E, Ferrucci JT Jr: Percutaneous drainage of 150 abdominal abscesses and fluid collections. Part II. Radiology 151:343, 1984
16. Sones PJ: Percutaneous drainage of abdominal abscesses. AJR 142:35, 1984
17. Bernardino ME, Berkman WA, Plemmons M, et al: Percutaneous drainage of multiseptated hepatic abscess. J Comput Assist Tomogr 8:38, 1984
18. Van Sonnenberg E, Wing VW, Casola G, et al: Temporizing effect of percutaneous drainage of complicated abscesses in critically ill patients. AJR 142:821, 1984
19. Neff CC, Mueller PR, Ferrucci JT Jr, et al: Serious complications following transgression of the pleural space in drainage procedures. Radiology 152:335, 1984
20. Jeffrey, RB Jr, Wing VW, Laing FC: Real-time sonographic monitoring of percutaneous abscess drainage. AJR 144:469, 1985
21. Kerlan RK Jr, Pogany AC, Jeffrey RB Jr et al: Radiologic management of abdominal abscesses. AJR 144:145, 1985
22. Kerlan RK Jr, Jeffrey RB Jr, Pogany AC, Ring EJ: Abdominal abscess with low-output fistulae: successful percutaneous drainage. Radiology 155:73, 1985

10 | Management of Endocarditis: Indications for Surgical Intervention

James W. Brooks, Jr.
William E. Dismukes

In the Gulstonian Lectures published in 1885, Sir William Osler reviewed his experience with patients afflicted with malignant endocarditis.[1] Osler was impressed with the clinical course, often marked by persistent fever, and by the finding of micrococci in cardiac vegetations at autopsy. He concluded that malignant endocarditis was caused by an infectious process involving the heart valves. Over the next 50 years investigators gained much insight into the pathogenesis of infective endocarditis (IE) and carefully recorded its clinical manifestations and complications. However, no progress was made toward effective therapy to reverse or arrest the disease process. Accordingly, up to the early 1940s IE inevitably resulted in death.

Successful medical treatment of patients with IE was first reported in 1944 when Loewe and associates described the cure of seven patients utilizing penicillin in doses of 40,000 to 200,000 units per day.[2] Despite the improvement in survival afforded by the use of penicillin and subsequent bactericidal antimicrobial agents, the mortality rate in patients with IE remained high. Effective antimicrobial therapy often prevented death from persistent infection; nevertheless, a significant proportion of patients eventually succumbed to congestive heart failure (CHF) caused by progressive and irreversible valvular damage.

In 1961 Starr and colleagues at the University of Oregon successfully implanted cardiac valvular prostheses in a series of patients with severe rheumatic heart disease.[3] Physicians were initially reluctant to apply this new technology to the therapy of patients with valvular damage from IE, fearing a prohibitively high incidence of persistence or relapse of infection on the implanted prosthesis. However, only 4 years later, in 1965, Wallace and associates at Duke University reported the first successful replacement of an aortic valve in a patient with active *Klebsiella* endocarditis.[4] Over the ensuing two decades, valve replacement has become an accepted and increasingly utilized modality of therapy in selected patients with IE. Here we will review issues dealing with the indications for surgical intervention and describe our recent experience with IE patients at the University of Alabama.

EPIDEMIOLOGY

Since the 1940s the epidemiology of IE has changed, and a variety of pathogenetic mechanisms now account for a more heterogeneous disease process. Whereas IE in the preantibiotic era was primarily a disease of young adults with underlying rheumatic heart disease, in recent years endocarditis has been observed more commonly in older patients. Degenerative valvular heart disease plays a more important role than rheumatic valvular disease as a predisposing factor for endocarditis in this older patient population. In addition, chronically ill elderly patients are predisposed to nosocomial endocarditis as more invasive diagnostic procedures and intravascular devices are utilized. Endocarditis continues to be an infectious complication in intravenous drug abusers, and since the 1960s IE has been recognized in patients who have undergone heart valve replacement with mechanical or bioprosthetic valves. In order to provide more meaningful analysis of complications, prognosis, and therapeutic interventions, IE is now generally divided into three types: native valve endocarditis (NVE), prosthetic valve endocarditis (PVE), and endocarditis associated with intravenous drug abuse (addict endocarditis).

The mortality rates of the different types of IE in patients from selected series over the past five decades (since the introduction of penicillin) are listed in Table 10-1. As noted, mortality rates vary according to the duration of follow-up after therapy. In general, in-hospital mortality rates are lowest. PVE is associated with the poorest prognosis, with mortality rates of 44 to 64 percent; in NVE mortality rates range from 15 to 42 percent. In general, addict endocarditis has the best prognosis, with mortality rates from 0 to 41 percent. In this latter group the widely varying rates depend on factors such as the etiologic microorganism and the specific valve involved. For example, addict endocarditis due to gram-negative bacilli or fungi is associated with higher mortality rates, and IE of the tricuspid valve, the most common site in addicts, is associated with a lower mortality rate than aortic valve disease. The indications for surgical intervention in the therapy of NVE, PVE, and addict en-

Table 10-1. Mortality Rates in Different Subgroups of Endocarditis

Series	Period of Study	NVE		PVE		ADDICT	
		No.	Mortality Rate (%)	No.	Mortality Rate (%)	No.	Mortality Rate (%)
Univ. Iowa Hospitals[5]	1944–49	59	26[a]				
	1950–63	130	30[a]				
St. Bartholomew's Hospital multicenter study, London[6]	1945–48	408	15[a] 42[b]				
Univ. Washington Hospitals[7]	1963–72	91	36[c]	16	44[c]	18	22[c]
Univ. Alabama Hospitals[8]	1967–77	135	26[a]	47	51[a]		
Claude Bernard Hospital, Paris[9]	1971–83	299	36[b]	79	61[b]		
Mayo Clinic[10]	1963–74			45	56[d]		
Massachusetts General Hospital[11]	1964–71			38	55[c]		
Univ. Alabama Hospitals[12]	1975–79			53	64[c]		
Hopital Cardio-Vasculaire et Pneumologique, Lyon, France[13]	1971–83			40	50[c]		
Washington, D.C. General Hospital[14]	1967–71					50	28[c]
Cook County Hospital[15]	1970–71					23	0[a]
Bronx Municipal Hospital Center[16]	1969–71					28	18[a]
San Francisco General Hospital[17]	1965–76					79	41[c]
National Collaborative[e] Endocarditis Study Group[18]	1976–79					48	2[a]

[a] In-hospital mortality.
[b] Six-month mortality.
[c] Extended follow-up mortality.
[d] Length of follow-up not stated.
[e] All patients had *Staphylococcus aureus* endocarditis.
(Adapted from Dismukes WE: Management of infective endocarditis. p. 189. In Rackley C (ed): Critical Care Cardiology (Cardiovascular Clinics 11/3) F. A. Davis Co., Philadelphia, 1981.)

Table 10-2. Procedures Useful in Monitoring Status of Patients with Endocarditis

Procedure	Significance
Serial blood cultures during therapy	Persistent bacteremia
Cardiac monitoring, especially during initial period of therapy	Arrhythmias
Serial electrocardiograms	Conduction defects (1°, 2°, 3° heart block, left bundle branch
Echocardiogram	Valvular insufficiency
	Vegetations
	Myocardial abscess
Cinefluoroscopy of prosthetic valve	Valve dehiscence or obstruction
Cardiac catheterization with angiography	Valvular insufficiency
	Extension of infection, e.g., fistulous tracts, aneurysms
	Multivalvular involvement
Computed tomography (CT) of head or abdomen	Emboli

docarditis are similar, but special considerations do exist for each of these groups.

MANAGEMENT

The cornerstone of medical management remains the prompt institution of bactericidal antimicrobial agents. Guidelines for optimal therapeutic regimens appropriate for the infecting pathogen have been recently reviewed.[19–25] Although many patients are cured by medical therapy alone, careful observation throughout hospitalization is mandatory, as patients with IE may deteriorate rapidly, necessitating emergent surgical intervention. Special monitoring procedures as outlined in Table 10-2 should be directed toward detecting: (1) changes in hemodynamic status; (2) evidence for persistence or spread of the local infectious process; (3) development of metastatic foci of infection; and (4) systemic embolic events. The frequency of obtaining each of these tests or procedures must be individualized and based on the patient's response to therapy and whether complications of IE are suspected.

INDICATIONS FOR SURGERY

One of the most difficult decisions to make when caring for patients with IE is whether or not to advise surgical intervention. A substantial proportion of patients with IE do poorly owing to complications of the disease process or to uncontrolled infection. As confidence in the effectiveness and safety of surgical intervention has increased, physicians have attempted to identify those patients with "complicated" IE who would most benefit from valve replacement. Recent reviews have focused on these complications and outlined generally accepted indications for surgery.[26–30] Table 10-3 assigns relative impor-

Table 10-3. Indications for Valve Replacement in the Management of Infective Endocarditis

	Accepted	Potential
Hemodynamic factors	Severe or progressive CHF due to native or prosthetic valvular dysfunction Unstable prosthetic valve by fluoroscopy or obstructed prosthesis	Mild to moderate CHF Paravalvular leak without CHF
Persistence or spread of infection	Persistent bacteremia despite appropriate "cidal" antimicrobial agents Fungal endocarditis	Persistent fever with negative blood cultures despite appropriate therapy Periannular or myocardial abscess or sinus of Valsalva aneurysm New or progressive cardiac conduction defect(s) Infection caused by organism other than penicillin-sensitive streptococcus Relapse after apparently successful treatment
Embolic complications	Recurrent major emboli	Single embolic event Echocardiographic evidence of vegetations

tance to these indications. In general, the development of one "accepted" indication warrants prompt surgery. In contrast, patients with only one "potential" indication for surgery may often be managed successfully by medical therapy alone. Similarly, the presence of two or more potential indications implies a stronger need for surgery. But most importantly, management must be decided on an individual basis.

Severe or progressive CHF is the most common indication for operative intervention in patients with IE; in several recent series, CHF was the major indication in at least 80 percent of patients.[8,9,31-34] Whereas irreversible valvular damage secondary to NVE or addict endocarditis is most commonly manifested as valvular insufficiency, in PVE valve incompetence is most often secondary to periannular infection with paravalvular leak. Acute valvular insufficiency may progress rapidly to significant CHF. Rarely, an acute change in a patient's hemodynamic status is caused by rupture of an intramyocardial abscess, creating a ventricular septal defect, or by rupture of an aneurysm of the sinus of Valsalva.

The prognosis for IE patients with moderate or severe CHF treated by medical therapy alone is poor, regardless of the cause. Richardson and associates at the University of Alabama Hospitals noted an in-hospital mortality rate of 66 percent for such a group of patients treated medically.[8] Similarly, for patients with moderate or severe CHF secondary to aortic insufficiency, results from two other series indicated an in-hospital mortality rate of approximately 80 percent when medical therapy alone was utilized.[35,36] In contrast, an improvement in survival has been observed in patients with moderate to severe CHF managed by valve replacement. An in-hospital mortality rate of only 9 percent was noted by Croft et al. for a group of patients whose primary indication for a combined medical-surgical approach was class III or class IV CHF; the in-hospital mortality for a similar group of patients treated medically was 51 percent.[37] In another study at the University of California at San Francisco-affiliated hospitals the 6-month mortality rate was 33 percent for patients with IE and severe CHF managed by combined medical-surgical therapy. In contrast, when medical therapy alone was used for a similar group of patients the 6-month mortality rate was 86 percent.[38]

Since operative mortality for valve replacement in patients with IE increases with the degree of heart failure, the presence of certain factors associated with progression of heart failure may facilitate a decision for early surgery under more favorable hemodynamic conditions. For example, aortic valve disease, specifically new aortic insufficiency, is more likely to be associated with progressive CHF than mitral valve disease.[9,38] Consequently the development of a new murmur of aortic insufficiency or premature closure of the mitral valve on echocardiogram demands very close observation.[39,40] Because progressive CHF, which eventually will require surgery, is sufficiently common in this setting, some experts advise early elective surgery for most patients with aortic insufficiency and mild CHF.[36,38,39] By contrast, mitral regurgitation can often be controlled medically. In patients with PVE a new regurgitation murmur usually implies infection involving the valve ring, with resulting paravavular leak. The frequent progression of heart failure in this setting and the difficulty in eradicating the periprosthetic infection should prompt consideration of early valve replacement.[8,41,42]

Regarding timing of surgery, patients with severe CHF should be operated on an urgent basis regardless of the length of prior antibiotic therapy. Delay of surgery in this situation in an attempt to stabilize the patient results in an even higher mortality. Similarly, the presence of an unstable prosthetic valve as revealed by cinefluoroscopy or the development of prosthetic valve obstruction requires immediate surgery. The optimal timing for surgery is unclear for patients with mild to moderate CHF, who can be temporarily hemodynamically stabilized but will ultimately need valve replacement; however, an argument can be made for a minimum of 7 days of antimicrobial therapy prior to surgery.

Although CHF or hemodynamic instability is the major indication for surgery in most patients, persistence or spread of infection is another important indication. Persistently positive blood cultures after 7 days of appropriate bactericidal antimicrobial therapy usually mean that medical therapy alone is ineffective. Boyd and associates showed that continuation of medical therapy alone in this situation was unlikely to result in cure and that subsequent delay in surgery was associated with a higher mortality rate.[43] We consider persistent bacteremia in the face of "adequate" antibiotic therapy an accepted indication for early valve replacement.

The etiologic microorganism may be an important predictor of the likelihood of cure with medical therapy alone. Since the mortality rate of fungal endocarditis approaches 100 percent with medical therapy alone, early valve replacement is usually recommended. Surgical intervention seems to improve survival; however, even with a combined approach of operation and antifungal therapy, the mortality rate remains about 50 to 60 percent.[44,45] In addition, bacteria other than penicillin-sensitive streptococci have been associated with a higher risk of complications in patients with IE. Gram-negative bacilli and *Staphylococcus aureus* have especially been incriminated. Despite the increased risk, most authorities recommend medical therapy alone for hemodynamically stable patients with uncomplicated IE due to bacteria other than penicillin-sensitive streptococci. However, in our opinion, once any complication, major or minor, develops, the threshold for early surgical intervention should be low.

Local spread of the infectious process into the valve annulus may result in a variety of complications, including aneurysm of the sinus of Valsalva, intramyocardial abscess, cardiac conduction defects, fistulous tracts, or pericarditis. These complications most frequently occur in patients with aortic valve endocarditis.[32,46,47] As noted earlier, serial electrocardiograms and echocardiograms may help to identify paravalvular spread of infection. In patients with PVE persistence of fever greater than 37.9°C has been associated with a persistent focus of paravalvular infection even when blood cultures are sterile.[48] Relapse after apparently successful therapy usually means persistence of infection on the involved valve (NVE) or around the valve (PVE). We consider factors or complications such as periannular or myocardial abscess, new or progressive conduction defects, persistent fever with negative blood cultures, infection caused by an organism other than a penicillin-susceptible streptococcus, and relapse as potential indications for operation.

In our opinion the presence of *recurrent* major systemic embolic events should mandate strong consideration of surgical intervention for valve debridement or replacement, even though data to support this approach are limited. Our recommendation is based on the concept of avoiding the high morbidity and mortality associated with major emboli.[8,26,27,31,34,43,49] For example, coronary artery emboli may be associated with a mortality rate as high as 70 percent,[8] and cerebral emboli may cause disabling neurological deficits and mortality rates of 30 to 50 percent.[8,49] Patients with a single major embolic event must be considered on an individual basis, although studies at the Massachusetts General Hospital have suggested that IE patients who appear to have only one embolus will, in many cases, have multiple emboli.[50]

In some studies the presence of vegetations on echocardiogram has been associated with an increased frequency of significant embolic events, CHF and subsequent need for surgery.[51-54] However, our current policy is not to view vegetations demonstrated by echocardiography as an absolute or accepted indication for valve replacement but rather to consider them as a potential indication, depending on a patient's overall clinical status.

Implantation of a mechanical prosthesis or bioprosthesis into a potentially infected and/or necrotic valve annulus creates concern about excessive surgical morbidity and mortality due to subsequent PVE or valve dehiscence. Table 10-4 reviews the outcome of surgery in patients with IE as reported in recent

Table 10-4. Outcome of Surgical Therapy for Infective Endocarditis

Series	Period of Study	No. of Patients Treated Surgically	Survivors with Persistent Infection of Prosthetic Valve (%)	Survivors with Paravalvular Leak Requiring Surgery (%)	In-Hospital Mortality Rate (%)
Review of early series; Jung JY, et al.[55]	1964–74	286 NVE	4	8	22
University of Alabama Hospitals[8]	1967–77	116 {NVE 81, PVE 35}	0	6	22
UCLA School of Medicine/ Wadsworth VA Hospital[34]	1967–81	42 {NVE 30, PVE 12}	3	3	10
Brompton Hospital, London[39]	1968–81	40 NVE	6	6	20
New York University Medical Center[43]	1970–75	54 {NVE 46, PVE 8}	5		19
Claude Bernard Hospital, Paris[9]	1971–83	150 {NVE 120, PVE 30}		9	28
Los Angeles County Harbor/ UCLA Medical Center[32]	1972–82	52 {NVE 47, PVE 5}	4	2	6
Medical College of Wisconsin Hospitals[31]	1974–80	80 {NVE 66, PVE 14}	1	3	10
University of Alabama Hospitals[12]	1975–79	33 PVE	8	24	36
University of the Witwatersrand and Baragwanath Hospital, Johannesburg[33]	1975–80	95 {NVE 86, PVE 9}	0	8	16

surgical series. In-hospital mortality rates range from 6 to 28 percent when series of NVE and PVE patients are combined. When PVE patients are analyzed separately, in-hospital mortality is generally higher, ranging from about 30 to 50 percent.[8,9,12,13,56]

Persistence of infection on the prosthetic valve due to the original microorganism is surprisingly uncommon. Rates of persistent PVE range from 0 to 8 percent. In addition, Young and associates in Houston[57] and Wilson and co-workers at the Mayo Clinic[58] reviewed a total of 37 surgical procedures during active IE, defined as positive blood cultures within 48 hours of surgery or positive culture or Gram stain of surgically removed valvular tissue. Only one of these 37 episodes was complicated by persistent infection. Hemodynamically significant paravalvular leak is also an uncommon complication of operation. Among patients with IE who survived operation, only 2 to 24 percent postoperatively developed a paravalvular leak that required another operation for

Table 10-5. Point System for Cardiac Surgery during Active Infective Endocarditis

Disorder	Point Rating[a] NVE	PVE
Heart failure		
Severe	5	5
Moderate	3	5
Mild	1	2
Fungal etiology	5	5
Persistent bacteremia	5	5
Organism other than "susceptible" streptococcus	1	2
Relapse	2	3
One major embolus	2	2
Two or more systemic emboli	4	4
Vegetations by echocardiography	1	1
Early mitral valve closure by echocardiography	2	N/A
Ruptured chordae tendineae or papillary muscle	3	N/A
Heart block	3	3
Ruptured sinus of Valsalva or ventricular septum	4	4
Unstable prosthesis	N/A	5
Early prosthetic valve endocarditis (<60 days)	N/A	2
Periprosthetic leak	N/A	2

[a] Accumulation of 5 or more points suggests the need for valve replacement.

N/A = not applicable

(Alsip SG, Blackstone EH, Kirklin JW, Cobbs CG: Indications for cardiac surgery in patients with active infective endocarditis. Am J Med: 78, suppl 6B, 138, 1985.)

hemodynamic reasons to repair the partial dehiscence. These data support the concept that surgery is a safe form of therapy in complicated IE.

In 1984, our colleagues, Gnann and Cobbs at the University of Alabama constructed a point system in an attempt to provide objective guidance for physicians faced with deciding whether or not to advise surgery for a patient with IE.[28] This point system, which underwent minor revisions in 1985, is reproduced in Table 10-5.[29] Gnann and Cobbs arbitrarily assigned a given point score to each complication of IE and proposed that an evaluation resulting in an accumulation of five or more points in a patient suggests the need for surgical intervention. The authors of this point system recognize that each case must be considered individually and only intended this algorithmic approach as a guide in the decision process.

RECENT ENDOCARDITIS EXPERIENCE, UNIVERSITY OF ALABAMA AT BIRMINGHAM

To assess the utility of the Gnann-Cobbs point system in predicting which patients will ultimately require valve replacement, we have retrospectively reviewed all patients with IE seen by a member of the Division of Infectious Diseases in University Hospital at the University of Alabama at Birmingham from July 1, 1983 through June 30, 1985. A total of 38 patients (39 separate

Table 10-6. Clinical Characteristics of Endocarditis Patients
University of Alabama Hospitals July 1983 to June 1985

	NVE[a]	PVE
No. of patients	28	10
Episodes of IE	29	10
Age: Range	7–91 yr	23–78 yr
Mean	49.1	49.9
Sex: Male	22	9
Female	6	1
Valves involved:		
Aortic	13	6
Mitral	7	1
Tricuspid	1	0
Aortic + mitral	1	1
Aortic + mitral + tricuspid	1	0
Tetralogy of Fallot repair	0	2
Unknown	6	0
Microorganism:		
Staphylococcus aureus	13	3
Penicillin-sensitive streptococci	7	1
Staphylococcus epidermidis	4	2
Enterococcus	2	1
Others	1	1
None identified	2	2

[a] Includes four patients with a history of intravenous drug abuse.

episodes of endocarditis) were identified (one patient had two separate episodes of IE due to different microorganisms). The clinical characteristics of these patients are detailed in Table 10-6, which shows that 28 patients had NVE (29 episodes) and 10 patients had PVE. The male/female ratio was 4.4:1, and the mean age was about 49 years. The aortic valve was most commonly involved. Right-sided endocarditis was uncommon, primarily as a consequence of the relatively small number of intravenous drug abusers in our population. *Staphylococcus aureus* was the most common etiologic microorganism and accounted for 16 of the 39 episodes. Penicillin-sensitive streptococci were second in frequency (eight episodes). There were no cases of fungal endocarditis and only one case of endocarditis due to a gram-negative bacillus (*Hemophilus influenzae*). No microorganism was identified in four patients, all of whom had clinical presentations highly suggestive of IE. Two of the four underwent surgery, which confirmed the suspicion of endocarditis.

A summary of the therapy and outcome of these 39 episodes of endocarditis is provided in Table 10-7. The median period of follow-up after completion of therapy was 17 months (range 4 to 24 months). Twenty-one (54 percent) of the episodes were managed by a combined medical-surgical approach. The most common indication for surgery was CHF, which was one of the major factors in 18 (86 percent) of the episodes requiring surgery; in 10 patients the indication for operation was CHF plus emboli. The overall survival rate was 77 percent (30 of 39). Among the survivors no patients relapsed, but two NVE patients developed reinfection with a different organism. A total of nine patients died; six deaths occurred in hospital and three occurred within 6 months after

Table 10-7. Therapy and Outcome of Endocarditis Patients
University of Alabama Hospital July 1983 to June 1985

	NVE	PVE
No. of episodes of IE	29	10
Medical therapy alone	14	4
Medical-surgical therapy	15	6
Indications for surgery		
CHF	5	3
CHF + emboli	9	1
Emboli	1	0
Relapse + unstable prosthesis	0	1
New conduction defect + persistent fever + paravalvular leak	0	1
Outcome		
Survived	21	9
Relapsed—same organism	0	0
Reinfection—different organism	2	0
Deaths		
In-hospital	5	1
Within 6 months	3	0
Overall mortality rate:	8/29 (28%)	1/10 (10%)
Medical therapy alone	4/14 (28%)	0/4 (0%)
Medical-surgical therapy	4/15 (27%)	1/6 (17%)

therapy. Among NVE patients the overall mortality rate was 28 percent, and the rates in the medically treated group and in the combined therapy group were similar. Among the 10 PVE patients the only death occurred in the combined medical-surgical group. The overall 6-month mortality rate for all patients was 23 percent, a notably low rate in this group of patients managed by an aggressive medical-surgical approach (compare with higher rates in earlier series, Table 10-1).

Each patient in our series was assigned points for each complication, as listed in the Gnann-Cobbs scoring system (Table 10-5). Analysis of our patients by the scoring system is given in Table 10-8. In only one patient with five or more points was surgery not done. This patient, who ultimately died, had moderate CHF and recurrent emboli but was felt not to be a candidate for aggressive

Table 10-8. Retrospective Analysis of Indications for Surgery in Endocarditis Patients[a]
University of Alabama Hospital July 1983 to June 1985

	Medical Therapy Alone	Combined Medical-Surgical Therapy
Episodes of IE	18	21
Total points for each episode of IE		
Range	−1 to 8	2 to 10
Mean	1.9	6.8
No. with 5 or more points	1	19
Six-month mortality (%)	1 (100%)	5 (26%)
No. with fewer than 5 points	17	2
Six-month mortality (%)	3 (18%)	0 (0%)

[a] For details of point system see Table 10-5.

surgical intervention because of underlying chronic debilitating illnesses. In contrast, two patients with fewer than 5 points had combined medical-surgical therapy. One of these had aortic valve NVE complicated by mild aortic insufficiency and a cerebral embolic event; the decision to operate was based on the single embolus. The other patient was operated because of severe preexisting calcific aortic stenosis. This patient's only potential indication for surgery was a retinal artery embolus.

Although the Gnann-Cobbs point system was not utilized prospectively to manage these patients, by our retrospective analysis the system correctly predicted in 36 of 39 episodes whether or not patients required surgery, as determined by the infectious diseases specialists and cardiovascular surgeons at our institution. Some authorities might question the arbitrariness of the scoring system and the inclusion or omission of specific indications or risks. Nonetheless, based on our experience, this system in conjunction with careful clinical assessment can provide helpful guidance in the management of patients with IE.

ILLUSTRATIVE CASES

The following two brief case histories serve to illustrate how the point system may be utilized when caring for patients with IE.

Case 1

A 78-year-old male, status post-aortic valve replacement with a porcine heterograft 5 years earlier, presented with a history of fever, chills, and malaise despite taking an oral cephalosporin for 2 days. He was hospitalized and treated with parenteral antibiotics for 5 days, with improvement in his symptoms. The day after discharge fever returned, and the patient suffered an arterial embolus to his left leg. Antimicrobial therapy was begun for suspected PVE. All blood cultures were negative, presumably as a consequence of prior antimicrobial therapy. Several days later the patient experienced a left hemispheric transient ischemic attack and was transferred to the University of Alabama Hospital. At our institution the patient developed mild aortic insufficiency with mild CHF. His hospital course over the next 10 days was complicated by a possible coronary artery embolus and a splenic infarction. At this point the patient underwent aortic valve replacement. Although the postoperative course was complicated by acute renal failure requiring temporary hemodialysis, the patient's renal function subsequently returned to normal, and he was reported doing well 6 months after discharge.

Comment. Despite initial reluctance to advise surgical intervention in this elderly patient, the consensus opinion of his physicians was that medical therapy alone would be unsuccessful. Valve replacement was therefore recommended based on mild CHF (2 points in PVE) and recurrent embolic events (4 points).

Case 2

A 54-year-old female, status post-mitral valve replacement with a Starr-Edwards prosthesis 8 years earlier, presented with fever, malaise, and *S. aureus* bacteremia. Appropriate antimicrobial therapy for PVE was instituted. Although blood cultures became negative within 6 days and good in vitro serum bactericidal activity was demonstrated, fever persisted throughout a 6-week course of therapy. Serial cinefluoroscopic examinations of the prosthesis documented normal valve function and no evidence of dehiscence. Serial echocardiograms revealed no evidence of extension of the infectious process into the surrounding myocardium. An abdominal computed tomographic scan was normal. Because no obvious source of persistent fever could be identified, the antibiotic regimen was altered because of suspected "drug fever," but daily fever continued. Antimicrobial therapy was discontinued after 6 weeks, whereupon blood cultures again became positive for *S. aureus* (same organism) within 3 days. Antibiotics were resumed, and on the same day the patient had a splenic infarction. A cardiac catheterization revealed no valvular insufficiency or other abnormalities. Mitral valve replacement was done, and at surgery a large 8 × 1 × 3 cm vegetation was found attached to the ventricular side of the prosthesis. Gram's stain revealed positive cocci in clusters, and the culture was positive for *S. aureus*. In the perioperative period the patient's course was further complicated by a mesenteric artery embolus, culminating in massive bowel infarction and death 2 days after surgery.

Comment   On the basis of the Gnann-Cobbs criteria the indications for surgery in this case included IE due to *S. aureus* (organism other than "susceptible" streptococcus, 2 points), relapse of infection (3 points), and an embolic event (2 points). In addition, we believe from past experience that persistent fever in patients with PVE is a potential indication for surgery.[48] In retrospect, earlier surgical intervention might have been warranted in this extraordinary case of PVE and might have provided a better chance for a successful outcome.

SUMMARY

Although many patients with IE can be successfully managed by medical therapy alone, surgical intervention is mandated by: (1) the development of severe or progressive CHF; (2) persistent bacteremia despite appropriate antimicrobial therapy; (3) fungal endocarditis; or (4) recurrent major emobli.

Delay in surgery in the presence of one of these four accepted indications adversely affects outcome. Experience over the past 20 years has shown that surgery in patients with IE is safe. Although persistent IE after surgery may occasionally occur, the incidence is low, even in the setting of active disease. The Gnann-Cobbs system was useful in predicting the need for surgical intervention in patients at our institution. We realize that rigid criteria are not always practical and that each patient with IE must be approached individually; nevertheless, the Gnann-Cobbs system may provide helpful guidance in the management of patients with IE.

REFERENCES

1. Osler W: Gulstonian lectures on malignant endocarditis. Lancet 1:415; 1:459; 1:505, 1885
2. Loewe L, Rosenblatt P, Greene HJ, Russell M: Combined penicillin and heparin therapy of subacute bacterial endocarditis. JAMA 124:144, 1944
3. Starr A, Edwards ML: Mitral replacement: clinical experience with a ball valve prothesis. Ann Surg 154:726, 1961
4. Wallace AG, Young WG, Osterhout S: Treatment of acute bacterial endocarditis by valve excision and replacement. Circulation 31:450, 1965
5. Rabinovich S, Evans J, Smith IM, January LE: A long-term view of bacterial endocarditis: 337 cases 1924 to 1963. Ann Intern Med 63:185, 1965
6. Cates JE, Christie RV: Subacute bacterial endocarditis. Q J Med 20(78):93, 1951
7. Pelletier LL, Petersdorf RG: Infective endocarditis: a review of 125 cases from the University of Washington hospitals, 1963–72. Medicine 56:287, 1977
8. Richardson JV, Karp RB, Kirklin JW, Dismukes WE: Treatment of infective endocarditis: a 10-year comparative analysis. Circulation 58:589, 1978
9. Witchitz S, Regnier B, Wolff M, et al: Surgery in infective endocarditis. Eur Heart J 5:suppl. C, 87, 1984
10. Wilson WR, Jaumin PM, Danielson GK, et al: Prosthetic valve endocarditis. Ann Intern Med 82:751, 1975
11. Dismukes WE, Karchmer AW, Buckley MJ, et al: Prosthetic valve endocarditis: analysis of 38 cases. Circulation 48:365, 1973
12. Ivert TSA, Dismukes WE, Cobbs CG, et al: Prosthetic valve endocarditis. Circulation 69:223, 1984
13. Gayet JL, Etienne J, Malquarti V, et al: Indices of effectiveness of medical and surgical treatment in 40 cases of prosthetic valve endocarditis. Eur Heart J 5:suppl. C, 133, 1984
14. Banks T, Fletcher R, Ali N: Infective endocarditis in heroin addicts. Am J Med 55:444, 1973
15. Menda KB, Gorbach SL: Favorable experience with bacterial endocarditis in heroin addicts. Ann Intern Med 78:25, 1973
16. Dreyer NP, Fields BN: Heroin-associated infective endocarditis: a report of 28 cases. Ann Intern Med 78:699, 1973
17. Hubbell G, Cheitlin MD, Rapaport E: Presentation, management, and follow-up evaluation of infective endocarditis in drug addicts. Am Heart J 102:85, 1981
18. Korzeniowski O, Sande MA, The National Collaborative Endocarditis Study Group: Combination antimicrobial therapy for *Staphylococcus aureus* endocarditis

in patients addicted to parenteral drugs and in nonaddicts. Ann Intern Med 97:496, 1982

19. Dismukes WE: Management of infective endocarditis. p. 189. In Rackley C (ed): Critical Care Cardiology (Cardiovascular Clinics 11/3). FA Davis Co. Philadelphia, 1981

20. Wilson WR, Geraci JE: Treatment of pencillin-sensitive streptococcal endocarditis. p. 101. In Sande MA, Kaye D, Root RK (eds): Endocarditis (Contemporary Issues in Infectious Diseases, Vol. 2). Churchill Livingstone, New York, 1984

21. Moellering RC: Treatment of enterococcal endocarditis. p. 113. In Sande MA, Kaye D, Root RK (eds): Endocarditis (Contemporary Issues in Infectious Diseases, Vol. 2). Churchill Livingstone, New York, 1984

22. Kaye D: Treatment of staphylococcal endocarditis. p. 135. In Sande MA, Kaye D, Root RK (eds): Endocarditis (Contemporary Issues in Infectious Diseases, Vol. 2). Churchill Livingstone, New York, 1984

23. Levison ME: Therapy of endocarditis due to gram-negative bacteria and fungi. p. 151. In Sande MA, Kaye D, Root RK (eds): Endocarditis (Contemporary Issues in Infectious Diseases, Vol. 2). Churchill Livingstone, New York, 1984

24. Karchmer AW: Treatment of prosthetic valve endocarditis. p. 163. In Sande MA, Kaye D, Root RK (eds): Endocarditis (Contemporary Issues in Infectious Diseases, Vol. 2). Churchill Livingstone, New York, 1984

25. Chambers HF, Mills J: Endocarditis associated with intravenous drug abuse. p. 183. In Sande MA, Kaye D, Root RK (eds): Endocarditis (Contemporary Issues in Infectious Diseases, Vol. 2). Churchill Livingstone, New York, 1984

26. Mills SA: Surgical management of infective endocarditis. Ann Surg 195:367, 1982

27. Dinubile MJ: Surgery in active endocarditis. Ann Intern Med 96:650, 1982

28. Cobbs CG, Gnann JW: Indications for surgery. p. 201. In Sande MA, Kaye D, Root RK (eds): Endocarditis (Contemporary Issues in Infectious Diseases, Vol. 2). Churchill Livingstone, New York, 1984

29. Alsip SG, Blackstone EH, Kirklin JW, Cobbs CG: Indications for cardiac surgery in patients with active infective endocarditis. Am J Med 78:suppl. 6B, 138, 1985

30. Karchmer AW, Stinson EB: The role of surgery in infective endocarditis. p. 124. In Remington JS, Swartz MN (eds): Current Clinical Topics in Infectious Diseases. Vol. 1. McGraw-Hill, New York, 1980

31. Perry LS, Tresch DD, Brooks HL, et al: Operative approach to endocarditis. Am Heart J 108:561, 1984

32. Nelson RJ, Harley DP, French WJ, Bayer AS: Favorable ten-year experience with valve procedures for active infective endocarditis. J Thorac Cardiovasc Surg 87:493, 1984

33. Lewis BS, Agathangelou NE, Colsen PR, et al: Cardiac operation during active infective endocarditis: results of aortic, mitral, and double valve replacement in 94 patients. J Thorac Cardiovasc Surg 84:579, 1982

34. Cukingnan RA, Carey JS, Wittig JH, Cimochowski GE: Early valve replacement in active infective endocarditis: results and late survival. J Thorac Cardiovasc Surg 85:163, 1983

35. Garvey GJ, Neu HC: Infective endocarditis—an evolving disease. A review of endocarditis at the Columbia-Presbyterian Medical Center, 1968–1973. Medicine 57:105, 1978

36. Griffin FM, Jones G, Cobbs CG: Aortic insufficiency in bacterial endocarditis. Ann Intern Med 76:23, 1972

37. Croft CH, Woodward W, Elliott A, et al: Analysis of surgical versus medical therapy

in active complicated native valve infective endocarditis. Am J Cardiol 51:1650, 1983

38. Mills J, Utley J, Abbott J: Heart failure in infective endocarditis: predisposing factors, course, and treatment. Chest 66:151, 1974

39. Kay PH, Oldershaw PJ, Dawkins K, et al: The results of surgery for active endocarditis of the native aortic valve. J Cardiovasc Surg 25:321, 1984

40. Mann T, McLaurin L, Grossman W, Craige E: Assessing the hemodynamic severity of acute aortic regurgitation due to infective endocarditis. N Engl J Med 293:108, 1975

41. Saffle JR, Gardner P, Schoenbaum SC, Wild W: Prosthetic valve endocarditis, the case for prompt valve replacement. J Thorac Cardiovasc Surg 73:416, 1977

42. Leport C, Vilde JL, Bricaire F, et al: Late prosthetic valve endocarditis. Bacteriological findings and prognosis in 29 cases. Eur Heart J 5:suppl. C, 139, 1984

43. Boyd AD, Spencer FC, Isom OW, et al: Infective endocarditis: an analysis of 54 surgically treated patients. J Thorac Cardiovasc Surg 73:23, 1977

44. Rubinstein E, Noriega ER, Simberkoff MS, et al: Fungal endocarditis: analysis of 24 cases and review of the literature. Medicine 54:331, 1975

45. Utley JR, Mills J, Roe BB: The role of valve replacement in the treatment of fungal endocarditis. J Thorac Cardiovasc Surg 69:255, 1975

46. Symbas PN, Vlasis SE, Zacharopoulos L, et al: Immediate and long-term outlook for valve replacement in acute bacterial endocarditis. Ann Surg 195:721, 1982

47. Arnett EN, Roberts WC: Valve ring abscess in active infective endocarditis: frequency, location, and clues to clinical diagnosis from the study of 95 necropsy patients. Circulation 54:140, 1976

48. Karchmer AW, Dismukes WE, Buckley MJ, Austen WG: Late prosthetic valve endocarditis: clinical features influencing therapy. Am J Med 64:199, 1978

49. Becker RM, Frishman W, Frater RWM: Surgery for mitral valve endocarditis. Chest 75:314, 1979

50. Pruitt AA, Rubin RH, Karchmer AW, Duncan GW: Neurologic complications of bacterial endocarditis. Medicine 57:329, 1978

51. Davis RS, Strom JA, Frishman W, et al: The demonstration of vegetations by echocardiography in bacterial endocarditis. Am J Med 69:57, 1980

52. Wong D, Chandraratna AN, Wishnow RM, et al: Clinical implications of large vegetations in infectious endocarditis. Arch Intern Med 143:1874, 1983

53. O'Brien JT, Geiser EA: Infective endocarditis and echocardiography. Am Heart J 108:386, 1984

54. Stewart JA, Silimperi D, Harris P, et al: Echocardiographic documentation of vegetative lesions in infective endocarditis: clinical implications. Circulation 61:374, 1980

55. Jung JY, Saab SB, Almond CH: The case for early surgical treatment of left-sided primary infective endocarditis: a collective review. J Thorac Cardiovasc Surg 70:509, 1975

56. Horstkotte D, Korfer R, Loogen F, et al: Prosthetic valve endocarditis: clinical findings and management. Eur Heart J:5suppl C, 117, 1984

57. Young JB, Welton DE, Raizner AE, et al: Surgery in active infective endocarditis. Circulation: 60suppl. 1, I-77, 1979

58. Wilson WR, Danielson GK, Giuliani ER, et al: Valve replacement in patients with active infective endocarditis. Circulation 58:585, 1978

11 | Abdominal Abscess— The Role of the Surgeon

Frank R. Lewis, Jr.

PREVENTION

The role of the surgeon in 1987 in the diagnosis and drainage of abdominal abscesses has been markedly reduced because of the greatly enhanced imaging techniques for the abdominal viscera and effective percutaneous drainage techniques developed during the last few years. For abscesses which are well defined and in accessible locations, percutaneous drainage is effective in more than 80 percent of cases, eliminates the morbidity associated with a surgical procedure, and allows more rapid recovery of the patient. The role of the surgeon is therefore primarily in two areas: prevention of abscesses by sound surgical techniques and surgical drainage when percutaneous drainage is inappropriate or unsuccessful.

Abscesses in the abdomen generally result from the simultaneous occurrence of two conditions: (1) the presence of bacteria from an exogenous or endogenous source of contamination; and (2) the provision of a culture medium in an area of dead space in which the organisms can flourish. Elimination of either of these conditions normally will prevent abscesses from developing, even if the other is present. The strategy of the surgeon should therefore be to prevent both wherever possible and at other times to reduce the likelihood of both coexisting.

Exogenous contamination in the abdomen usually results from skin flora or from breaks in technique during draping or during the operative procedure itself. It should be recognized that it is impossible to sterilize the skin and that organisms will always remain in the hair follicles and other skin appendages. Nevertheless, several details which will reduce the skin flora are important. First, there should be no breaks in the skin in the region of the operative site. If skin lesions, furuncles, or ulcers are present, surgery should be deferred until these have either healed or resolved for several days unless the operation is emergent. Skin flora can be further reduced by having the patient bathe or shower with an antibacterial soap for a few days before surgery.

Shaving of the operative site should either be avoided altogether if hair growth is sparse, or not carried out until immediately before or after the patient is transferred to the operating room. Shaving of the skin the night before surgery leads to large increases in the skin flora due to the microscopic skin trauma induced and should always be avoided.

The operative site itself should be scrubbed for 10 minutes if the patient has not been able to shower or bathe with antibacterial soap preoperatively. Finally, a paint-on antiseptic skin prep is used prior to draping. The most effective prep is one containing iodine, either a dilute solution of inorganic iodine or one of the organic iodine complexes.

Draping of the wound is the next source of possible contamination, and care should be taken to drape the operative field as narrowly as possible. Drapes which are waterproof should always be used, and care should be taken to avoid moving the drapes after they have been placed on the patient to prevent carrying bacteria from unprepped to prepped areas.

Endogenous contamination when working in the abdomen usually results from bowel contamination due either to perforations of a viscus or intentional opening of the bowel during the procedure. The relative contamination from this source depends on the site of perforation as well as the time during which perforation has been present. Perforations of the stomach and duodenum normally produce minimal contamination owing to the low density of microorganisms present in the patient who has normal acid production. When the stomach is full, when the patient has blood in the stomach or duodenum, or when he is achlorhydric, the relative contamination will be increased.

The small bowel down to the terminal ileum normally has low bacterial counts as well, typically 10^5 organisms per milliliter or less, and this is not a major source of contamination even when the bowel has been perforated preoperatively, as with penetrating trauma.

In contrast, the bacterial flora rises dramatically in the distal few feet of ileum and in the colon is of the order of 10^{10} organisms per milliliter. Perforation of the colon, like a perforated diverticulum or perforative appendicitis, must therefore be viewed as a special hazard, with a high risk of abscess formation.

Two points are important to remember in this regard. The first is to anticipate possible need to open the colon in elective procedures and to provide a mechanical and oral antibiotic prep preoperatively for this possibility. The second is to remember that the peritoneal cavity is very effective in dealing with a single bacterial contamination episode; what it does not tolerate is ongoing contamination. Thus, when the latter is a possibility, as with repair of enteric fistula or a suture line repair in the gut, every possible technical maneuver should be employed to prevent secondary spillage. Such measures include operative control of fistulas, catheter decompression of the bowel, use of omental or serosal patches over suture lines, exteriorization of sutured bowel, or diversion of the fecal stream proximal to suture lines.

Finally, the second prerequisite for abscess formation is a culture medium and dead space in which bacterial growth can occur. This typically results from hematoma or seroma formation in the peritoneal cavity, which tends to occur in the dependent areas such as the subphrenic and subhepatic spaces and in the pelvis. These are best avoided by meticulous hemostasis whenever possible and by wide drainage when hematoma formation is unavoidable, as with severe blunt liver injury. In addition, if one can reasonably anticipate postoperative fluid drainage, as with pancreatic injury, wide drainage should be provided in a dependent location, and sump drains should be additionally used. Sump drains are not effective for removal of blood but work quite well for bile and for pancreas and bowel drainage. When drainage of bleeding is necessary, it is only done effectively with a large external opening in a dependent location such that clots can escape. For major liver injury, a 6- to 9-cm opening in the bed of the twelfth rib is typically provided, and several large Penrose drains are inserted.

At the same time that the need to drain aggressively is recognized when fluid accumulation is anticipated, one should also recognize those situations in which drainage is unnecessary or counterproductive. Such instances include splenectomy, cholecystectomy, and the usual bowel anastamosis, including the colon. In these situations the use of drains is more likely to induce abscesses by allowing ingress of organisms along the drain tract than it is to prevent infection. When drains are placed in doubtful situations, they should always be removed quickly if no significant drainage is seen in the immediate postoperative period.

DIAGNOSIS

The specific diagnostic maneuvers for localization of abdominal abscesses today are almost the exclusive province of the radiologist, and the clinical skills of most surgeons in defining the presence of an intra-abdominal abscess are relatively moribund. Anyone who is suspected of having an abscess because of fever, leukocytosis, and abdominal findings is typically subjected to ultrasonography or computerized tomography (CT) to provide the definitive answer. While the diagnostic accuracy and reliability of ultrasound appears to be markedly dependent on the experience, effort, and expertise of the ultrasonographer, this is not equally true for CT, which provides cross-sectional images of exceptional anatomic accuracy, which can be read with reliability for abscess presence by virtually all radiologists. Thus, a CT scan of good quality, with the resolution of current generation machines, is essentially 100 percent reliable in proving or disproving the presence of an abdominal abscess and precisely defining its anatomic relationships.

Nuclear scanning techniques have largely been abandoned for diagnosis of abscesses because of the superiority of CT, although the use of indium labeling of platelets or white blood cells is still championed by some in difficult cases.

The role of the surgeon, then, is to identify the clinical situations in which abscesses may be present, either in patients initially presenting or in those who are postoperative, and to order the appropriate diagnostic test, usually CT, to confirm them or rule them out.

INDICATIONS FOR SURGICAL DRAINAGE

As discussed elsewhere in this volume, drainage of most abscesses is possible today by percutaneous techniques. However, there are a few defined situations in which that is not appropriate or is unsuccessful. In these instances the surgeon must utilize classical operative approaches if the patient is to be successfully treated. While the boundaries of percutaneous versus operative techniques of drainage are not always well defined and may depend to some extent on local expertise and tradition, the following situations are generally the ones in which operative drainage will be needed.

Presence of Phlegmon Rather than Abscess

In the developing stages of most abscesses there will be a mixture of inflammatory debris, necrotic tissue, and white cell exudates that is referred to by the term *phlegmon*. After several days the central portion of the phlegmon liquefies as a result of bacterial and white cell enzymatic action, and the perfused boundary of the area progressively organizes and fibroses, forming a wall which limits the process. As the process evolves, a stage is reached at which there is a well-defined abscess, which can be drained. Earlier than this, the tissue is not sufficiently liquefied to drain via catheter, and open surgical drainage will be necessary to evacuate and possibly debride the inflammatory debris.

Extensive Multilocular or Ill-Defined Abscesses

Abscesses with multiple cavities that are not intercommunicating will generally be poorly drainable with catheters because multiple placements will be necessary and often not all the cavities will be entered. At times the anatomic extent and boundaries of the abscess will also not be precisely definable. In such situations surgical exposure and direct operative definition and debridement of the area may be necessary.

Viscous Debris/Necrotic Tissue

At times even when the walls of the abscess have become well developed and are easily definable, the contents will not have liquefied completely. This situation is often seen in pancreatic pseudocysts and abscesses. Catheter drainage of such cavities, while it allows withdrawal of some pus, will not provide for complete decompression, and the patient may continue to be septic owing to the incomplete removal of infected material.

Abscesses Due to Enteric Fistulas or Anastomotic Leaks

Abscesses due to these causes cannot be adequately treated by catheter drainage because they are continually seeded by ongoing drainage from the bowel. In such cases sepsis can only be controlled by wide surgical drainage to open the abscess cavity and sometimes by diversion of the enteric stream in addition. Attempts at catheter drainage may achieve easy fluid drainage but will not control the patient's sepsis.

Inaccessible Locations

To be drainable by catheter, abscesses must be accessible from some point on the surface of the trunk without passing the catheter through the solid or hollow organs in the abdomen. Since the catheters introduced tend to be 6 to 10 Fr in size, they make sizable perforations in whatever they pass through and are capable of causing significant problems of their own. Fortunately, this is not a major problem, as most abscesses are accessible from the surface without difficulty, but occasionally, particularly with centrally located abscesses, surgical exposure will be necessary.

Abscesses More Easily Drained Surgically

Some abscesses which present superficially and can be drained with a direct incision placed over them are nevertheless better drained surgically than with a catheter because the procedure is more easily and more surely done. In addition, pelvic abscesses which present on rectal examination are more easily drained transrectally than via catheter. On the other hand, abscesses which will require formal laparotomy with a transabdominal approach to the abscess and resultant widespread contamination of the peritoneal cavity are better drained percutaneously if they are accessible.

Extremely Large Abscesses

Very large abscesses, although they can be decompressed by catheter, arc probably better drained surgically because it is impossible to fully drain all the recesses of the cavity by a single centrally placed cathctcr. In such situations the patients typically remain indolently septic because the inflammatory exudate and bacteria can continue to exist and be absorbed into the circulation.

SURGICAL APPROACHES

One of the two classical approaches to abdominal abscesses is to incise more or less directly over the collection and drain it extraperitoneally if the abscess is in a location accessible to this technique. The advantage of this approach is that it avoids peritoneal contamination and the systemic bacteremia which usually follows. The second approach, which was previously used when the diagnosis of abscess was uncertain and the need for thorough abdominal exploration was felt to be present, is the transabdominal approach, usually through a midline laparotomy. The need for total abdominal exploration is minimal today as a result of the advances in imaging techniques but still occurs on occasion. Thus, the major use of laparotomy is in the situations described above in which percutaneous drainage is ineffective or unusable. In such instances, although the bacteremic insult to the patient is greater than if an extraperitoneal approach were used, it is usually well tolerated with the potent antibiotics that are available. Most of the time the patient will experience bacteremia and signs of systemic sepsis during the first 24 to 48 hours after the surgical procedure, but after that these conditions subside and recovery is the rule.

SUMMARY

The need for surgical drainage of abdominal abscesses has decreased dramatically in the last 10 years with the advent of precise radiologic procedures for localizing the collections and equally sophisticated catheter techniques for entering and draining the abscesses. The field continues to be in evolution, and more aggressive and experienced radiologists will no doubt continue to expand the indications. Overall, the patient has been the beneficiary in this change because the percutaneous techniques are effective in approximately 80 percent of abscesses and they avoid the risks of general anesthesia and surgery. On the other hand, there are defined instances in which surgical drainage is more appropriate and effective than catheter drainage, and one should always be aware that catheter drainage, if less than complete, may inadequately control the sepsis. In such cases, allowing the patient to remain persistently septic rather than to undergo a surgical procedure which would fully decompress the abscess cavity will certainly result in a higher mortality.

SUGGESTED READINGS

Aeder MI, Wellman JL, Haaga JR, et al: Role of surgical and percutaneous drainage in the treatment of abdominal abscesses. Arch Surg 118:273, 1983

Ferraris VA: Exploratory laparotomy for potential abdominal sepsis in patients with multiple organ failure. Arch Surg 118:1130, 1983

Gerzof SG, Robbins AH, Johnson WC, et al: Percutaneous catheter drainage of abdominal abscesses. N Engl J Med 305:653, 1981

Halasz NA, vanSonnenberg E: Drainage of intra-abdominal abscesses. Am J Surg 146:112, 1983

Johnson WC, Gerzof SG, Robbins AH, et al: Treatment of abdominal abscesses. Ann Surg 194:510, 1981

Martin EC, Karlson KB, Fankuchen EI, et al: Percutaneous drainage of postoperative intra-abdominal abscesses. AJR 138:13, 1982

Porter JA, Loughry CW, Cook AJ: Use of the computerized tomographic scan in the diagnosis and treatment of abscesses. Am J Surg 150:257, 1985

vanSonnenberg E, Ferrucci JT Jr, Mueller PR, et al: Percutaneous radiographically guided catheter drainage of abdominal abscesses. JAMA 247:190, 1982

12 | Infectious Complications Following Trauma

Donald D. Trunkey

Death following trauma has a trimodal distribution, with approximately 50 percent of the deaths occurring within minutes of the accident.[1] These patients die primarily of lacerations to the brain, brain stem, spinal cord, and aorta and rupture of the myocardial chambers. The second death peak occurs within hours of the injury, and these deaths are usually due to head injury (epidural, subdural, and intracerebral hematomas) and hemorrhage from torso viscera. The third death peak, which constitutes approximately 20 percent of the total, occurs within days to weeks of the injury, and the great majority (78 percent) are due to sepsis and multiple organ failure. Burn patients seem to be at a particularly high risk, with 38 percent dying from sepsis; in some series this approaches 75 percent.[2] In contrast, only 5 percent of patients with penetrating trauma and 8 percent of those with blunt trauma die from sepsis[3] (Table 12-1). Most of the patients who die from sepsis have orthopedic injuries, but other risk factors include the presence of shock on admission, contamination of the peritoneal cavity from associated small bowel or colon injuries, and head injuries.

There are a great number of factors that contribute to infection following a traumatic injury. These include the area of the body wounded, the kinetic energy involved in wounding, contamination of the wound, virulence of the organisms introduced, and subsequent treatment. In general, it is uncommon to have major infection associated with the primary wounds, yet it is quite common to develop a nosocomial infection as the major infectious complication following trauma. In a study performed by Schimpff et al.,[4] it was observed

Table 12-1. Incidence of Fatal Sepsis (1985)

(147,257 trauma deaths, total)		
Type of trauma	Number of deaths from sepsis	Percent of total
Burn injuries	4500	75
Penetrating injuries	3000	5
Blunt injuries	7900	8

that 48 percent of patients with severe trauma developed one or more noso-comial infections. This was in contrast to only 3 percent of those with less severe injuries. Although the injuries were not quantified in terms of injury severity score, severity was grossly quantified by the length of stay in the intensive care unit. Patients who remained in the intensive care unit longer than 5 days had an infection rate of 60 percent, with a mortality rate of 16 percent.

It is difficult to ascertain the exact number of deaths caused by infectious complications after trauma. If one assumes that 6,000 of the 165,000 trauma deaths annually are due to burns and that 75 percent of these patients die from infectious complications, this would result in 4,500 deaths. Clearly, the majority of homicides and suicides are due to penetrating trauma, which has an infectious death rate of 5 percent,[3] resulting in 3,000 total deaths. The remaining trauma victims die primarily from blunt trauma, in which the infectious death rate is 8 percent, or 7,900 deaths.[3] This is a total of somewhat over 15,000 deaths, which correlates relatively well with data from the Centers for Disease Control.[5] Although this represents a very rough analysis, it does emphasize the seriousness and magnitude of the infection problem following major injury.

RISK FACTORS

Alexander has arbitrarily divided the predisposing factors to infection after trauma into intrinsic and extrinsic, which we have modified.[6] The intrinsic factors primarily relate to the host defense system, which can be further divided into the specific and the nonspecific host defense, the latter including the inflammatory mediators.

Intrinsic Factors

Nonspecific Host Defense

Many nonspecific inflammatory host defense mechanisms involve removing bacteria from the system and then destroying these organisms in some manner. The mechanical barriers to bacterial invasion are often included as components of this nonspecific host defense system and include the skin, respiratory mucosa, and gastrointestinal mucosa. The major components of the nonspecific inflammatory system that affect bacteriocidal activity include neutrophils, eosinophils, macrophages, the plasma proteins of the coagulation cascade, the proteins of the complement system, interferon, and other plasma proteins with chemotactic, pyrogenic, or opsonic action. Many of these substances constitute mediators of the inflammatory process.

Specific Host Defense

The specific immune system is composed primarily of three interacting cellular components, the monokines and lymphokines that they produce, and specific antibodies.[7] The cellular components are the thymus-derived lymphocytes (T cells), commonly associated with cell-mediated immunity; bursal equivalent or bone marrow–derived lymphocytes (B cells), which as precursors to plasma cells are responsible for the production of antibodies; and a heterogenous monocyte population, which processes antigens and initiates stimulation of the immune system. This discussion of host factors in surgical infection is covered in greater detail in Chapter 4.

Extrinsic Factors

The extrinsic risk factors can be further divided into iatrogenic and noniatrogenic factors. Although this is a useful classification in order to emphasize prevention, there is obvious crossover between the two groups if therapy is inappropriate.

The most common noniatrogenic extrinsic factor is contamination of the wound. In theory, this risk factor should be a nonproblem if proper surgical treatment is provided. If the wound is relatively small and tidy with minimal contamination, primary surgical closure might be warranted. If the wound is untidy, however, proper surgical treatment includes irrigation, debridement of all devitalized tissue and foreign bodies, and delayed primary closure. The importance of this treatment cannot be overemphasized and if properly adhered to, it should lead to minimal infectious complications.

The iatrogenic extrinsic risk factors include catheters and tubes associated with invasive monitoring and treatment, malnutrition, the intensive care unit milieu (personnel and equipment hygiene), and changes in the host flora caused by the injudicious use of broad-spectrum prophylactic antibiotics.

Catheters and Lines

It has been my impression, based on 12 years of experience in caring for the critically injured patient, that catheters (intravenous, intra-arterial, intratracheal, and urinary) contribute significantly to infectious complications. This can be minimized by removing and replacing as indicated all catheters and lines placed in the emergency room during the resuscitation. It should be assumed that all such lines are contaminated and have been inserted under less than desirable aseptic techniques. Ideally, catheters placed in the operating room and intensive care setting should have meticulous aseptic technique and should therefore be less susceptible to infectious complications. In practice, however, this may or may not be true, and in most series[4] catheters represent a significant source of major infection. Ironically, the incidence of skin infection and significant thrombophlebitis or pyophlebitis is relatively low as compared with the more distant infections, predominantly of the lungs, associated with catheter sepsis. Nasogastric tubes contribute to significant infection by causing continued nasopharyngeal irritation, which then leads to sinusitis. Endotracheal tubes are a common source of pulmonary sepsis, including tracheitis, bronchitis, and bronchopneumonia. Indwelling urinary catheters left in long enough will all cause bacteriuria, and some patients will go on to develop clinically apparent urinary tract infections, including prostatitis. Surgical drains are notorious for introducing hospital organisms into body cavities. Although this can be minimized by the use of closed systems and in-line micropore filters, it is best to avoid drains unless their advantages outweigh their disadvantages.

Malnutrition

Although malnutrition can be present when the patient is injured, it is more commonly an iatrogenic problem. An increase in tissue catabolism following major injury is universal and is proportional to the severity of the trauma. Burn injuries are associated with the worst catabolic states, but any patient with an injury severity score of greater than 30 can be assumed to be in negative nitrogen balance immediately following the injury. This becomes a vicious circle with the onset of sepsis. Since malnutrition is such a common problem following severe injury, it should be anticipated, and a nutritional plan including enteral and/or parenteral hyperalimentation must be instituted within 48 hours of injury. Although some calories are provided with the maintainence intravenous fluids following the resuscitation, it is inadequate to meet the total caloric needs of the severely catabolic patient, and it does not address the calorie/nitrogen ratios. In general, we feel that the enteral nutrition route is optimal but parenteral hyperalimentation should be considered when this is not feasible. The presence of ileus should not deter the enteral route since even in this setting patients can absorb significant amounts of calories and protein when provided as an elemental diet.

Intensive Care Unit Conditions

The third iatrogenic extrinsic factor is the intensive care unit milieu. Hygiene of personnel, including physicians, nurses, and respiratory therapists, cannot be overemphasized. The washing of hands between patients is critical.

Similarly, equipment, bedding, floors, walls, windows, and even the patient must be cleaned on a regular basis to minimize the spread of opportunistic organisms. Isolation techniques should be introduced in appropriate instances to protect immunocompromised patients or to prevent the epidemic spread of specific organisms.

Inappropriate Antibiotic Use

The last iatrogenic extrinsic factor is the change in the host flora caused by the injudicious use of broad-spectrum prophylactic antibiotics. This will be covered in more detail below.

PROPHYLACTIC ANTIBIOTICS

Use in Specific Injuries

Head Injuries

The role of antibiotic prophylaxis in traumatic head injuries remains somewhat controversial. Most investigators agree that penicillin prophylaxis is of no benefit in minor traumatic wounds.[8-10] In a randomized case control study done by Ignelezi and VanderArk,[11] patients with basilar skull fracture were shown not to benefit from prophylactic antibiotics. Their results further suggested that those patients who were placed on antibiotics acquired gram-negative organisms resistant to these antibiotics.

A remaining controversial area is the treatment of compound fractures of the cranium. Multiple studies designed to examine the efficacy of antibiotics have not shown an advantage for prophylaxis. Current rationale for antibiotic use is provided by experiences in orthopedic surgery[12]; however, the application of these findings to cranial fractures remains questionable.

Maxillofacial

In general, maxillofacial injuries do not require prophylactic antibiotics[13]; exceptions would be destructive wounds or particularly untidy wounds. There may be instances in which cosmetic considerations override optimal surgical management such as delayed primary closure. In these instances prophylactic antibiotics may be warranted to help promote primary closure. Controlled randomized studies have not provided the scientific evidence to support such a management, however.

Neck

Injuries to the neck do not require prophylactic antibiotics even when the esophagus is injured. Standard surgical management of exploration, irrigation, debridement, and drainage when indicated suffices.

Thorax

The use of prophylactic antibiotics as an adjunctive treatment measure in injuries to the chest is controversial. In a double-blind, prospective study Grover, et al.[14] showed that patients treated with clindamycin had a lower incidence of radiographically diagnosed pneumonia, fever, and a positive pleural or wound cultures. Although there was a trend for treated patients to have less clinical empyema, this was not statistically significant. Cost-benefit analysis indicated that the use of prophylactic antibiotics in this study was marginal; statistical significance was not achieved between the antibiotic-treated and placebo groups.

More recently a double-blind study by LoCurto et al.[15] showed that patients who had a tube thoracostomy performed for trauma had less infectious complications when treated prophylactically with cefoxitin as compared with placebo. It should be pointed out, however, that 30 percent of those patients who had tube thoracostomy and were treated with placebo had wound infections, which is much higher than that reported in the literature.

In contrast, a study performed by LeBlanca[16] showed no statistical difference when patients were randomized between antibiotic and placebo. It is my feeling that antibiotics should be used only when there is gross contamination of the pleural cavity by rupture of a hollow viscus, such as the esophagus, or contamination of the pleural cavity by gastric or bowel contents and associated violation of the diaphragm.

Abdomen

Most surgeons agree that trauma to the abdominal viscera causing contamination by small bowel or colon requires therapeutic use of antibiotics.[17–25] Multiple studies show a higher incidence of wound and intraperitoneal infectious complications when antibiotics are withheld. When antibiotics are used with peritoneal toilet and delayed primary wound closure, infectious complications can be kept to a minimum. Ideally, the antibiotics should be started as soon after the injury as possible and preferably before surgery. The use of antibiotics for other visceral injuries has not been proved efficacious in prospective randomized clinical trials.

Fractures

The most frequently cited randomized study showing the efficacy of antibiotics in compound fractures was reported in 1974.[12] Patzakis and his coworkers showed that untreated patients had an infection rate of 13.9 percent, while patients treated with penicillin and streptomycin had a 9.7 percent infection rate and patients receiving cephalothin had a significantly lower infection rate of 2.3 percent. Most orthopedic surgeons use prophylactic antibiotics for compound fractures.

A more recent study by Bergman[26] classified wounds as grade 1, 2, and 3, based on degree of soft tissue–associated injury, grade 3 being the worst. Grade 1 wounds, which had minimal soft tissue lesions, showed no statistical difference in infection rates between saline and antibiotic. Grade 2 and 3 wounds, however, were best managed with antibiotics, and statistical significance was achieved. I believe this study emphasizes that not all compound fractures need be treated with antibiotics, and it further emphasizes that irrigation, debridement, and delayed primary closure of wounds still constitute the hallmark for treatment of traumatic wounds.

Soft Tissue

Two recent prospective randomized trials have shown no difference in the use of antibiotics in soft tissue injuries of the hand and simple lacerations elsewhere on the body.[27,28] Again, emphasis was placed in both studies on standard wound management. More controversial is the management of untidy or grossly contaminated wounds, crush wounds, and wounds with extensive soft tissue destruction. The adjunctive use of prophylactic antibiotics appears to be warranted in these instances but is not a substitute for removal of all devitalized tissue, irrigation, debridement, and *delayed primary closure*.

Choice of Antibiotics for Prophylaxis

In general, it is far better to start the patient on an antibiotic with a narrow spectrum as compared with one with a broad spectrum. This is particularly true in the patient with an injury severity score greater than 30, in whom there is a high chance of compromise to the immune system. Broad-spectrum antibiotics will simply select out opportunistic organisms, which may be more devastating in the long run. Compound fractures and soft tissue wounds necessitating antibiotics are probably best treated with a first-generation cephalosporin or nafcillin. Gram stains and cultures should be obtained in all soft tissue wounds and compound fractures prior to treatment. Antibiotic selection for wounds invading the small bowel and colon should include coverage for anaerobes and aerobes commonly found in the intestinal flora. We prefer an aminoglycoside such as gentamicin plus clindamycin or a second-generation cephalosporin such as cefoxitin.[18]

DIAGNOSIS OF WOUND INFECTIONS

Most wounds are classified according to the standards developed by the Committee on Trauma of the National Research Council.[29] The diagnosis of wound infection can be more difficult in some instances since infections in the operative site are sometimes very subtle and surgeons speak in terms of "febrile morbidity." Most of the time, however, inflammation, cellulitis, and frank suppuration with failure to heal are the hallmarks of wound infection. Abscess formation, particularly within a body cavity, can be extremely difficult to diagnose by clinical signs alone. The use of the computed tomography (CT) scan has been a major advance in the clinician's ability to localize and even treat abscesses.

Bacteremia or fungemia may be transient and of no clinical consequence. In contrast, *sepsis* refers to symptomatic invasion of the host tissues and *septicemia* implies the presence of organisms in the blood that are usually associated with overt and sometimes severe signs and symptoms. *Septic shock* is the hemodynamic instability that may arise as a result of septicemia.

Sepsis is usually associated with constitutional symptoms of fever, malaise, leukocytosis, and multiple metabolic and physiologic abberations, including glucose intolerance, negative nitrogen balance, and ileus. Septicemia, on the other hand, may be relatively asymptomatic or may produce rigors, high fever, and leukocytosis. Septic shock may present in one of two ways. The most common syndrome is the hyperdynamic state in the normovolemic patient that is characterized by an increased cardiac output, decreased peripheral vascular resistance, hypotension, normal or increased central venous pressure, hyperventilation, respiratory alkalosis, and warm, dry extremities.[30] Chills and fever are nonspecific findings which imply septicemia but are dependent on the patient's ability to mount a febrile response. The hypodynamic form of septic shock is common in septic patients who are also hypovolemic, either from overt blood loss or from covert "third space" loss secondary to multiple cellular defects and interstitial edema. Plasma volume depletion is common in peritonitis and may contribute to third space losses. It is not uncommon for a patient to present with a hyperdynamic state and progress to the hypodynamic state, which carries a worse prognosis. Hypodynamic septic shock is characterized by decreased cardiac output, increased peripheral resistance, hypotension, decreased central venous pressure, and cold, cyanotic extremities. Metabolic acidosis rapidly ensues, since hyperventilation alone can no longer compensate for the progression of metabolic derangement.

The triad of unexplained mild hyperventilation, respiratory alkalosis, and altered sensorium may herald the development of sepsis and should lead to a search for a source of infection. The dilemma is to identify or predict sepsis as soon as possible in order to prevent its sequelae. The array of laboratory tests is vast, and the choice of a specific test is dependent on the probable site(s) of disease harboring the underlying infection. When sepsis manifests itself, the clinician usually has an indication of probable source based on history and physical examination. Chest x-ray, which may be helpful in following progression of pulmonary disease, frequently lags behind the clinical picture. Diminished pulmonary function, as evidenced by hypoxemia and decreased arterial-venous oxygen difference, implicates the pulmonary circuit as a possible source of infection but may frequently reflect the same changes when the focus of infection is outside the lungs. Blood cultures may identify the organism(s) involved and therefore may be helpful in localizing the infection. The white blood cell count and hematocrit may be of use but could be misleading, depending on the volume status and bone marrow reserves of the patient. Platelet count has been found to be a fairly sensitive indicator of impending sepsis in response to therapy.[31] A decreased platelet count can be helpful along with the appearance of fibrin degradation products and a decreased fibrinogen to determine if disseminated intravascular coagulation is present. Recently there has been a trend to attempt to grade and develop prognosticators in sepsis. Acute-phase reactants such as C-reactive protein, haptoglobin, fibrinogen, ceruloplasmin, and transferrin are increased at different intervals after trauma and sepsis and may prove useful for monitoring and determining the prognosis of septic patients.[32]

Some of the more obvious studies that should be conducted regularly in the post-trauma period are daily Gram stains of the sputum, which should be examined not only for a predominant organism but also for the presence of white cells. These findings should be correlated with the chest x-ray and oxygenation to establish a diagnosis of pneumonia. Similarly, the urine should be frequently examined for pyuria and bacteriuria and should be cultured when appropriate. If the septic patient has had abdominal surgery, the presence of intraperitoneal abscess should be assumed until proved otherwise. We have found that ultrasound is a good screening test but that the CT scan has better sensitivity and specificity. Both can be used to guide drainage of selected abscesses by percutaneous catheter, but surgical drainage is still the most accepted approach. Other sources of sepsis that are not infrequent in the post-trauma period are sinusitis secondary to nasopharyngeal tubes, prostatitis secondary to indwelling Foley catheters, and pyophlebitis secondary to indwelling venous lines. Any drainage from a wound should be Gram-stained. Casts should be removed when necessary and the wounds examined.

TREATMENT

Treatment of wound infections is relatively straightforward. Appropriate antibiotics based on initial Gram stain and subsequent cultures should be instituted. Foreign bodies including sutures, should be removed when possible, debridement carried out when necessary, and the wounds dressed with clean dressings that are frequently changed. Wet-to-dry dressings are a useful adjunct but in general nothing should be placed in the wound that you would not put onto the human cornea.

The treatment of abscess after diagnosis is again straightforward. Drainage either by surgery or percutaneous catheters under CT or ultrasound guidance is mandatory. Appropriate antibiotics should be based on the Gram stain and subsequent cultures. Failure of clinical symptoms to resolve should alert the clinician to the possibility of multiple abscesses or an incompletely drained abscess. Continuous irrigation of abscess cavities with antibiotic solution is probably not as effective as appropriate systemic levels of antibiotic.

The primary goal in treatment of sepsis and septic shock is to remove the septic focus and to support any failing organs or systems until sepsis and its sequelae are eradicated. Necrotic tissue may constitute an ongoing source of septicemia and therefore must be *drained or debrided as quickly as possible.* This may require an urgent operation on a critically ill patient, since it is impossible to quell the symptoms of sepsis despite other supportive measures without elimination of the septic source. The importance of this approach cannot be overemphasized.

The septic patient should be quickly prepared for surgery, if necessary. Preoperative antibiotics are given on the basis of Gram stain results or of an educated guess based on location. Intravenous fluids are given to replete large third-space volume losses and to fill the greatly dilated vascular bed. The patient is monitored with a urinary catheter, and all patients in shock should have, at the minimum, a centrally located intravenous line for monitoring intravenous pressure. A Swan-Ganz catheter for monitoring left atrial pressures is an option, especially in patients with pre-existing cardiac or pulmonary disease or in patients not responding hemodynamically to volume replacement.

At surgery thorough exploration is necessary, with complete drainage of any abscess cavities and thorough debridement of necrotic areas down to viable bleeding tissue. If the patient's condition does not improve within 6 to 12 hours, remaining septic foci should be suspected and identified.

If no surgical areas are found as a source of infection, cultures should be taken of all accessible body fluids, including sputum, urine, oral pharyngeal secretions, and spinal fluid. Additionally, fluid from paracentesis or thoracentesis may need to be evaluated.

When possible, antibiotics should be started after the cultures are taken. A Gram stain gives the best clue as to the infecting source if material is obtained and it takes only a few minutes to perform. If no culturable material is available, one has to rely on judgment as to the most likely source of infection. For infections of the abdominal or pelvic cavities, an aminoglycoside for gram-negatives and clindamycin, chloromycetin, or metronidazole for anaerobic organisms are chosen. Genitourinary infections may require an aminoglycoside but are frequently covered with sulfonamides or doxycycline. Soft-tissue infections are frequently caused by gram-positive organisms unless involving decubiti or necrotizing fasciitis; these can be covered by penicillin, with additional coverage for anaerobic growth if suspected. Lung infections are usually amenable to sputum Gram stain prior to antibiotic coverage. A wide variety of organisms can invade lung, and broad-spectrum coverage with penicillin, cephalosporins, or aminoglycosides is indicated. One must also remember that anaerobic infections can be found in the lung, typically in a lung abscess.

The septic patient should be monitored in an intensive care setting. Central venous pressure and urine output should be monitored frequently. In patients with underlying disease, a pulmonary artery line should be inserted, if possible, and the patient monitored to prevent fluid overload, with its potential for causing sepsis-related adult respiratory distress syndrome. The pulmonary wedge pressure should be maintained around 8 to 12 mmHg to maintain adequate filling pressure while preventing pulmonary edema and overloading the cardiovascular system.

If these measures fail to restore hemodynamic stability, the use of ionotropic agents is warranted. The best agent is probably dopamine, which has a beta-adrenergic stimulatory effect in low doses, generally under 10 μg/kg/min. Above this level the alpha-adrenergic effects take over; its peripheral vasoconstrictive effect decreases peripheral perfusion and should be avoided.

The use of corticosteroids is controversial. Studies have shown a wide spectrum of results, with no effect whatsoever in significantly decreasing mortality[33,34]; to wit, any benefit to be derived is realized only when administration precedes the onset of septic shock. Conceptually, the idea of stabilizing lysozomal membranes and inhibiting the inflammatory reactions sounds good, but the adverse effects of immune suppression and potentiation of upper gastrointestinal hemorrhage outweigh the potential benefits.

Some centers now routinely administer naloxone to patients in shock. This is based on experimental studies in animals, which showed that shock survival rates in 24 hours were increased by blocking the endorphin response.[35] Clinical trials in humans have yet to show any significant improvement in outcome. Other substances, such as glucose, potassium, insulin and cryoprecipitate infusions, also lack prospective randomized clinical trials showing their efficacy.

In summary, wound infections, abscesses, sepsis and septic shock are common problems in the post-injury state. The pathophysiology of sepsis is secondary to disturbances of cell function. If the cell or groups of cells are severely altered, this in turn affects organ function. If the organ dysfunction cannot be corrected or treated, death to the organism may occur. The primary goals of treatment are surgical drainage of all sources of pus when possible, administration of appropriate antibiotics, prudent fluid resuscitation, and support of specific organ dysfunction.

REFERENCES

1. Trunkey DD: Trauma. Sci Am 249:28, 1983
2. Polk HC, Stone HH: *Pseudomonas* and other gram negative bacteria. p. 303. In Stone H, Polk HC (eds): Contemporary Burn Management, Little Brown, Boston, 1971
3. Baker CC, Oppenheimer L, Stevens B, et al: Epidemiology of trauma deaths. J Surg 140:144, 1980

4. Schimpff SC, Miller RM, Polakavetz S, Hornick RB: Infection in the severely trau-matized patient. Ann Surg 179:352, 1974
5. Carmona R, Catalano R, Trunkey DD: Septic shock. p. 156. In Shires GT (ed): Shock and Related Problems. Churchill Livingstone, Edinburgh, 1984
6. Alexander JW: Prophylactic antibiotics in trauma. Am Surg 48:45, 1982
7. Miller SE, Miller CL, Trunkey DD: The immune consequences of trauma. Surg Clin North Am 62:167, 1982
8. Hutton PAN, Jones BM, Law DJW: Depopenicillin as prophylaxis in accidental wounds. Br J Surg 65:549, 1978
9. Robert AHN, Teddy TJA: A prospective trial of prophylactic antibiotics in hand lacerations. Br J Surg 64:394, 1977
10. Samson RH, Altman SF: Antibiotic prophylaxis for minor lacerations: controlled clinical trial. NY State J Med 77:1728, 1977
11. Ignelezi RJ, VanderArk GD: Analysis of the treatment of basilar skull fractures with and without antibiotics. J Neurosurg 43:721, 1975
12. Patzakis MJ, Harvey PJ, Ivler D: Role of antibiotics in the management of open fractures. J Bone Joint Surg [Am] 56:532, 1974
13. Guglielmo JB, Hohn DC, Koo PJ, et al: Antibiotic prophylaxis in surgical proce-dures. Arch Surg 118:943, 1983
14. Grover FL, Richardson DJ, Fewel JG, et al: Prophylactic antibiotics in the treat-ment of penetrating chest wounds: a prospective double-blind study. J Thorac Car-diovasc Surg 74:528, 1977
15. LoCurto JA, Swan KG, Tischler CD, et al: Tube thoracostomy and trauma: anti-biotics or not? Presented at 45th Ann Mtg. American Association for the Surgery of Trauma
16. LeBlanc KA, Tucker WY: Prophylactic antibiotics and closed tube thoracostomy. Surg Gynecol Obstet 160:259, 1985
17. Fullen WD, Hunt J, Altemeier WA: Prophylactic antibiotics in penetrating wounds of the abdomen. J Trauma 12:282, 1972
18. Nichols RL, Smith JW, Klein DB, et al: Risk of infection after penetrating abdom-inal trauma. N Engl J Med 311:1065, 1984
19. Rowlands BJ, Ericcson CD: Comparative studies of antibiotic therapy after pen-etrating abdominal trauma. Am J Surg 148:791, 1984
20. Moore FA, Moore EE, Mill MR: Preoperative antibiotics for abdominal gunshot wounds: a prospective randomized study. Am J Surg 146:762, 1983
21. Mbawa NC, Rose RA, Schumer W: Evaluation of efficacy of cefoxitin in the pre-vention of abdominal trauma infections. Am Sur 49:582, 1983
22. Gentry LO, Feliciano DV, Lea AC, et al: Perioperative antibiotic therapy for pen-etrating injuries to the abdomen. Ann Surg 200:561, 1984
23. Hofstetter SR, Pachter HL, Bailey AA, Coppa GF: A prospective comparison of two regimens of prophylactic antibiotics in abdominal trauma: cefoxitin vs. triple drug. J Trauma 24:307, 1984
24. Crenshaw C, Glanges E, Webber C, McReynolds DB: A prospective random study of a single agent vs combination antibiotics as therapy in penetrating injuries of the abdomen. Surg Gynecol Obstet 156:289, 1983
25. Oreskovich MR, Dellinger EP, Lennard ES, et al: Duration of preventive antibiotic administration for penetrating abdominal trauma. Arch Surg 117:200, 1982
26. Bergman B: Antibiotic prophylaxis in open and closed fractures: a controlled clin-ical trial. Acta Orthop Scand 53:57, 1982
27. Haughey RE, Lammers RL, Wagner DK: Use of antibiotics in the initial manage-ment of soft tissue hand wounds. Ann Emerg Med 10:187, 1981

28. Thirlby RC, Blair AJ, Thal ER: The value of prophylactic antibiotics for simple lacerations. Surg Gynecol Obstet 156:212, 1983
29. Ad Hoc Committee of the Committee on Trauma, Division of Medical Sciences, National Academy of Sciences National Research Council: Postoperative wound infections: the influence of ultraviolet radiation of the operating room and various other factors. Ann Surg 160:23, 1964
30. MacLean LD, Mulligan W, McClean A: Patterns of septic shock in man: a detailed study of 56 patients. Ann Surg 166:543, 1967
31. Rowe MI, Buckner NS: Early diagnosis of gram negative septicemia in the pediatric surgical patient. Ann Surg 182:280, 1975
32. Koh A: Synthesis and Turnover of Acute Phase Reactants: Energy Metabolism in Trauma. p. 79. Churchill Livingstone, Edinburgh, 1970
33. Hinshaw LB, Beller-Todt BK, Archer LT: Current management of the septic shock patient: experimental basis for treatment. Circ Shock 9:543, 1982
34. Ottosson J: Experimental septic shock: effects of corticosteroids. Circ Shock 9:571, 1982
35. Faden AJ, Holladay JW: Opiate antagonists: a role in the treatment of hypovolemic shock. Science 205:317, 1979

13 | Acute Pelvic Inflammatory Disease

Daniel V. Landers
Richard L. Sweet

Acute pelvic inflammatory disease (PID), or more specifically, acute salpingitis, continues to be a major health concern in the United States and abroad. An estimated 1 million women are treated for acute PID annually in the United States at a cost of over 700 million dollars.[1] In addition, there are significant medical consequences arising from these infections. Approximately 20 percent of women who have had PID are infertile, and among those who do conceive there is a 6- to 10-fold increased risk of ectopic pregnancy.[2,3]

Tubo-ovarian abscess, another important complication of PID, is reported to occur in as many as one-third of patients hospitalized for acute PID.[4] Abscess formation, ectopic pregnancy, infertility, pelvic adhesions, and chronic pelvic pain are all sequelae of PID that may require surgical intervention, with the associated increase in morbidity and cost. Early diagnosis and aggressive therapy using antimicrobial agents that are effective against the pathogens known to have an etiologic role in PID may reduce the incidence of recurrences and surgical intervention.

ETIOLOGY

The polymicrobial nature of PID has been recognized and a variety of different etiologic agents identified. The conventional separation of PID into gonococcal and nongonococcal disease, based on endocervical cultures, has been found to be grossly inadequate. Fallopian tube and peritoneal fluid cultures from patients with acute PID have demonstrated the true nature of the

Table 13-1. Organisms Commonly Isolated
from Patients with Acute PID

Sexually transmitted organisms
  Chlamydia trachomatis
  Neisseria gonorrhoeae
  Mycoplasma hominis
  Ureaplasma urealyticum
Facultative-aerobic organisms
  Nonhemolytic streptococci
  Alpha-hemolytic streptococci
  Group B streptococci
  Coagulase-negative staphylocci
  Gardnerella vaginalis
  Escherichia coli
Anaerobic organisms
  Peptostreptococci
  Bacteroides bivius
  Bacteroides capillosus
  Other *Bacteroides* spp

disease.[5–8] A variety of aerobic and anaerobic organisms have been isolated from the peritoneal cavity and fallopian tubes of patients with acute PID.[9–11] Despite isolation of *Neisseria gonorrhoeae* from the endocervix, this organism has been recovered from only 6 to 70 percent of peritoneal and/or fallopian tube cultures.[5–10] Thus, although the role of *N. gonorrhoeae* in the pathogenesis of acute PID is significant, a variety of other organisms may also contribute. *Chlamydia trachomatis*, an even more common sexually transmitted organism, has been implicated in the pathogenesis of acute PID. Scandinavian studies have provided considerable evidence for an etiologic role of *C. trachomatis* in acute PID[11–15]; more than one-half of PID cases in Scandinavia are attributed to *C. trachomatis*. In addition, both *Mycoplasma hominis* and *Ureaplasma urealyticum* have been considered potential pathogens in patients with acute PID, although their exact role has yet to be determined.[9,13,15] Thus, acute PID is a polymicrobial infection involving combinations of sexually transmitted organisms and the mixed aerobic and anaerobic endogenous genital tract flora. Table 13-1 summarizes the organisms most frequently isolated from the upper genital tract of PID patients. The anaerobic gram-negative bacilli, such as *Bacteroides bivius, Bacteroides disiens*, and *Bacteroides fragilis*, are of particular concern because of the resistant nature of their antimicrobial sensitivity patterns. *B. bivius* and *B. disiens* are similar to *B. fragilis* in their tendency to be resistant to penicillin G, ampicillin, and first-generation cephalosporins by way of beta-lactamase production. All three of these organisms have been recovered from the site of infection in patients with upper genital tract infections. It has been demonstrated in both clinical and animal model studies that early treatment with antimicrobial agents effective against anaerobic as well as facultative organisms, with particular focus on the resistant anaerobic gram-negative bacilli, results in improved response rates and reduction in bacteremia, abscess formation, and septic pelvic thrombophlebitis.[16–20]

Table 13-2. Diagnostic Criteria for Acute Pelvic Inflammatory Disease

Direct abdominal tenderness with or without rebound tenderness
  plus
Uterine and/or cervical motion tenderness
  plus
Adnexal tenderness
  plus
One or more of the following:
  Leukocytosis (WBC > 10,000 per mm^3)
  Temperature > 38°C
  Pelvic abscess or inflammatory mass on exam or ultrasound
  Purulent material from peritoneal cavity by culdocentesis
  Gram stain of endocervix positive for gram-negative intracellular diplococci

(Hager WD, Eschenbach DA, Spence MR, Sweet RL: Criteria for diagnosis and grading of salpingitis. Obstet Gynecol 61:113, 1983. Reprinted with permission from the American College of Obstetricians and Gynecologists.)

DIAGNOSIS OF ACUTE PID

The diagnosis of acute PID has for years lacked standardization and accuracy. Jacobson and Westrom reported results on 814 women with a clinical diagnosis of acute salpingitis who underwent diagnostic laparoscopy.[21] They confirmed the diagnosis in only 65 percent of the cases. Chaparro and coworkers[22] diagnosed acute PID at laparoscopy in 45 percent of patients who were not clinically suspected to have PID. Thus, the sensitivity and specificity of the diagnosis of acute PID on clinical grounds was unacceptably low. In an effort to improve the accuracy of the clinical diagnosis Hager et al. formulated the diagnostic criteria listed in Table 13-2.[23] However, the use of these criteria would still exclude a significant number of patients who actually have PID. Laparoscopy has been the only reliable method for making the diagnosis of acute PID, but for logistic and economic reasons, this technique may be impractical in many settings. Recent evidence suggests that histologic evaluation of an endometrial biopsy specimen for inflammatory cell infiltration may be a useful tool in confirming the diagnosis of acute PID, particularly in patients suspected to have PID on clinical grounds who also have endocervical *C. trachomatis* or *N. gonorrhoeae*.[24] The present difficulty in diagnosing acute PID on clinical grounds may force clinicians to overtreat the disease to avoid missing the diagnosis.

TREATMENT

The optimal therapy for patients with acute PID requires early diagnosis and prompt treatment, with antimicrobial agents effective against the major pathogens known to be involved in the disease process. This goal is difficult, if not impossible, to achieve. Since the sexually transmitted organisms such as *C. trachomatis* and *N. gonorrhoeae* must be treated in addition to the endogenous facultative and anaerobic microorganisms, combination antimicro-

Table 13-3. Centers for Disease Control Treatment Recommendations for Acute Pelvic
Inflammatory Disease (1985)

Inpatient Treatment
1. Doxycycline 100 mg I.V. twice daily plus cefoxitin 2.0 g I.V. 4 times daily. Continue drugs I.V. for at least 4 days and at least 48 hours after the patient improves. Then continue doxycycline 100 mg by mouth twice daily to complete 10 to 14 days total therapy.
2. Clindamycin 600 mg I.V. 4 times daily plus gentamicin 2.0 mg/kg I.V. followed by 1.5 mg/kg 3 times daily in patients with normal renal function. Continue drugs I.V. for at least 4 days and at least 48 hours after patient improves. Then continue clindamycin 450 mg by mouth 4 times daily to complete 10 to 14 days total therapy.

Ambulatory treatment
Cefoxitin 2.0 g I.M.
      or
Amoxicillin 3.0 g by mouth
or Ampicillin 3.5 g by mouth
      or
Aqueous procaine penicillin G 4.8 million units I.M.
      or
Ceftriaxone 250 mg I.M.
(Each of these regimens except ceftriaxone accompanied by probenecid 1.0 g by mouth)
      followed by
Doxycycline 100 mg by mouth twice daily for 10 to 14 days

bial regimens are being employed. The Centers for Disease Control (CDC), recognizing the need for broad-spectrum coverage, has recommended several regimens for the treatment of patients with acute PID.[25] These regimens, listed in Table 13-3, include cefoxitin plus doxycycline and clindamycin plus gentamicin. The goal of these recommendations is to provide effective therapy against *N. gonorrhoeae, C. trachomatis*, and the facultative and anaerobic bacteria of the genital tract, including the resistant anaerobic gram-negative bacilli. The importance of providing coverage for all the potential pathogens was demonstrated by Sweet et al.,[26] who found persistent *C. trachomatis* in the endometrium of patients with upper genital tract infections treated with broad-spectrum antibiotics not effective against *C. trachomatis*. As more information on the pathogenesis and microbiology of these infections becomes available and newer, more effective antimicrobial regimens are developed, these treatment recommendations will continue to undergo revision.

Considerable controversy exists over the appropriateness of outpatient therapy for acute PID. Virtually no good data are available to evaluate the comparative efficacy of outpatient and inpatient antimicrobial regimens. Unfortunately, logistic and economic considerations have resulted in 75 percent of the cases in the United States being treated on an outpatient basis. The major weakness of the outpatient regimens, listed in Table 13-3, is the inadequacy of antimicrobial coverage for all the suspected pathogens.

The commonly accepted indications for hospitalization of patients with acute PID include temperature greater than 38°C, uncertainty of the diagnosis, nausea and vomiting (which preclude use of oral medication), pregnancy, upper peritoneal signs, and suspicion of a pelvic or tubo-ovarian abscess. If outpatient therapy is used, however, the patient's status must be reassessed within 48 hours to ensure the adequacy of response. The presence of an intrauterine device (IUD) in a patient with acute PID may also be an indication for inpatient therapy, and the device should be removed after adequate levels of antimicrobials have been achieved. Adolescent patients with PID may also benefit from inpatient treatment because of the high rate of noncompliance, nulliparity, and desire for preserved fertility in this patient population.

Surgical Treatment

Although the vast majority of patients with acute PID will respond to the antimicrobial regimens described above, occasionally surgical intervention is necessary to effect a cure. Most cases of PID that require surgical intervention either are deep-seated infections involving tubo-ovarian abscesses, pyosalpinx, or inflammatory complexes or are chronic, recurrent cases in which intractable pain persists despite eradication of microorganisms. This pain probably relates to persistent inflammation or scarring and adhesion formation.

It may be difficult to distinguish a tubo-ovarian abscess from a pyosalpinx, ovarian abscess, or other inflammatory complex, but current trends in the management of these masses are similar: aggressive antimicrobial therapy, with surgical intervention reserved for those failing to respond. The principles applied in the management of tubo-ovarian abscess are equally applicable to any patient presenting with acute PID complicated by an inflammatory complex mass in the pelvis.

Tubo-ovarian abscess has been reported to occur in as many as one-third of hospitalized patients with acute PID, although most series report a 10 to 15 percent incidence.[27-32] Since the presenting clinical findings for patients with uncomplicated PID and those with tubo-ovarian abscesses are essentially the same, differentiation requires the identification of an inflammatory adnexal mass. Physical examination may be insufficient to make this identification because pain and tenderness may preclude an adequate pelvic examination. Several relatively noninvasive imaging techniques, including ultrasound, computed tomography (CT), and magnetic resonance imaging, may be used to aid in the diagnosis of pelvic abscesses. Ultrasound is the most commonly used modality in the evaluation of PID patients; it is a relatively inexpensive, yet accurate, method of evaluating PID patients for pelvic masses. A number of investigators have looked at the accuracy of ultrasound in the diagnosis of pelvic abscesses.[28,33,34] Taylor et al. noted that 36 of 40 abdominal and 32 of 33 pelvic abscesses were correctly identified, while 112 of 113 suspected abdominal and 33 of 34 suspected pelvic abscesses were correctly ruled out.[33] Our current approach is to use ultrasound as the initial diagnostic aid in patients with PID and reserve the other, more expensive imaging modalities for those patients in whom ultrasound fails to provide adequate information.

The controversy in the management of tubo-ovarian abscesses revolves around the dictum that abscesses require surgical drainage or extirpation for cure. However, several studies have now shown that tubo-ovarian abscesses can be treated conservatively, without significant risk to the patient, in hopes of preserving fertility and/or ovarian function. These studies have shown that nearly two-thirds of tubo-ovarian abscess patients will have a favorable initial response to antibiotics alone.[28,31,32,35] One smaller study did not confirm this finding.[30] A major disadvantage in the majority of these studies was the lack of detailed analysis comparing responses to particular antimicrobial regimens. Since pelvic infections are associated with anaerobic gram-negative bacilli such as *B. fragilis*, which have a propensity to form abscesses, improved results should be seen in patients treated aggressively with antimicrobial agents effective against these organisms. There are, however, insufficient data available as yet to confirm this suspicion for tubo-ovarian abscesses.

In a series of 167 patients treated initially with antibiotics alone[28] we found a reduction in mass size and symptomatic improvement in 25 percent of patients treated only with penicillin, 49 percent of patients treated with penicillin and an aminoglycoside, and 68 percent of patients treated with regimens that included clindamycin ($P < .01$). A total of 104 patients who were available for follow-up had been treated with regimens that did not include clindamycin or other antimicrobial agents effective against the resistant gram-negative anaerobic bacteria. The response rate was 36.5 percent, compared with the 68 percent response rate of the 63 patients treated with regimens that included clindamycin.

The opposite trend was noted on examination of those with an increase in mass size. Surgical extirpation of an abscess was required during the initial hospitalization for failure to respond to antibiotics in 42 patients. Of these, 64 percent had been treated with regimens not containing clindamycin compared with the 36 percent that received clindamycin-containing regimens. There were 134 patients who returned 2 to 4 weeks after discharge following conservative treatment of tubo-ovarian abscesses. In 86 percent of the clindamycin-treated patients the masses were decreased in size or absent, compared with 46 percent of the non-clindamycin-treated group. The superior response seen in clindamycin-treated patients may well reflect its superior activity against resistant gram-negative anaerobes, such as *B. fragilis* and *B. bivius*, and its documented ability to penetrate abscesses in the animal model.[37] Animal models have been used extensively to demonstrate antibiotic penetration and activity within the abscess environment. As research continues to reveal the characteristics of antibiotics such as clindamycin, metronidazole, and cefoxitin, we begin to see plausible explanations for the improved response of tubo-ovarian abscesses to some antimicrobial treatment regimens.

Prior to the advent of antibiotic preparations, pelvic abscesses were treated with bedrest, fluids, heat, and if accessible, colpotomy drainage. Even with the addition of antibiotics to the armamentarium, surgical removal of infected pelvic organs remained the predominant mode of therapy. In recent years, with the improvement in available antibiotics and the enhanced awareness of infection-related infertility, an increasing number of investigators has encouraged conservative medical management of the unruptured tubo-ovarian abscess.[4,28,31,32] The approach we currently use in the management of suspected tubo-ovarian abscess is outlined in Figure 13-1. If a ruptured tubo-ovarian ab-

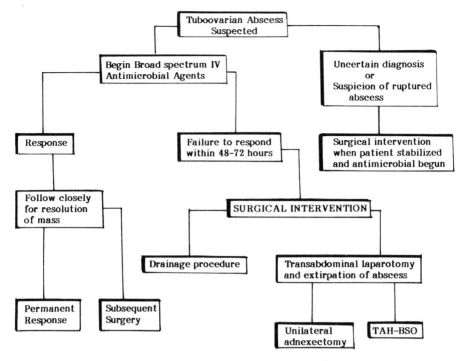

Fig. 13-1 Management scheme for tubo-ovarian abscess.

scess is suspected, the patient is stabilized, antibiotics are begun, and immediate surgical intervention is undertaken. The only other situation in which immediate surgery is indicated is that in which the diagnosis is in question and there is a reasonable suspicion of a surgical emergency. Otherwise, the patient is begun on a regimen of intravenous antibiotics, which includes coverage against the resistant gram-negative anaerobes as well as the other facultative and anaerobic organisms found in these infections. On our service patients with tubo-ovarian abscesses are usually treated with clindamycin and an aminoglycoside. If despite appropriate antimicrobial therapy the patient fails to respond within a reasonable amount of time (48 to 72 hours), we then proceed with surgical intervention. The term *respond* does not mean complete cure but rather evidence of improvement, such as defervescence or decrease in pain, white blood cell count, or abscess size. During the initial antibiotic therapy the clinician must be alert to the possibility of abscess rupture, which may become a surgical emergency. Once a decision to operate has been made, there should be no further delay.

Certain factors may be of some predictive value in determining which patients are more likely to fail antibiotic therapy alone. Adnexal masses larger than 8 cm and/or bilateral adnexal involvement has been found to be predictive of failure to respond to medical therapy.[32] This does not mean that all such patients will fail medical therapy but rather that they are at increased risk for failing this approach. Surprisingly, the presence of fever, the degree of leukocytosis, or a past history of PID could not be shown to be predictive of patients who would fail antibiotic therapy alone.

Abscess rupture can be a serious complication associated with tubo-ovarian abscess. Intra-abdominal rupture is a surgical emergency, and unnecessary delay of surgical intervention may increase the mortality risk. In 1964 Pedowitz and Bloomfield[27] reported on 143 cases of ruptured adnexal abscesses. They found that the very high mortality rate for patients treated prior to 1947 was dramatically reduced with a more aggressive surgical approach combined with available medical adjuvants. They also reported that there were 235 published cases after 1945 at centers using an operative approach. In analyzing the 14 deaths that occurred, they felt that 10 might have been prevented and cited physician delay in establishing the diagnosis as the most common cause of preventable death. Collins and Jansen[37] also reported a dramatic reduction in mortality rate after adopting an aggressive surgical approach in addition to antibiotic therapy. In 1969 Mikal and Sellmann[38] reported a 3.7 percent mortality rate from 1959 to 1966. Rivlin and Hunt[39] in 1977 reported a 7.1 percent mortality in 113 patients with ruptured tubo-ovarian abscess. This study was unique in that hysterectomy was performed in only 3 percent of patients, with hormonal and menstrual function being retained in 73.5 percent. Prior to this study the standard practice was complete removal of uterus, tubes, and ovaries following abscess rupture. Furthermore, Rivlin and Hunt reported that only 17.5 percent of patients required further surgery at a later date in the 1- and 5-year follow-up period. We have since successfully treated four patients with ruptured unilateral tubo-ovarian abscess by extirpation of the affected adnexa.[29] In the 2- to 10-year follow-up none of these patients required further surgery, and one patient carried a subsequent intrauterine pregnancy to term. In current practice, with the availability of the newer, improved antimicrobial agents, the mortality rate following abscess rupture is very low. However, prompt surgical intervention may reduce unnecessary morbidity following abscess rupture. Furthermore, it appears that ruptured unilateral tubo-ovarian abscesses can be safely treated with a conservative surgical approach such as unilateral adnexectomy, aimed at preserving hormonal and reproductive function.

When an unruptured tubo-ovarian abscess fails antibiotic therapy, surgical intervention is indicated. There is no general consensus as to the appropriate technique to use, although there seems to be a general trend toward a more conservative approach in patients concerned about future fertility. Over the years these abscesses have been treated by extraperitoneal drainage; posterior colpotomy drainage; percutaneous, transabdominal, and laparoscopic drainage; unilateral adnexectomy; and total abdominal hysterectomy with bilateral salpingo-oophorectomy. Drainage via a posterior vaginal colpotomy incision has been used for many years. This procedure can be effective when combined with antimicrobial therapy and restricted to patients with fluctuant abscesses in the midline which dissect the rectovaginal septum and are firmly attached to parietal peritoneum. These requirements reduce the number of cases of tubo-ovarian abscess that can be safely drained by this procedure. If these requirements are not met, the morbidity can be significantly higher. In 1982 Rivlin and coworkers[39] reported 348 cases of colpotomy drainage resulting in 23 cases (6.5 percent) of diffuse peritoneal sepsis. There were 6 deaths (23 percent) among these 23 cases. In 1983 Rivlin[40] reported on 59 patients treated with colpotomy drainage, of whom 13 required further operation during the same admission; additional surgery was required at a later date in 11 patients. We rarely use vaginal colpotomy to drain tubo-ovarian abscesses because most tubo-ovarian abscesses do not meet our requirements (midline, adherent to peritoneum, dissecting the rectovaginal septum) and because of the high proportion of these patients needing additional surgery. In general, in view of the significant number of abscesses that are unilateral, an adnexectomy with extirpation of infected tissue may offer a significantly better fertility prognosis than colpotomy drainage, which leaves behind the abscess wall. When a transabdominal approach is taken extirpation of the abscesses is usually the most effective treatment. In the past surgical extirpation usually involved removing the uterus, tubes, and ovaries. Several investigators have since reported favorable results with unilateral excision of one-sided tubo-ovarian abscesses. These data indicate that approximately 17 percent of patients[28,32,38,39] treated with unilateral adnexectomy will require additional surgery at a later date.

Surgical extirpation of a tubo-ovarian abscess may be a difficult procedure because of distorted anatomy and involvement of contiguous structures, including bowel, bladder, and ureter. Considerable exposure may be needed, and a generous incision is recommended. Careful exploration of the entire abdomen for other concealed pockets of pus should be performed. Large-bore, closed-suction drains should be left in place, exiting either through the vaginal cuff (if hysterectomy is performed) or a colpotomy incision. A strong fascial closure technique, such as a Smead-Jones, and a delayed primary closure of the skin is the procedure of choice.

The success of percutaneous drainage of intra-abdominal abscesses guided by CT has led investigators to apply this technique to tubo-ovarian abscesses. We must await future reports with large numbers in order to evaluate the success of this technique. Investigators have, however, reported on laparoscopically directed percutaneous drainage of tubo-ovarian abscesses with encouraging results,[41,42] but large numbers with long-term follow-up of future surgery and fertility will be needed to fully evaluate the usefulness of this approach.

SUMMARY

In summary, the diagnosis and management of acute pelvic inflammatory disease has undergone significant changes over the past decade. These changes have been based primarily on data collected at the time of laparoscopy. Although the inaccuracy of the clinical diagnosis has led investigators to propose more selective criteria for the diagnosis of acute PID, these criteria still fall short of enabling clinicians to identify PID patients in order to reduce the incidence of the major sequelae associated with acute infection. Treatment regimens have been improved dramatically on the basis of microbiologic data from the fallopian tube, endometrium, and peritoneal cavity. These improved treatment regimens may reduce the incidence of some of the major sequelae leading to the need for surgical intervention. However, a great deal more information about etiology, diagnosis, treatment, and prevention of the disease process will be needed in order to dramatically reduce the incidence of infertility, ectopic pregnancy, pyosalpinx, tubo-ovarian abscesses, and the tubal scarring and obstruction associated with acute PID.

REFERENCES

1. Curran JW: Economic consequences of pelvic inflammatory disease in the United States. Am J Obstet Gynecol 138:848, 1980
2. Westrom L: Effect of acute pelvic inflammatory disease on fertility. Am J Obstet Gynecol 122:707, 1975
3. Westrom L: Incidence, prevalence and trends of acute pelvic inflammatory disease and its consequences in industrialized countries. Am J Obstet Gynecol 138:880, 1980
4. Landers DV, Sweet RL: Current trends in the diagnosis and treatment of tubo-ovarian abscess. Am J Obstet Gynecol 151:1098, 1985
5. Eschenbach DA, Buchanan T, Pollock H et al: Polymicrobial nature of acute pelvic inflammatory disease. N Engl J Med 293:166, 1975
6. Sweet RL, Mills J, Hadley WK, et al: Use of laparoscopy to determine the microbiologic etiology of acute salpingitis. Am J Obstet Gynecol 134:68, 1979
7. Lip J, Burgoyne X: Cervical and peritoneal bacterial flora associated with salpingitis. Obstet Gynecol 28:561, 1966
8. Thompson SE, Hager WD, Wong KH, et al: The microbiology and therapy of acute pelvic inflammatory disease in hospitalized patients. Am J Obstet Gynecol 136:179, 1980
9. Sweet RL, Draper DL, Schachter J, et al: Microbiology and pathogenesis of acute salpingitis as determined by laparoscopy: What is the appropriate site to sample? Am J Obstet Gynecol 138:985, 1980
10. Monif GRG, Welkos SL, Baer H, et al: Cul-de-sac isolates from patients with endometritis-salpingitis-peritonitis and gonococcal endocervicitis. Am J Obstet Gynecol 1126:158, 1981
11. Mardh P-A, Ripa T, Svensson L, Westrom L: *Chlamydia trachomatis* infection in patients with acute salpingitis. N Engl J Med 298:1377, 1977
12. Osser S, Persson K: Epidemiology and serodiagnostic aspects of *Chlamydia* salpingitis. Obstet Gynecol 59:206, 1982
13. Moller BR, Mardh P-A, Ahrons S, Nussler E: Infections with *Chlamydia trachomatis*, *Mycoplasma hominis* and *Neisseria gonorrhoeae* in patients with acute pelvic inflammatory disease. Sex Transm Dis 8:198, 1981
14. Gjonnaess H, Dalaker K, Anestad G, et al: Pelvic inflammatory disease: etiologic studies with emphasis on chlamydial infection. Obstet Gynecol 59:550, 1982
15. Mardh P-A, Lund I, Svensson L, et al: Antibodies to *Chlamydia trachomatis*, *Mycoplasma hominis* and *Neisseria gonorrhoeae* in sera from patients with acute salpingitis. Br J Vener Dis 57:125, 1981

16. Gall SA, Kohan MT, Ayers OM, et al: Intravenous metronidazole or clindamycin with tobramycin for therapy of pelvic infections. Obstet Gynecol 57:51, 1981

17. Joiner K, Lowe B, Dzink J, Bartlett JG: Comparative efficacy of ten antimicrobial agents in experimental *Bacteroides fragilis* infections. J Infect Dis 145:561, 1982

18. Bartlett JG, Louie TJ, Gorbach SL, Onderdonk AB: Therapeutic efficacy of 29 antimicrobial regimens in experimental intraabdominal sepsis. Rev Infect Dis 3:535, 1981

19. Ledger WJ: Selection of antimicrobial agents for treatment of infections of the female genital tract. Rev. Infect Dis suppl., 5:98, 1983

20. DiZerga G, Yomekura L, Roys S, et al: A comparison of clindamycin-gentamicin and penicillin-gentamicin in the treatment of post cesarean section endomyometritis. Am J Obstet Gynecol 134:238, 1979

21. Jacobson L, Westrom L: Objective diagnosis of acute pelvic inflammatory disease. Am J Obstet Gynecol 105:1088, 1969

22. Chaparro MV, Ghosh S, Nashed A, et al: Laparoscopy for the confirmation and prognosstic evaluation of PID. Int J Gynaecol Obstet 15:307, 1978

23. Hager WD, Eschenbach DA, Spence MR, Sweet RL: Criteria for diagnosis and grading of salpingitis. Obstet Gynecol 61:113, 1983

24. Kiviat NB, Wolner-Hanssen P, Eschenbach DA, et al: Development of histopathologic criteria for endometritis and salpingitis caused by *Neisseria gonorrhoeae* and/or *Chlamydia trachomatis* (Abstract No. 270). Presented at Interscience Conference on Antimicrobial Agents and Chemotherapy, Minneapolis, Sept. 30, 1985

25. 1985 STD Treatment Guidelines. Morbidity Mortality Weekly Rep, suppl. 34: No. 4S, Oct. 18, 1985

26. Sweet RL, Schachter J, Robbie MO: Failure of beta-lactam antibiotics to eradicate *Chlamydia trachomatis* in the endometrium despite apparent clinical cure of acute salpingitis. JAMA 150:2641, 1983

27. Pedowitz P, Bloomfield RD: Ruptured adnexal abscess with generalized peritonitis. Am J Obstet Gynecol 88:721, 1964

28. Landers DV, Sweet RL: Tubo-ovarian abscess: contemporary approach to management. Rev Infect Dis 5:876, 1983

29. Nebel WA, Lucas WE: Management of tubo-ovarian abscess. Obstet Gynecol 32:381, 1968

30. Hager WD: Follow-up of patients with tubo-ovarian abscess(es) in association with salpingitis. Obstet Gynecol 61:680, 1983

31. Franklin EW, Hevron JE, Thompson JD: Management of the pelvic abscess. Clin Obstet Gynecol 16:66, 1973

32. Ginsberg DS, Stem JL, Hamod KA, et al: Tubo-ovarian abscess: a retrospective review. Am J Obstet Gynecol 138:1055, 1980

33. Taylor KJK, DeGraaft MCI, Wasson JF, et al: Accuracy of grey-scale ultrasound diagnosis of abdominal and pelvic abscesses in 220 patients. Lancet 1:83, 1978

34. Spirtos NJ, Bernstine RL, Crawford WL, Rayle J: Sonography in acute pelvic inflammatory disease. J Reprod Med 27:312, 1982

35. Scott WC: Pelvic abscess in association with intrauterine contraceptive devices. Am J Obstet Gynecol 131:149, 1978

36. Joiner KA, Lowe BR, Dzink JL, Bartlett JG: Antibiotic levels in infected and sterile subcutaneous abscesses in mice. J Infect Dis 143:487, 1981

37. Collins CA, Jansen FW: Treatment of pelvic abscess. Clin Obstet Gynecol 2:512, 1959

38. Mickal A, Sellmann AN: Management of tubo-ovarian abscess. Clin Obstet Gynecol 12:252, 1969

39. Rivlin ME, Hunt JA: Ruptured tubo-ovarian abscess: Is hysterectomy necessary? Obstet Gynecol 50:518, 1977
40. Rivlin ME, Golan A, Darling MR: Diffuse peritoneal sepsis associated with colpotomy drainage of pelvic abscess. J Reprod Med 27:406, 1982
41. Adducci JE: Laparoscopy in the diagnosis and treatment of pelvic inflammatory disease with abscess formation. Int Surg 66:359, 1981
42. Henry-Suchet J, Soler A, Loffreda V: Laparoscopic treatment of tubo-ovarian abscesses. J Reprod Med 29:579, 1984

14 | Urosepsis: The Role of the Urologist

Sheldon D. Roberts
Martin I. Resnick

Urinary tract infections are common and are routinely treated by physicians in various specialties. Although nonbacteremic urinary infections are not generally difficult to treat, they can develop into serious systemic gram-negative septicemias. The term *urosepsis* has traditionally been used in the urologic community to describe any febrile urinary tract infection associated with bacteremia. Most often these infections occur in hospitalized patients who have been compromised by debilitating illness or urologic instrumentation. Urosepsis is difficult to treat and is associated with a high mortality, especially when it is accompanied by septic shock. The prevention and treatment of urosepsis is an important public health problem and has remained a challenge in compromised patients.

In the preantibiotic era gram-negative bacteremia was an uncommon entity,[1] but at present it constitutes the most frequent type of bacteremia in this country.[2] In several studies the urinary tract has been found to be the most frequent site of origin of gram-negative bacteremia, and, not surprisingly, bacteremia caused by gram-negative bacilli is a frequently encountered infection in urologic patients.[2-7] It is therefore important to identify those factors which place patients at risk for developing these infections, and it is also important to identify those clinical characteristics of patients suffering from bacteremic urinary tract infections.

HISTORICAL BACKGROUND

Physicians have long observed severe illness in patients following genitourinary manipulation or surgery. In the prebacteriology era the causative mechanism of these reactions was speculative at best. Clark postulated that

201

"urinary fever" was the result of disturbance in renal function with a concomitant pathologic renal lesion.[8] Weir believed that "catheter fever" was caused by a poisoning of the wound with an ascending urinary inflammation caused by a change in the condition of the urine.[9] The first reported association of urethral fever with bacilli was made by Clado, who in 1887 identified a long, spore-forming bacillus in three patients with urethral fever. The bacilli were obtained twice by splenic punctures and once in a postmortem examination of the spleen and liver.[10] Also in 1887, Hallé discovered a bacterium in the urine, blood, and renal abscess from a patient with a rapidly fatal course.[11]

In 1916 Crabtree reported seven patients with positive blood cultures after urethral catheterization and four additional instances of positive blood cultures in association with pyelonephritis. In the late 1920s Winfield W. Scott began the practice of obtaining routine blood cultures in febrile urology patients and reported the characteristics of 82 septicemic patients detected over 2 years.[13] In most cases the septicemia was associated with either open surgical procedures or some form of endourologic instrumentation. Scott reported 15 fatalities in his series (a quite respectable 18 percent!) and recognized the importance of host factors as determinants of survival. Enteric organisms were most frequently the pathogens involved. Scott also stressed that postoperative bacteremia was often of no clinical significance. In 1930 Barrington and Wright drew routine blood cultures on patients undergoing urethral operations such as internal urethrotomy and urethral dilatation and found evidence of bacteremia 1 to 2 minutes postoperatively in 13 of 23 patients.[14] They concluded that invasion of bacteria into the circulation must occur directly through abraded tissues and not via some other circuitous route, such as lymphatic channels. They stressed that the magnitude of bacterial invasion must be due both to the numbers of organisms in the urethra and urine and to the degree of damage caused by the urethral procedure.

ETIOLOGIC AGENTS

In all studies that have addressed this issue, *Escherichia coli* has been found to be the most common organism of urinary origin to cause bloodstream infection. Almost all bacteria in this group are the gram-negative organisms that cause septicemic urinary tract infections (Table 14-1)[15] Septicemic patients treated for recurrent urinary tract infections who have chronic indwelling urinary catheters or who have undergone numerous genitourinary manipulations are more likely to be infected by *Proteus* spp., *Pseudomonas aeruginosa*, and other bacteria that are resistant to the more commonly used antimicrobial agents. There is a tendency for better prognosis (lower mortality) in those instances of urosepsis caused by *E. coli* than those caused by other enteric organisms.[16] This may be because of the tendency of patients with less chronic disease to first develop infections with *E. coli* and for more debilitated patients to become infected with more resistant organisms. The poorest prognoses are associated with mixed infections.[7,16] It must be emphasized that the chance of

Table 14-1. Bacterial Agents of Bacteremic Urinary
Tract Infection

Agent	Number	Percent
Escherichia coli	94	45.0
Klebsiella pneumoniae	26	12.4
Enterobacter spp.	13	6.2
Serratia marcescens	3	1.4
Pseudomonas	18	8.6
Proteus and *Providencia*	31	14.8
Other aerobic organisms	1	<1.0
Mixed or polymicrobic organisms	23	11.0
TOTAL	209	100%

(Kreger BE, Craven DE, Carling PC, et al: Gram-negative bacteremia.
III. Reassessment of etiology, epidemiology and ecology in 612 patients.
Am J Med 68:332, 1980.)

survival is most affected by the underlying medical condition of the host and
not by any virulence factors present in the infecting organism.

There is an association between stool colonization of gram-negative bacilli
and subsequent gram-negative bacteremia.[17] The gastrointestinal tract is a reservoir from which urinary tract colonization originates, and, with the exception
of *E. coli*, most gram-negative urinary pathogens appear in the stool during
hospitalization.[18] Greater frequency of hospitalization can presumably predispose to infection with a greater array of resistant organisms. In studies by Bryan
and Reynolds of 221 episodes of hospital-acquired bacteremic urinary tract
infections, of 28 patients whose deaths were thought to be directly attributable
to the bacteremic urinary tract infection, 19 (68 percent) had diffuse central
nervous system disease, malignancy, alcoholic liver disease, advanced arteriosclerosis with renal failure, or diabetes mellitus.[16]

Serratia marcescens is a nosocomial urinary pathogen which may be associated with increased risk for spread to the bloodstream. Krieger and associates found that although only 2.7 percent of patients developed bacteremia,
those patients with hospital-acquired *S. marcescens* bacteriuria were at a markedly increased risk (16 percent) for developing bacteremia.[19] Shaberg and colleagues found that 9.0 percent of all patients with *S. marcescens* developed
bacteremia and that there is an associated 6 percent mortality.[20]

PATHOGENESIS

Because urinary tract infections are such common occurrences in hospitalized patients, bacteremia from urinary sources accounts for most cases of
gram-negative bacteremia. In fact, up to 0.1 percent of all hospitalized patients
will develop bacteremic urinary tract infections during their hospitalization.[19,21]
In both children and adults the most common portal of entry of bacteria into
the bloodstream is the urinary tract.[7] Of those patients with nosocomial urinary
tract infections the development of bacteremia is positively correlated with
males but is not affected by age or race.[19]

BACTERIURIA ASSOCIATED WITH GENITOURINARY MANIPULATION

Fever and rigors associated with the passage of urethral catheters have been recognized for many decades, and it has been observed that these symptoms are more likely to occur in the presence of infected rather than sterile urine.[14] Although the bacteremia associated with genitourinary manipulation is generally transient and harmless, septicemia may develop in the compromised host. Fatal bacteremia following urologic procedures, however, is uncommon.[16,23]

Bacteremia following transurethral resection of the prostate gland is common,[23,24] and it is that form of manipulation that is most likely to be associated with urosepsis.[24,25] Many patients who develop bacteremia have sterile, not infected, urine preoperatively. Within 3 to 4 hours after the operation blood cultures will be positive, and often a urinary tract infection will later develop from the same organism.[26,27]

Table 14-2 summarizes data concerning bacteremia associated with transurethral resection of the prostate. This complication occurs in 1.6 to 66.7 percent of patients undergoing the procedure.[24,25,28,29,30] It is unclear why there is such a large variation among the published reports that address this topic, but factors that differ from one urologic practice to another are the use of perioperative antibiotics, different practices of sterile technique, and length of resection time. In all instances the percentage of patients who became bacteremic in the presence of a sterile urine was less than for patients with infected urine.

Sullivan and associates[23] sought to identify those factors which would predispose patients undergoing transurethral prostatectomy to septicemia (Table 14-3) and found that preoperative urinary tract infection, preoperative Foley catheterization, and prostatitis were all positively correlated with septicemic episodes. Age, amount of preoperative residual urine, duration of resection, and the amount of tissue resected had no impact on the propensity towards septicemia. Almost all the patients with positive blood cultures demonstrated systemic manifestations of septicemia.

Bacteremia has also been seen in association with other manipulations of the genitourinary tract. Both cystoscopy and urethral dilation have been shown

Table 14-2. Bacteriuria Associated with Transurethral Resection of the Prostate

Reference	No. Cases	Percent Bacteremia	Pts. with Preop Bacteriuria/ Postop Bacteremia
Biorn et al.[24]	106	12.2	7/10
Bulkley et al.[25]	125	1.6	1/2
Creevy et al.[28]	356	44.1	—
Kidd et al.[29]	47	6	3/3
Last et al.[30]	18	66.7	—

Table 14-3. Factors Affecting Septicemia in Prostatectomy Patients

Factor	Negative Blood Culture (n = 53)	Positive Blood Culture (n = 24)	P
Age	64.8	66.3	NS[a]
Residual urine	265.1	301.3	NS[a]
Preoperative UTI[a]	29%	67%	P < .01
Duration of procedure (min.)	62	59.3	NS[a]
Amount of gland removed (grams)	13.3	17.3	NS[a]
Prostatitis noted pathologically	31%	60%	P < .05
Preoperative Foley catheter	21%	50%	P < .01

[a] NS = not significant; UTI = urinary tract infection.

to cause transient bacteremia. The chief predisposing factor in appearance of bacteremia in both procedures is the presence of urinary tract infection.[23] Indwelling urethral catheters alone can predispose to urosepsis in compromised patients.[31,32]

The pathogenesis of catheter-associated bacteriuria in patients who are given closed urinary drainage devices is not entirely understood and may, in fact, depend on the particular drainage device that is used. The retrograde migration of bacteria may be either intraluminal from the collection bag[33] or extraluminal in the periurethral mucous sheath present from the urethral meatus to the bladder.[34,35] Thompson and colleagues[36] were able to demonstrate prior collection bag contamination with the same organism responsible for bacteriuria in only 5 of 68 patients with catheter-associated bacteriuria. It is therefore not surprising that antibiotic or peroxide irrigations of indwelling catheters have not been of value in eradication of this problem.[36,37] Efforts to reduce meatal colonization with daily meatal care have also been unsuccessful (see chapter 2).[38]

It is evident that the greatest determinant in the acquisition of urosepsis is the adequacy of host defenses. Quintiliani and associates[39] found that urosepsis associated with genitourinary manipulation was generally symptomatic only in the presence of obstructive uropathy or an impairment of host defenses

Table 14-4. Associated Conditions in Patients with Bacteremia Definitely Related to Urinary Tract (UT) Instrumentation

Condition	No. Cases
Preexisting UT disease alone	23
Preexisting UT disease and diabetes	4
Preexisting UT disease and cirrhosis	2
Preexisting UT disease, diabetes, and cirrhosis	1
No preexisting UT disease	0
	30

(Quintiliani R, Cuhha BA, Klimek J, et al: Bacteriaemia after manipulation of the urinary tract. The importance of preexisting urinary tract disease and compromised host defences. Postgrad Med J 54:668, 1978.)

Table 14-5. Sepsis Associated with Urinary Tract Infection

	Obstructive Uropathy	Nonobstructive Uropathy
Improved or cured	5	24
Died	2	1
Total	7	25

(Tunn UW, Thieme H: Sepsis associated with urinary tract infection: antibiotic treatment with peperacillin. Arch Intern Med 142:2035, 1982.)

(most often diabetes and/or cirrhosis). No patient in their series who was free or urinary tract disease developed sustained bacteremia associated with urinary tract instrumentation (Table 14-4). For instance, patients who required perioperative indwelling urinary catheters were free of septic complications.

Tunn and Thieme[40] studied 32 patients with urosepsis, of whom 7 (21 percent) had an associated obstructive uropathy (Table 14-5). All seven of these patients had urinary stone disease as the cause of the obstruction, and operative intervention was uniformly necessary and was performed. Four of these patients had frank sepsis and three patients had sepsis with mild hypotension. Two patients in whom operative therapy was initiated in the more unstable phases of septicemia died. Of the 25 patients with nonobstructive uropathy, 24 responded well to intensive medical therapy, and 1 patient died of multiple organ failure. Hence, in this series those patients with bacteremia associated with obstructive uropathy tended to have serious clinical syndromes.

COMMUNITY-ACQUIRED BACTEREMIC URINARY TRACT INFECTION

Bryan and Reynolds[41] reviewed the records of 313 patients with community-acquired septicemia associated with urinary tract infections. The urinary tract was the primary site of orgin in 21 percent of all community-acquired bacteremic infections, and although the overall mortality rate for these patients was 13.7 percent, the cause of death in the majority was thought to be due to other debilitating medical illnesses. The mortality attributed directly to bacteremic urinary tract infection (which was defined as deaths which occurred within 7 days of the last positive blood culture and in which there were no other more obvious explanations for death) was 4.8 percent. Of the 15 deaths attributable to septicemia 13 occurred in patients on medical services. All these patients had serious underlying medical diseases, such as alcoholic liver disease, malignancy, or chronic neurologic disease. The only patient who died on a urology service had sustained urethral trauma from improper insertion of an indwelling catheter at home. The authors stressed the importance of host factors as determinants of death in community-acquired septicemic urinary tract infections.

Esposito and associates[42] studied 100 consecutive cases of community-acquired bacteremia in patients 65 years of age or older and found that in this geriatric population the urinary tract was the most frequent source (34 percent). Of these 34 patients, 8 had an indwelling urethral catheter at time of admission. These patients only occasionally had classic manifestations of urinary tract infection, such as dysuria, urgency, or flank pain, but more commonly presented with generalized symptoms associated with septicemia, such as anorexia, malaise, and mental status changes. Of the 34 patients, 5 died. This same group later studied another 34 patients with community-acquired bacteremic urinary tract infection. Of these 34, 11 had sustained some mechanical insult to the urinary tract, such as obstruction or manipulation of an indwelling urethral catheter, within 72 hours prior to the onset of symptoms; the other 23 patients had experienced no preceding mechanical manipulation. In these 23 patients, a number of urologic abnormalities were detected, including bladder outlet obstruction, renal calculi, and renal abscesses. There were three mortalities in the study group.

HOSPITAL-ACQUIRED BACTEREMIC URINARY TRACT INFECTION

Hospital-acquired urinary tract infections are among the most common nosocomial infections. Approximately 2 of every 100 patients admitted to hospitals in the United States will acquire a urinary infection, and this results in about 500,000 infections each year (about one-third of all nosocomial infections.[31,34] It has been estimated that between 1 and 3 percent of these cases may be associated with bacteremia, with an associated fatality rate greater than 30 percent.[16,31] Data can therefore be easily extrapolated to demonstrate that nosocomial bacteremic urinary tract infections are either directly causative or indirectly associated with thousands of deaths in the United States each year.

Bryan and Reynolds[16] studied 221 episodes of septicemia attributed to hospital-acquired urinary tract infection. This represented 7.3 episodes per 10,000 patient admissions. A full 71 percent of the patients involved had had an indwelling urinary catheter prior to the onset of the bacteremia. The overall mortality rate for patients experiencing hospital-acquired septicemic urinary tract infection was 30.8 percent, and the mortality rate directly attributed to septicemic urinary tract infection was 12.7 percent. The chance of a septicemic infection causing death was related to the severity of the underlying disease but not to age, sex, or the infecting microorganism. All the patients whose deaths were thought to be attributable to hospital-acquired septicemic urinary tract infection had serious medical disorders such as neurologic disease, malignancy, alcoholism, or liver disease. Shock was associated with a mortality rate of 49 percent.

Siroky and associates reviewed 175 cases of metastatic infections originating from the genitourinary tract.[45] They found that the most common sites of metastatic infection are bone (especially spine) and endocardium. A wide range of organisms was isolated, but gram-negative infections were most common (59 percent). Men accounted for 86 percent of the patients, and 81 percent had some urologic pathologic entity.

CLINICAL FEATURES

The severity of the symptoms associated with urosepsis falls along a continuum, which ranges from a mild febrile urinary tract infection to profound septic shock. Spiking fevers and shaking chills with or without hypotension had been considered the classic mode of presentation of gram-negative septicemia, but these findings have been observed in only 30 percent of all such patients. Other patients will present with less specific symptoms (Table 14-6).[2] Mental status changes, metabolic acidosis, hypotension, and oliguria are common presentations which should alert the clinician to the possibility of septicemia. Although fever is usually present, failure to mount a febrile response within 24 hours is associated with a poor prognosis.[5]

A variety of dermatologic manifestations can be present in gram-negative septicemias, but one lesion which is pathognomonic is ecthyma gangrenosum, which can be associated with *Pseudomonas* septicemia (Fig. 14-1).[2] This can manifest as either a black necrotic lesion or a vesicular lesion with an erythematous margin.

Hematologic findings include leukocytosis, and approximately 60 percent of patients will have thrombocytopenia or other disorders of coagulation. About 10 percent of patients will develop disseminated intravascular coagulation (DIC). Coagulation abnormalities seem to occur more frequently in the debilitated host, but DIC occurs irrespective of host condition.[5]

The presence of findings associated with gram-negative septicemia concomitantly with bacteriuria and clinical findings associated with infection of the urinary tract is the usual mode of presentation of urosepsis. The underlying uropathy can be either nonobstructive or obstructive, and because relief of

---

Table 14-6. Clinical Findings Suggestive of Gram-Negative Bacteremia

Chills, fever, and hypotension
Fever only (particularly in patients with granulocytopenia, neoplastic and hematologic diseases, and intravascular or urinary catheters)
Hyperpnea, tachypnea, and respiratory alkalosis
Hypotension
Oliguria or anuria
Acidosis
Hypothermia
Change in mentation (confusion, stupor, agitation, etc.)
Thrombocytopenia
Disseminated intravascular coagulation
Adult respiratory distress syndrome
Evidence of urinary tract infection
Evidence of pulmonary infection
Ecthyma gangrenosum

(McCabe WR, Treadwell TL: Gram-negative bacteremia. Monogr Urol 4:193, 1983.)

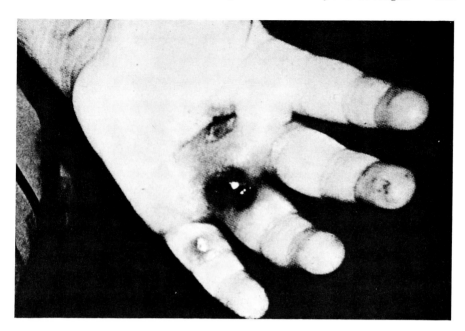

Fig. 14-1 The two types of skin lesions typical of ecthyma gangrenosum, which is suggestive of *Pseudomonas aeruginosa* bacteremia. The black, necrotic lesion is more typical, but the vesicular lesion with an erythematous margin (on the little finger) also may be seen. Similar lesions are infrequently observed in bacteremia caused by *Aeromonas* spp and certain other species. (McCabe WR, Treadwell TL: Gram-negative bacteremia. Monog Urol 4:193, 1983.)

urinary obstruction is mandatory in the latter instance, attempts should be made to differentiate the two radiographically. Intravenous urography has traditionally been the diagnostic procedure of choice for identifying obstruction, but if this modality cannot be used (usually because of allergy to contrast medium or increased risk of contrast nephropathy due to renal insufficiency), ultrasonography has been demonstrated to be an accurate study to detect upper urinary tract dilatation.

The association of obstructive uropathy, urinary tract infections, and bacteremia is well known. The rise in intraluminal pressure within the renal collecting system may result in changes which provide access for infected urine into the renal parenchyma.[46] Nonobstructive uropathy may cause urosepsis in many ways, but pyelonephritis and iatrogenic etiologies are most common.

The association of shock with gram-negative sepsis has long been known to carry a high mortality rate. The genitourinary tract is the leading source of septicemia responsible for septic shock, and an obstructed system is usually present.[47] Most cases are due to single gram-negative organisms, although 10 to 20 percent of cases of septic shock are caused by mixed infections. The normovolemic patient will have an increased cardiac output, with associated hypotension and peripheral vasodilatation as manifested by warm and dry skin. A more morbid presentation is seen in the relatively hypovolemic patient, who presents with low cardiac output, peripheral vasoconstriction, and increased peripheral vascular resistance.

TREATMENT

Initial antibiotic therapy is usually undertaken before the availability of culture and sensitivity results and is therefore empiric. In these cases both gram-positive and gram-negative pathogens should be covered by the antibiotic regimen. Combination antibiotic therapy of an aminoglycoside with either a penicillin or cephalosporin displays synergistic effects when administered in therapeutic doses. Gram stain of urine, pus, or the buffy coat is helpful in selecting optimal therapy. When culture results are available, the therapeutic regimen can be appropriately altered, and often single-agent therapy can be instituted.

The crucial element in the treatment of septic shock is the early identification of the etiology of the septicemia. Patients must be resuscitated rapidly, and emergency interventional therapy is mandated if urinary obstruction or abscess is present. Appropriate monitoring with a Swan-Ganz catheter in an intensive care setting is often indicated. A Foley catheter should be placed to measure urinary output on an hourly basis. Arterial blood gases should be frequently studied, and an arterial line for continuous arterial blood pressure monitoring should be placed.

Crystalloid such as saline and Ringer's lactate is of value in restoration of cardiac output, and fluid can be administered generously in the early fluid resuscitation of patients with septic shock. The speculation that lactated Ringer's solution can aggravate the lactic acidosis present in such patients is unproven. The use of colloids as volume expanders is controversial.

Vasopressors can be used to improve tissue perfusion in those cases in which organ dysfunction is evident. Hypotension is not necessarily bad if the end organs are being adequately perfused. Dopamine is one pressor which does not diminish renal blood flow. It may have a beneficial effect on myocardial metabolism.

Decompression of the Obstructed Urinary Tract

When urinary obstruction is present in association with urosepsis, emergency management is mandated. The simplest procedure which adequately drains the urinary tract proximal to the point of obstruction will improve the patient's conditions, and definitive treatment can be undertaken at a later time. Although the value of temporary drainage is accepted in the urologic community, the interval between such drainage and definitive therapy is controversial.

Percutaneous nephrostomy was first described by Goodwin and associates in 1953[50] and is easy to perform under local anesthesia and relatively safe when performed under ultrasound[51] or fluoroscopic guidance.[52] Adequate drainage can usually be achieved with small polyethylene pigtail catheters that are provided in commercially available percutaneous nephrostomy kits, but occasionally tract dilatation and insertion of an 18 Fr or larger indwelling catheter is necessary to drain viscous purulent material.

Ureteral stents are usually placed cystoscopically in order to bypass any obstruction. A variety of products utilizing a wide range of designs and materials has been developed in efforts to avoid both encrustation of the catheter and stent migration resulting from the peristalsing ureter.

Urinary obstruction with associated sepsis can also occur at the level of the bladder outlet or urethra. This is more common in men with either prostatic (benign hyperplasia, carcinoma) or urethral stricture disease and can often be managed with urethral catheterization. If this cannot be acomplished, suprapubic catheter placement can easily be performed by utilizing many of the techniques developed for placing percutaneous nephrostomy tubes.

Prophylactic Antibiotics in Urologic Surgery

When performing relatively simple transurethral procedures such as cystoscopy, urethral dilatation, and resection of bladder tumors in the presence of sterile urine, no antibiotics are indicated (Table 14-7). If a urinary tract

Table 14-7. Prophylactic Antibiotics in Urologic Surgery

Procedure	Category	Recommendations
1. Transurethral procedure (cystoscopy, urethral dilatation, transurethral resection of bladder tumors)	Clean	1. Sterile preoperative urine culture 2. If culture infected, sterilize prior to procedure 3. One ampule of neosporin sulfate (40 mg); polymyxin B sulfate (200,000 units) solution in irrigating solution or instilled in bladder at end of procedure
2. Prostatectomy: preoperative catheter	Clean Contaminated	1. Preoperative urine in culture; if infected, treat appropriately 2. If preoperative urine sterile, administer broad-spectrum antibiotic: cefazolin 1 g I.M. or I.V. (or equivalent first-generation cephalosporin) $\frac{1}{2}$ hr prior to surgery and continue 24 hr postop
3. No preoperative catheter	Clean	1. With sterile preop urine culture antibiotic prophylaxis optional (see above) 2. Treat infected urine prior to prostatectomy

(Russo P, Packer MG, Fair WR: Antibiotic prophylaxis in urologic surgery. AUA Update Ser 4:1, 1985.)

Table 14-8. Prophylaxis for Bacterial Endocarditis

Patients at risk are those with suspected congenital or acquired heart disease, prosthetic heart valves, ventriculoseptal patches, prior history of infective endocarditis, mitral valve prolapse, and/ or transvenous pacemakers.

Parenteral
  Ampicillin 2 g I.M. or I.V. *plus*
  Gentamicin[a] (1.5 mg/kg—not to exceed 80 mg) I.M. or I.V.
Initial dose $\frac{1}{2}$ to 1 hr preoperative. Give same doses of gentamicin[a] and ampicillin once each 8 hr postoperative
For patients allergic to penicillin:
  Vancomycin[a] 1 g over 1 hr, starting 1 hr prior to surgery, repeat once 8 hr later
                                      plus
  Gentamicin (1.5 mg/kg) I.M. or I.C. $\frac{1}{2}$–1 hr preoperative, repeat once 8 hr later

Oral (outpatient procedures)
  Amoxicillin 3 g P.O. 1 hr preoperatively and 1.5 g 6 hr later

If procedure is prolonged, additional perioperative doses may be necessary.

[a] In cases of impaired renal function adjust doses and/or schedule appropriately.
  (Russo P, Packer MG, Fair, WR: Antibiotic prophylaxis in urologic surgery. AUA Update Ser 4:1, 1985.)

infection is present, however, it is imperative to eradicate it prior to the operative procedure. Administration of broad-spectrum antibiotics prior to transurethral resection of the prostate gland is advised if an indwelling catheter is in place before the procedure. If the patient has not had an indwelling catheter and the urine is sterile, antibiotic prophylaxis is optional. We must emphasize that all identified urinary tract infections should be appropriately treated preoperatively.

Prophylaxis of Endocarditis

The most common urinary pathogens are usually not causative agents in bacterial endocarditis, and gram-negative endocarditis is an uncommon entity. Prophylaxis (Table 14-8) should therefore be designed to cover enterococci.[54] Bacteremia usually precedes endocarditis, and the initial event in the pathogenesis of this disease entity is the adherence of blood-bone bacteria to foreign bodies or to damaged or otherwise abnormal cardiac surfaces. Patients who have congenital or acquired valvular heart disease, prosthetic valves, or a previous history of bacterial endocarditis should therefore be given prophylactic antibiotic treatment. Patients with mitral valve prolapse or transvenous pacemakers are also at increased risk and should have preoperative treatment. Parenteral therapy with gentamicin in combination with either ampicillin or vancomycin is recommended for inpatient treatment,[55] and those patients undergoing outpatient treatment can be treated with oral amoxicillin.[56]

CONCLUSION

Urosepsis remains a common clinical challenge in urologic practice. The dramatic increase in incidence of bacteremia and sepsis in this country[57] and the high percentage of bacteremic episodes of urinary etiology emphasize the continued presence of urinary tract–associated bacteremia as a public health problem.

REFERENCES

1. Waisbren BA: Bacteremia due to gram-negative bacilli other than *Salmonella*. A clinical and therapeutic study. Arch Intern Med 88:467, 1957
2. McCabe WR, Treadwell TL: Gram-negative bacteremia. Monog Urol 4:193, 1983
3. Hodgin UG, Sanford DP: Gram-negative rod bacteremia. Am J Med 39:952, 1965
4. McCabe WR, Jackson GG: Gram-negative bacteremia. I. Etiology and ecology. Arch Intern Med 110:845, 1962
5. Kreger BE, Craven DE, McCabe WR: Gram-negative bacteremia. IV. Re-evaluation of clinical features and treatment in 612 patients. Am J Med 68:344, 1980
6. Fried MA, Vosti KL: The importance of underlying disease in patients with gram-negative bacteremia. Arch Intern Med 121:418, 1968
7. DuPont HL, Spink WW: Infections due to gram-negative organisms: an analysis of 860 patients with bacteremia at the University of Minnesota Medical Center, 1958–1966. Medicine (Baltimore) 48:307, 1969
8. Clark A: The discussion on catheter or urinary fever. Lancet 1:137, 1884
9. Weir AF: Catheter fever. New York Med J 34:15, 1984
10. Clado A: Bacteriologie de la fièvre urineuse. Bull Soc Anat Paris 13:631, 1887
11. Hallé B: Recherches bacteriologiques sur un cas de fièvre urineuse. Bull Soc Anat Paris 13:610, 1887
12. Crabtree EG: Observations on the etiology of renal infections. Lancet Clin Cincinnati 115:96, 1916
13. Scott WW: Blood stream infections in urology: a report of eighty-two cases. J Urol 21:527, 1929
14. Barrington FJF, Wright HD: Bacteriaemia following operations on the urethra. J Pathol Bacteriol 33:871, 1930
15. Kreger BE, Craven DE, Carling PC, et al: Gram-negative bacteremia. III. Reassessment of etiology, epidemiology and ecology in 612 patients. Am J Med 68:332, 1980
16. Bryan CS, Reynolds KL: Hospital-acquired bacteremic urinary tract infections: epidemiology and outcome. J Urol 132:494, 1984
17. Selden R, Lee S, Wang WL, et al: Nosocomial *Klebsiella* infections. Intestinal colonization as a reservoir. Ann Intern Med 74:657, 1971
18. Seidenfeld SM, Luby JP: Urologic sepsis. Urol Clin North Am 9:259, 1982
19. Krieger JN, Kaiser DL, Wenzel RP: Urinary tract etiology of bloodstream infections in hospitalized patients. J Infect Dis 148:57, 1983
20. Schaberg DR, Weinstein RA, Stamm WE: Epidemics of nosocomial urinary tract infection caused by multiple resistant gram-negative bacilli: epidemiology and control. J Infect Dis 133:363, 1976
21. Clemmensen O, Aggar P, Krarup T: Urological septicemia. Scand J Urol Nephrol 13:313, 1979

22. Powers JH: Bacteremia following instrumentation of the infected urinary tract. NY State Med J 36:323, 1936
23. Sullivan NM, Sutter VL, Mim MM, et al: Clinical aspects of bacteremia after manipulation of the genitourinary tract. J Infect Dis 127:49, 1973
24. Biorn CL, Browning WH, Thompson L: Transient bacteremia immediately following transurethral prostatic resection. J Urol 63:155, 1950
25. Bulkley GJ, O'Conner VJ, Sokol JA: A clinical study of bacteremia and overhydration following transurethral resection. J Urol 72:1205, 1954
26. Allan WR, Kumar A: Prophylactic mezlocillin for transurethral prostatectomy. Br J Urol 57:46, 1985
27. Slade N: Bacteremia and septicemia after urologic operations. Proc R Soc Med 51:331, 1958
28. Creevy CD, Feeney MS: Routine use of antibiotics in transurethral prostatic resection: a clinical investigation. J Urol 71:615, 1954
29. Kidd EE, Burnside K: Bacteriaemia, septicaemia and intravascular hemolysis during transurethral resection of the prostate gland. Br J Urol 37, 551, 1965
30. Last PM, Harbison PA, Marsh JA: Bacteriaemia after urological instrumentation. Lancet 1:74, 1966
31. Turck M, Stamm W: Nosocomial infection of the urinary tract. Am J Med 70:651, 1981
32. Gleckman R, Blagg N, Hibert et al: Catheter-related urosepsis in the elderly: a prospective study of community-derived infections. J Am Geriatr Soc 30:255, 1982
33. Thornton GF, Andriole GT: Bacteriuria during indwelling catheter drainage. II. Effect of a closed sterile drainage system. JAMA 214:339, 1970
34. Kass EH, Schneiderman LJ: Entry of bacteria into the urinary tracts of patients with inlying catheters. N Engl J Med 256:556, 1957
35. Garibaldi RA, Burke JP, Britt MR, et al: Meatal colonization and catheter associated bacteriuria. N Engl J Med 303:316, 1980
36. Thompson RL, Haley CE, Searey MA, et al: Catheter-associated bacteriuria: failure to reduce attack rates using periodic instillations of disinfectant into drainage systems. JAMA 251:747, 1984
37. Warren JW, Platt R, Thomas RJ, et al: Antibiotic irrigation and catheter-associated urinary infections. N Engl J Med 299:570, 1978
38. Burke JP, Garibaldi RA, Britt MR, et al: Prevention of catheter-associated urinary tract infections. Efficacy of daily meatal care regimens. Am J Med 70:655, 1981
39. Quintiliani R, Cuhha BA, Klimek J, et al: Bacteriaemia after manipulation of the urinary tract. The importance of pre-existing urinary tract disease and compromised host defences. Postgrad Med J 54:668, 1978
40. Tunn UW, Thieme H: Sepsis associated with urinary tract infection: antibiotic treatment with peperacillin. Arch Intern Med 142:2035, 1982
41. Bryan CS, Reynolds KL: Community-acquired bacteremic urinary tract infection: epidemiology and outcome. J Urol 132:490, 1984
42. Esposito AL, Gleckman RA, Cram S, et al: Community-acquired bacteremia in the elderly: analysis of one-hundred consecutive episodes. J Am Geriatr Soc 28:315, 1980
43. Gleckman RA, Blagg N, Hibert D, et al: Community-acquired bacteremic urosepsis in the elderly patients: a prospective study of 34 consecutive episodes. J Urol 128:79, 1982
44. Wenzel RP, Osterman CA, Henting KJ: Hospital-acquired infections. II. Interior rates by site, service and common procedures in a university hospital. Am J Epidemiol 104:845, 1976

45. Siroky MG, Moylan RA, Austen G, et al: Metastatic infection secondary to genitourinary tract sepsis. Am J Med 61:351, 1976
46. Richard C: Les septicemies en urologie. J Urol Nephrol:1, suppl. 82, 1, 1976
47. Schwartz RA, Cerra FB: Shock: a practical approach. Urol Clin North Am 10:89, 1983
48. Carson CC: Gram-negative sepsis and urinary tract infections. Drug Ther 4:41, 1982
49. Sladen A: Methylprednisolone pharmacology doses in shock lung syndrome. J Thorac Cardiovaso Surg 71:800, 1976
50. Goodwin WE, Casey WC, Woolf W: Percutaneous trocar (needle) nephrostomy in hydronephrosis. JAMA 157:891
51. Stables DP: Percutaneous nephrostomy: technique, indications, and results. Urol Clin North Am 9:15, 1982
52. Anson K, Smith AD: Emergency management of obstructive uropathy. Urol Clin North Am 10:161, 1983
53. Russo P, Packer MG, Fair WR: Antibiotic prophylaxis in urologic surgery. AUA Update Ser 4:1, 1985
54. Finn JJ, Kane LW: Enterococcal endocarditis as a complication of urologic instrumentation. J Urol 68:933, 1952
55. Kaplan EL, Anthony BF, Bisno A, et al: Prevention of bacterial endocarditis. Circulation 56:139, 1977
56. Medical Lett Drugs Ther 26:4, 1984
57. Centers for Disease Control: National nosocomial infections study report. p. 2–14. Nov. 1979

15 | Osteomyelitis

Jon T. Mader
George Cierny III

On the basis of etiologic and clinical considerations, bone infections have traditionally been classified as either hematogenous osteomyelitis or osteomyelitis secondary to a contiguous focus of infection. Contiguous focus osteomyelitis has been further subdivided into osteomyelitis in patients who have a relatively normal vascular system and that occurring in patients with generalized vascular insufficiency.

Osteomyelitis may be an acute or a chronic process. Acute osteomyelitis is characterized by a suppurative infection accompanied by edema, vascular congestion, and small vessel thrombosis. The vascular supply to the bone is compromised as the infection extends into the marrow and/or the surrounding soft tissues. Large areas of dead bone or sequestra result when both the medullary and periosteal vessels thrombose. Viable colonies of bacteria may be harbored within the necrotic and ischemic tissues even after an intense host response and/or therapeutic antibiotics. Thus, early in the course of the acute infection the stage is set for a chronic process. The hallmarks of chronic osteomyelitis are a nidus of infected dead bone or scar tissue, an ischemic soft tissue envelope, and a refractory clinical course.

PATIENT EVALUATION

A sedimentation rate, complete blood count, x-rays, a technetium bone scan, gallium or indium abscess scans, and computed tomography (CT) can be useful in initially evaluating and staging suspected osteomyelitis.[1] These studies assist in the diagnosis, assess the extent of infection, aid in site selection for a bone biopsy, and are useful in the patient follow-up.

Radiographic changes in acute hematogenous osteomyelitis are often difficult to interpret and lag at least 2 weeks behind the evolution of the infection.[2] The earliest radiographic changes are soft tissue swelling, periosteal thickening and/or elevation, and focal osteopenia. These findings are subtle and may be missed. The more diagnostic lytic changes are delayed and often associated with an indolent infection of several months duration. Later, when the patient is receiving appropriate antimicrobial therapy, radiographic improvement may lag behind the clinical recovery. In contiguous focus and chronic osteomyelitis the radiographic changes are even more subtle, are often found in association with other nonspecific radiographic findings, and require a careful clinical correlation to achieve diagnostic significance.

Radionuclide imaging has proved useful in diagnosing osteomyelitis before radiologic changes occur. The technetium polyphosphate ^{99m}Tc scan will demonstrate increased isotope accumulation in areas of increased blood flow and reactive new bone formation.[3] In biopsy-confirmed cases of hematogenous osteomyelitis, the ^{99m}Tc scan is usually positive as early as 48 hours following the initiation of the bone infection.[4] Negative ^{99m}Tc scans have been reported in documented osteomyelitis and may relate to impaired blood supply in the infected area.[5]

Other radiopharmaceuticals used for the evaluation of osteomyelitis include gallium citrate and indium chloride. Gallium and/or indium scans show increased isotope uptake in areas of concentrated polymorphonuclear leukocytes, macrophages, and malignant tumors.[6,7] In contrast to gallium citrate, indium chloride can be used to selectively label polymorphonuclear leukocytes and macrophages and is not found to accumulate in areas of reactive bone.[8] Since these scans do not show bone detail well, it is often difficult to distinguish between bone and soft tissue inflammation; a comparison with a ^{99m}Tc scan may help to resolve this problem.[9]

Indium-labeled leukocyte scans have been used for the evaluation of osteomyelitis. Proctor[10] demonstrated indium leukocyte scans to be positive in 42 percent of patients with acute osteomyelitis and 65 percent of patients with septic arthritis. Patients who had chronic osteomyelitis, bony metastases, and degenerative arthritis often had negative scans.

Although CT may be used to help define areas of necrotic bone and assess the status of the soft tissue envelope, CT scans are not indicated in all cases of osteomyelitis; however, in the difficult patient they can help in planning the surgical approach and ensure a thorough debridement[11,12] One disadvantage of this study is the scatter phenomenon occurring when metal is present in or near the area of bone infection. This scatter results in a significant loss of image resolution.

The diagnosis of bacterial osteomyelitis ultimately requires isolation of bacteria from the bone or the blood. In acute osteomyelitis associated with diagnostic radiographic or radionuclide scan findings, positive blood cultures can often obviate the need for a bone biopsy. However, chronic osteomyelitis rarely leads to a bacteremia unless there is an acute exacerbation of the infection in the soft tissues. Sinus tract cultures are not reliable for predicting which organism(s) will be isolated from infected bone.[13] In these cases a bone biopsy for aerobic and anaerobic cultures is mandatory. The selection of the

Table 15-1. Systemic or Local Factors That Affect Immune Surveillance, Metabolism, and Local Vascularity[a]

Systemic (B$_s$)	Local (B$_1$)
Malnutrition	Chronic lymphedema
Renal, liver failure	Venous stasis
Alcohol abuse	Major vessel compromise
Immune deficiency	Arteritis
Malignancy	Extensive scarring
Diabetes mellitus	Radiation fibrosis
Extremes of age	
Steroid therapy	
Tobacco abuse	

[a] According to the Cierny-Mader classification system of adult osteomyelitis.[1,16]

biopsy site is guided by the clinical, radiographic, and isotope scan findings. Organisms are successfully isolated from patients with suspected osteomyelitis 95 percent of the time at the University of Texas Medical Branch (UTMB) by use of these guidelines.

Sedimentation rates and leukocyte counts are frequently elevated prior to therapy in the acute disease although the white blood cell count rarely exceeds 15,000 per cubic millimeter. The leukocyte count is usually normal in patients with chronic osteomyelitis. The sedimentation rates and leukocyte counts may fall with appropriate therapy. However, both values may rise acutely around each debridement surgery. A sedimentation rate which returns to normal during or after the course of therapy is a favorable prognostic sign. However, this laboratory determination is not reliable in the compromised host since these patients are constantly challenged by minor illnesses and peripheral lesions, which may elevate this index.

The integrity of the local and systemic host defenses must be evaluated. Host deficiencies influence treatment options, prognosis, and the assessment of treatment results. Following debridement surgery, the patient must be able to impede infection, resist contamination, heal surgical wounds, and tolerate the metabolic stress of sequential surgeries. A list of factors influencing the ability of the host to elicit an effective response to infection and treatment is found in Table 15-1. Local factors lead to a vascular compromise of bone and soft tissue. Systemic compromise affects immune surveillance, metabolism, and leukocyte function and may lead to large and/or small vessel disease. Local and systemic factors may combine in diseases such as diabetes mellitus. Whenever possible, a host compromise should be improved or corrected before or during therapy, for example by nutritional support for the malnourished patient.

THERAPY

Acute Hematogenous Osteomyelitis

In children acute hematogenous osteomyelitis is primarily a medical disease. In the adult, however, debridement and drainage procedures are often required. Identification of the causative pathogen is essential, as the infection is usually controllable with specific antimicrobial therapy. Mismanagement with inappropriate antibiotic(s) can result in disease extension, sequestra formation, and a refractory infection. Surgical intervention is indicated for those patients who do not respond to specific antimicrobial therapy within 48 hours or who have evidence of persistent soft tissue abscesses or suspected joint sepsis.

The first step toward treatment is to obtain appropriate culture material. A bone biopsy is necessary unless the patient has positive blood cultures, along with x-ray or bone scan findings consistent with acute hematogenous osteomyelitis. After cultures are obtained, a parenteral antimicrobial treatment regimen for the clinically suspected pathogens is initiated. Once the organism has been obtained, the antibacterial activity of different antibiotic classes can be determined by appropriate sensitivity methods. The disk diffusion method is often a sufficient guideline for antibiotic therapy. However, many consider quantitative antibiotic sensitivity testing by the macrodilution or microdilution techniques on all aerobic bone isolates to be a prerequisite. This is necessary to determine the minimum inhibitory concentration (MIC) and the minimum bactericidal concentration (MBC) of the antibiotics chosen for the pathogenic organism(s). It is best to choose an antibiotic or antibiotic combination that has a low MIC and MBC relative to its expected serum concentration. We prefer the MIC of the treatment antibiotic for the infecting organism(s) to be at least eight times less than the expected serum concentration, if possible. The original antibiotic regimen may be continued or modified on the basis of sensitivity results. The patient is treated for 4 to 6 weeks with appropriate parenteral antimicrobial therapy dated from the initiation of therapy or from the last major debridement surgery. The goal of the therapy is to prevent a refractory infection. If the initial medical management fails and the patient is clinically compromised by a recurrent infection, medullary and/or soft tissue debridement will be necessary in conjunction with another course of antibiotics. The decision to surgically intervene may be made at any time during therapy, which supports the need for a team approach to these problems.

Occasionally oral antibiotic therapy can be utilized for treatment of childhood osteomyelitis.[14,15] However, it is recommended that the patient first receive 2 weeks of parenteral antibiotic therapy prior to beginning an oral regimen. In addition, the patient and family must be compliant and agree to close outpatient follow-up. Absorption and activity of the orally administered antibiotic should be monitored by the measurement of the serum bactericidal activity against the causative pathogen. A peak bactericidal dilution (SBT) of at least 1:8 or greater should be present and maintained. Oral therapy is possible in hematogenous osteomyelitis in pediatric patients because of an increased bone blood flow and the aggressive mesenchymal and immunologic responses found in this age group.

Chronic Osteomyelitis Secondary to Contiguous Focus Infection

These types of chronic osteomyelitis that are secondary to contiguous focus infection share the common features of infected necrotic bone and poorly perfused soft tissue enveloping the bone. Adequate drainage, thorough debridement, obliteration of dead space, and specific antimicrobial coverage are the mainstays of therapy. Following patient evaluation a bone biopsy is performed and sent for aerobic and anaerobic cultures. Ideally the patient begins antibiotic therapy only after the results of the cultures and their sensitivities are known. However, if debridement surgery is immediately required, the patient may receive antibiotics to cover the clinically suspected pathogens before the bacteriologic data are reported. These antibiotics may be modified when results of the debridement cultures and sensitivities are determined.

Adequate debridement surgery is the cornerstone of therapy in these infections. Careful preoperative planning is critical to achieve a high rate of success and to minimize wound complications. When possible, debridement surgery is performed after specific antibiotic therapy has begun. Antimicrobial therapy initiated before surgery decreases the risk of bacteremia at surgery, helps marginate the wound, and produces more supple soft tissues at the time of surgery.[16] The debridement is direct, atraumatic, and executed with reconstruction in mind. If necessary, the wound is debrided every 48 to 72 hours until all nonviable tissue and superfluous hardware such as plates, pins, and screws have been removed. Whenever possible, the incisions are placed between myocutaneous territories, with disregard at times of old surgical scars. Sinus tracts are excised if present for more than 1 year.

All dead or ischemic hard and soft tissues are excised unless a more limited palliative procedure has been chosen from the start. The extent of the debridement is predictable from the preliminary assessment. If complete excision will threaten stability, external fixation and/or a bypass graft may be necessary prior to or during debridement surgery. The instruments we use in the debridement procedures include scalpels, curettes, straight-stem and angled dental mirrors, and a pneumatic bone scalpel. Because of the speed and gentle efficiency of this pneumatic system, osteotomes are rarely used. The debridement process begins in a centrifugal fashion. This technique helps maintain an outer ring of bone that shares its circulation with the attached soft tissues. The cortical and cancellous bone remaining in the wound after debridement surgery must bleed uniformly to ensure antibiotic perfusion and avoid continued sequestration. Definitive wound management usually takes place 5 to 7 days after the last debridement. In the interim, the wound usually is left open.

Appropriate obliteration of the dead space created by debridement surgery (Fig. 15-1). is mandatory to arrest the disease and maintain the integrity of the skeletal part involved.[17] The goal of dead space management is to replace dead bone and scar with durable vascularized tissue. Secondary intention healing is discouraged. The scar tissue that fills the defect later becomes avascular and may form a new nidus of infection within the contaminated zone. Suction irrigation systems are rarely used because of the high incidence of associated nosocomial infections[18,19] and the unreliability of these setups. Complete wound closure is attained whenever possible. Local tissue flaps or free flaps may be used to fill dead space,[20,21] and cancellous bone grafts may be placed beneath local or transferred tissues when structural augmentation is necessary. Open cancellous grafts without soft tissue coverage as described by Papineau[22] are used sparingly, as the epithelial coverage is not durable and may lead to su-

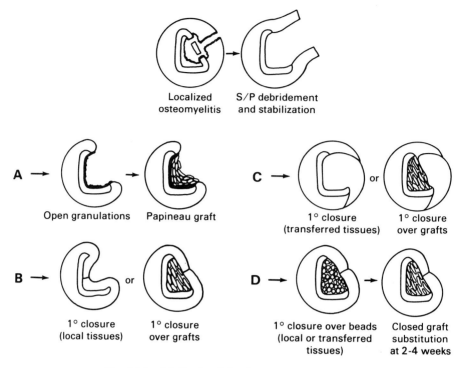

Localized
osteomyelitis

S/P debridement
and stabilization

A →

Open granulations   Papineau graft

C →   or

1° closure
(transferred tissues)

1° closure
over grafts

B →   or

1° closure
(local tissues)

1° closure
over grafts

D →

1° closure over beads
(local or transferred
tissues)

Closed graft
substitution
at 2-4 weeks

Fig. 15-1   Methods of dead space management.

perficial ulceration following minor trauma or persistent venous stasis. Open cancellous grafts are simple, effective, and useful when a free tissue transfer is not a treatment option and local tissue flaps are inadequate. Regardless of the methods used, careful preoperative planning is crucial to make efficient use of the patient's limited cancellous bone reserves.

Antibiotic-impregnated acrylic beads have been used to sterilize and/or temporarily maintain a dead space created by debridement surgery.[1,16,23] In our experience any patient-compatible, powdered antibiotic may be safely delivered in this manner. The antibiotic first must be adequately pulverized and then uniformly mixed with the powdered cement prior to adding the monomer. Thermal stability of the antibiotic(s) is not necessary when the beads are fashioned in the dough phase. Two or three antibiotics may be combined in a single mix. Before using this technique, the debridement must be thorough and the wound flora susceptible to the antibiotics.

The five antibiotics we use most commonly in beads and their mixing ratios are listed in Table 15-2. If the volumetric ratio of the powders exceeds 24 ml/ 120 ml (antibiotic/40 g cement), the cement will not harden reliably. In our experience, antibiotic-impregnated polymethylmethacrylate (PMMA) beads have streamlined patient management by eliminating open wound care, decreasing surgical morbidity, and enhancing the therapeutic options in dead space management. The beads are usually removed within 2 to 4 weeks and

Table 15-2. Antibiotic Bead Cocktail: Amount[a] of Antibiotic Placed in One Package of PMMA[b] Powder

Cephalosporins	
Cefazolin	3.0–6.0 g
Moxalactam	3.0–6.0 g
Cefotaxime	5.0–10.0 g
Tobramycin	4.8–9.6 g
Vancomycin	2.0–4.0 g
Ticarcillin	6.0–12.0 g

[a] Lower dosages used in antibiotic combinations.
[b] PMMA = polymethylmethacrylate.

replaced with a cancellous bone graft. The evolution of local antibiotic therapy is rapidly taking place.[24–26] In a series of 50 patients at UTMB, the indications for antibiotic-impregnated beads were: dead space maintenance followed by cancellous bone grafting (68 percent), debridement and closure (15 percent), combined debridement–internal fixation procedures (14 percent), and systemic intraoperative compromise (3 percent). Of the 50 wounds, 48 healed uneventfully.[27]

The length of systemic antibiotic administration remains controversial. Six weeks has become the standard length of antibiotic therapy, but this time frame has no documented superiority over other time intervals. In our experience the systemic antibiotic coverage should span the time needed to revascularize debridement surfaces and/or applied cancellous bone grafts. The patient is given 4 to 6 weeks of parenteral antimicrobial therapy, usually dated from the last major debridement surgery.[16,17] Clinical trials are underway to evaluate local antibiotic therapy in combination with short courses of parenteral antibiotics for certain types of osteomyelitis. Outpatient intravenous therapy is now possible and feasible. The long-term intravenous access catheters (Hickman-Broviac catheters) make outpatient intravenous treatment possible and decrease the hospitalization time.[28] At UTMB 105 Hickman catheters were inserted in 96 patients with a diagnosis of osteomyelitis[29]; 65 percent of these catheters were used for outpatient therapy. The overall complication rate was 20 percent (21/105 catheters); the infectious complication rate was 11/105 (10.5 percent), or 0.16 per 100 catheter days; and the noninfectious complication rate was 10/105 (9.5 percent) or 0.14 per 100 days. The catheter had to be removed prematurely before the completion of antibiotic therapy in only 5 of the 105 (4.8 percent) catheter insertions. The Hickman catheter is a safe and effective intravenous access device for long-term antibiotic therapy. Inpatient management with intravenous antibiotic therapy is facilitated by the stable long-term venous access, and a responsible patient or visiting nurse can be trained to administer the antibiotic at home via the implanted catheter.

Chronic Osteomyelitis Secondary to Contiguous Focus Infection with Vascular Disease

Therapy of osteomyelitis associated with vascular insufficiency is difficult owing to the relative inability of the host to participate in the eradication of the infectious process. The infection is usually insidious in onset and beyond simple salvage by the time the patient seeks medical therapy. Conservative debridement and parenteral antibiotics followed by oral antibiotic coverage often fail to eradicate the infection.[30] In time most of these patients require some type of ablative surgery. Digital and ray resections, transmetatarsal amputations, and midfoot disarticulations allow the patient to ambulate without a prosthesis. The amputation level is determined by the vascular status of the tissues proximal to the site of infection and the requirements for a thorough debridement. Cutaneous oxygen tensions correlate with the adequacy of tissue perfusion and a careful measurement of this parameter is often helpful in selecting a surgical site where wound healing can be expected.[31] A conservative debridement and parenteral or oral antibiotics may be used to suppress the infection when a more definitive surgical procedure would lead to unacceptable patient morbidity or disability.

PATIENT FOLLOW-UP

The term *cure* is not appropriate when describing successful treatment of osteomyelitis. Quiescent disease may become reactivated up to 30 years later. Instead, we use the term *arrested osteomyelitis* to describe clinically inactive disease.

Following the completion of the initial surgery and course of antibiotics, the patients are evaluated monthly for 6 months, every 3 months for the remainder of the year, and biannually for 2 years. A sedimentation rate, complete blood count, and radiograph are obtained on each visit, and an indium scan is performed every 6 months. In most uncomplicated and adequately treated cases of adult osteomyelitis, the sedimentation rate returns to normal in the uncompromised patient population. In our experience this occurs within 3 to 18 months, depending on the complexity of the disease and its treatment.[1,16] In the compromised host the sedimentation rate is an unreliable indicator since these patients are constantly plagued by illnesses and lesions which can affect this laboratory index. A more sensitive indicator for the arrest of the infection is the indium scan; this indicator returns to normal 6 months to 2 years after treatment. We have not had a relapse among patients who had a negative indium scan.[1,8,16]

STAGING OF OSTEOMYELITIS

There are four major factors influencing the treatment and prognosis of osteomyelitis: (1) the degree of necrosis, (2) the condition of the host, (3) the site and extent of involvement, and (4) the disabling effects of the disease itself. Without reference to these factors it is difficult to compare treatment results or the effectiveness of new treatment modalities. Few classification systems of osteomyelitis have been published (Table 15-3). The classification scheme offered by Waldvogel[30] was the first to identify the host as a separate problem.

Table 15-3. Classification Systems for Osteomyelitis

Waldvogel et al.[30] (1970)	Hematogenous osteomyelitis
	Contiguous focus osteomyelitis
	Osteomyelitis associated with vascular disease
Kelley et al.[32] (1975)	Chronic hematogenous osteomyelitis
	Osteomyelitis with fracture union
	Osteomyelitis with fracture nonunion
	Post-traumatic or postoperative osteomyelitis
	Vertebral osteomyelitis
	Osteomyelitis of small bones of the foot
	Osteomyelitis of the skull, facial bones, or phalanges of the foot or hand

Kelley[32] recognized the deleterious effects of motion and sequestered hardware in the long bone and considered infections of the axial and appendicular skeleton separately. Except for Kelley's regional segregation, these two systems simply list the different etiologies of osteomyelitis.

The Waldvogel and Kelley classifications of osteomyelitis are useful but do not define the anatomic nature of the disease, take into account the quality of the host, determine treatment, or identify prognostic factors. An alternate classification was developed by Cierny and Mader[1,16] to include these factors (Table 15-4). In this approach the infection and host are staged according to four anatomic types and three physiologic classes. The system is governed by the status of the disease process regardless of its etiology. The anatomic types of osteomyelitis are designated as medullary, superficial, localized, or diffuse infection. *Medullary osteomyelitis* denotes infection confined to the intramedullary surfaces of the bone. Hematogenous osteomyelitis and infected intramedullary rods are examples of this anatomic type. *Superficial osteomyelitis* is a true contiguous focus infection of bone. An exposed, infected, necrotic

Table 15-4. Cierny and Mader Classification System

Anatomic type
Type 1: Medullary osteomyelitis
Type 2: Superficial osteomyelitis
Type 3: Localized osteomyelitis
Type 4: Diffuse osteomyelitis

Physiologic class
A Host: Normal host
B Host: Systemic compromise (B_s)
           Local compromise   (B_l)
C Host: Requires suppressive or no treatment; minimal disability; treatment worse than the disease; or not a surgical candidate

Clinical stage
Type + class = clinical stage
Example: Stage $4B_s$ osteomyelitis = a diffuse lesion in a systemically compromised host

(Data from refs. 1 and 16.)

outer surface of the bone lies at the base of a soft tissue wound. *Localized osteomyelitis* is a stable, well-demarcated lesion characterized by a full-thickness cortical sequestration and/or cavitation, which can be removed surgically without compromising bony stability. An infected fracture union or pin tract infection are common examples of these lesions. *Diffuse osteomyelitis* is a through and through and/or permeative process which usually requires an intercalary resection of the bone for cure. Diffuse osteomyelitis is mechanically unstable at presentation or after debridement surgery. An infected nonunion and septic necrosis of the femoral head are examples of diffuse osteomyelitis. Both localized and diffuse types usually represent an infection with both superficial and medullary components.

The condition and disability of the host are designed by one of three physiologic classes; the patient is classified as an A, B, or C host. A patient with a normal response to infection and surgery is an A host. The B host is a compromised patient with local, systemic, or combined deficiencies in wound healing (Table 15-1). When the treatment or results of treatment are potentially more compromising than the presenting condition(s), the patient is classified a C host. In our series 100 percent of the deaths, 94 percent of the treatment failures, and 88 percent of all wound complication occurred in the B hosts.[1,16,17] However, compromised patients undergoing successful reversal of their deficiencies responded to therapy similarly to A hosts. Therapy from the onset must include a program designed to gain and maintain a maximum host response.

To classify the disease and host, the anatomic type is combined with a physiologic class to designate one of 12 clinical stages of osteomyelitis. The terms *acute* and *chronic* osteomyelitis are not used in this staging system; areas of macronecrosis must be surgically removed regardless of the acuity or chronicity of the infection if a nonrefractory course is to be expected. The stages are dynamic and interact according to the pathophysiology of the disease; they may be altered by successful therapy, host alteration, or treatment. The Cierny-Mader staging system provides a framework for describing and developing experimental models of osteomyelitis, planning medical and surgical treatments, and comparing the results of therapy from institution to institution. As more interest and research is focused in the area of bone infection, shared nomenclature and an appropriate classification system become essential.

ACKNOWLEDGMENTS

The authors wish to thank Aurora Galvan and Joan Mader for manuscript preparation.

REFERENCES

1. Cierny G, Mader JT, Penninck JJ: A clinical staging system of adult osteomyelitis. Contemp Orthop 10:17, 1985
2. Butt WP: The radiology of infection. Clin Orthop 96:20, 1973

3. Jones AG, Francis MD, Davis MA: Bone scanning: radionuclidic reaction mechanisms. Semin Nucl Med 6:3, 1976
4. Treves S, Khettry J, Broker FH, et al: Osteomyelitis: early scintigraphic detection in children. Pediatrics 57:173, 1976
5. Russin LD, Stabb EV: Unusual bone-scan findings in acute osteomyelitis: case report. J Nucl Med 17:617, 1976
6. Deysine M, Rafkin H, Teicher I, et al: Diagnosis of chronic and postoperative osteomyelitis with gallium 67 citrate scans. Am J Surg 129:632, 1975
7. Sayle B, Cierny G, Mader JT: Indium-111 chloride imaging in the detection of osteomyelitis. J Nucl Med 24:72, 1983
8. Sayle BA, Fawcett HD, Wilkey DJ, et al: Indium-111 chloride imaging in chronic osteomyelitis. J Nucl Med 26:225, 1985
9. Lisbona R, Rosenthall L: Observations of the sequential use of ^{99m}Tc phosphate complex and ^{67}Ga imaging in osteomyelitis, cellulitis, and septic arthritis. Radiology 123:123, 1977
10. Propst-Proctor SL, Dillingham MF, McDougall IR, Goodwin D: The white blood cell scan in orthopedics. Clin Orthop 168:157, 1982
11. Kuhn JP, Berger PE: Computed tomographic diagnosis of osteomyelitis. Radiology 130:503, 1979
12. Seltzer SE: Value of computed tomography in planning medical and surgical treatment of chronic osteomyelitis. J Comput Assist Tomogr 8:482, 1984
13. Mackowiak PA, Jones SR, Smith JW: Diagnostic value of sinus tract cultures in chronic osteomyelitis. JAMA 239:2772, 1978
14. Nelson JD: A critical review of the role of oral antibiotics in the management of hematogenous osteomyelitis. p. 64. In Remington RS, Swartz MN (eds): Current Clinical Topics in Infectious Diseases. Vol 4. McGraw-Hill, New York, 1983
15. Prober CG: Oral antibiotic therapy for bone and joint infections. Pediatr Infect Dis 1:8, 1982
16. Cierny G, Mader JT: Adult chronic osteomyelitis. Orthopedics 7:1557, 1984
17. Cierny G, Mader JT: The surgical treatment of adult osteomyelitis. p. 10. In Evarts CMC (ed): Surgery of the Musculoskeletal System. Churchill Livingstone, New York, 1983
18. Clawson DK, Davis FJ, Hansen ST: Treatment of chronic osteomyelitis with emphasis on closed suction-irrigation technic. Clin Orthop 96:88, 1973
19. Letts RM, Wong E: Treatment of acute osteomyelitis in children by closed-tube irrigation: a reassessment. Can J Surg 18:60, 1975
20. Ruttle PE, Kelley PJ, Arnold PG, et al: Chronic osteomyelitis treated with a muscle flap. Orthop Clin North Am 15:451, 1984
21. May JW, Gallico GG, Lukash FN: Microvascular transfer of free tissue for closure of bone wounds of the distal lower extremity. N Engl J Med 306:253, 1982
22. Papineau LJ, Alfageme A, Dalcourt JP, Pilon L: Osteomyelite chronique: Excision et greffe de spongieux à l'air libre après mises à plat extensives. Int Orthop 3:165, 1979
23. Wilson KJ, Anastasio TJ, Cierny G, Mader JT: Diffusion of antibiotics from polymethylmethacrylate beads. Paper H-6, National Student Research Forum, Galveston, 1984
24. Hedstrom S, Lidgren L, Torholm C, Onnerfalt R: Antibiotic containing bone cement beads in the treatment of deep muscle and skeletal infections. Acta Orthop Scand 51:863, 1980
25. Becker RO, Spadaro JA: Treatment of orthopaedic infections with electrically generated silver ions. J Bone Joint Surg 60A:871, 1978

26. Kawashima M, Tamura H: Topical therapy in orthopedic infection. Orthopedics 7:1592, 1984
27. Cierny G, Couch LA, Mader JT: Clinical evaluation of antibiotic-impregnated polymethylmethacrylate beads in patients with osteomyelitis. Abstract 872, 25th Interscience Conference on Antimicrobial Agents and Chemotherapy, 1985
28. Hickman RO, Buckner CD, Clift RA, et al: A modified right atrial catheter for access to the venous system in marrow transplant recipients. Surg Gynecol Obstet 148:871, 1979
29. Couch LA, Cierny G, Mader JT: Inpatient and outpatient use of the Hickman catheter for adults with osteomyelitis. Abstract 902, 25th Interscience Conference on Antimicrobial Agents and Chemotherapy, 1985
30. Waldvogel FA, Medoff G, Swartz MM: Osteomyelitis: a review of clinical features, therapeutic considerations, and unusual aspects. N Engl J Med 282:198, 260, 316, 1970
31. Matsen FA, Wyss CR, Pedegana LR, et al: Transcutaneous oxygen tension measurement in peripheral vascular disease. Surg Gynecol Obstet 150:525, 1980
32. Kelley JP, Wilkowske CJ, Washington JA: Chronic osteomyelitis in the adult. p. 120. In Ahstrom, JP (ed): Current Practice in Orthopaedic Surgery. Mosby, St Louis, 1975

16 Infections of Prosthetic Joints

Mary P. Pugsley
W. Eugene Sanders, Jr.

To a patient with severe arthritis, total joint replacement offers cessation of pain and return of normal function, goals often not achievable with any other therapeutic modality. Because of the overall success of total joint replacements, an estimated 100,000 total hip[1] and 50,000 total knee arthroplasties are performed each year in this country. Arthroplasties of other joints are being performed frequently as well. With the implantation of any prosthetic device, one of the most dreaded complications is infection. It decreases the likelihood of a favorable clinical result, is costly and time-consuming to treat, and may result in prolonged illness and even death. In this chapter we will review the problem of infections of prosthetic joints, particularly hips and knees. Epidemiology, pathogenesis, and clinical, bacteriologic, and radiographic features will be described. Currently employed methods for prevention and treatment will be compared and contrasted.

HIPS

Early in the experience with total hip arthroplasty (THA) infection rates as high as 5 to 11 percent were reported.[2-7] Other investigators, especially in more recent series, have noted infection rates of only 0 to 4 percent.[7-21] The development of an infection in a prosthetic hip involves a complex interaction between host and bacterial factors. Documented risk factors for infection include rheumatoid arthritis, prior surgery on the hip, and postoperative complications following THA that require operative intervention. Phenomena observed in vitro which may influence the development of infection in prosthetic joints include local tissue necrosis, due to drilling of bone and polymerization of acrylic cement, and abnormalities in the morphology and function of macrophages when exposed to methyl methacrylate.

Surprisingly in view of their frequent association with other infections, diabetes mellitus,[15,18] steroid therapy,[15,18] liver disease,[15] malignancy,[15] and obesity[15,18] have not been implicated as risk factors for infection following THA in prospective studies. On the other hand, patients with rheumatoid arthritis have a substantially increased risk of infection as compared with patients with osteoarthritis.[7,15,22] This increased risk may result from local factors in the hip itself from the immunological abnormalities associated with rheumatoid arthritis, or from both.

In a THA necrotic tissue results from dissection and drilling[23] as well as from heat generated by the polymerization of methyl methacrylate.[23] Necrotic tissue and hematoma may serve as foci for bacterial survival and replication. Excessive manipulation of the joint during the operative and perioperative period appears to enhance the likelihood of infection. Among the best-documented risk factors is a previous surgical procedure on the hip:nailing, endoprosthesis, or prior THA, for example. This increases the chance of infection two- to eightfold above that for surgery on a previously unmanipulated hip.[7,12,15,16,18,22,24] The presence of scar tissue, which requires more operative manipulation and impairs wound healing, and antecedent occult infection[15] may account in part for the increased risk in these patients. Postoperative complications requiring surgical intervention[18] and traumatic disease of the hip[7,15] also increase the risk of infection.

Methyl methacrylate, the cement used in most THAs, impairs chemotaxis of polymorphonuclear cells[25] and changes the morphology of rabbit macrophages and human monocytes from their normal spreading configuration to a spherical shape.[26] Both phenomena may impair the effectiveness of local host defenses at the site of a THA. Recently some prosthetic joints have been designed which do not require cement but instead are stabilized by ingrowth of bone into the prosthesis.[19–21] This type of device circumvents the deleterious effects of cement on local host defenses. Bacteria on the surface of a prosthetic hip may have an additional advantage. In vivo bacterial adhesion is enhanced by the formation of a polysaccharide glycocalyx, which is thought to enclose bacteria in a protective environment that is relatively resistant to the antibacterial activity of complement and antibiotics.[27] Recently, using electron microscopy of tissue specimens from patients with infected orthopedic prosthetic devices, Gristina and Costerton have demonstrated bacteria embedded in such biofilms.[28] The presence of this relatively impermeable biofilm may not only impair access of local antibacterial factors to infecting organisms, increasing their chances of survival, but may also make recovery of bacteria for diagnostic purposes unreliable if only small amounts of fluid are obtained, as with aspiration of the joint.

Clinical Manifestations

Infections of prosthetic joints have been classified according to presumed pathogenetic mechanisms and clinical presentation of the illness. Both early and subacute late infections are thought to result from the introduction of bacteria into the wound at the time of surgery. In contrast, hematogenous infections of prosthetic joints result from infection elsewhere and can occur at any time after the joint is inserted. Most authors classify infections as "early" if they occur within 3 months of surgery and as "late" if symptoms begin thereafter. From 15 to 40 percent of infections in prosthetic joints occur after 1½ to 2 years postoperatively,[7,10,22,29,30] some as long as a decade later.[7,22,30] Therefore, patient follow-up must extend for prolonged periods in order to generate meaningful data in clinical studies.

Pain is the most common symptom in patients with deep infections of THA.[15,30] Pain is often, but not invariably, accompanied by fever or signs of local inflammation with early infection.[31] Commonly a draining hematoma or other abnormality of wound healing precedes the diagnosis of an early periprosthetic infection.[3,15,16,18]

Pain on weight bearing, with or without pain at rest, is also the most frequent complaint of patients with subacute late deep infections. Postoperative pain may fail to subside completely or hip discomfort may gradually recur. Unfortunately, pain is often the only evidence of a problem in these patients. Abnormal amounts of pain coupled with radiographic evidence of loosening of the prosthesis may in fact prompt surgical exploration, during which previously unsuspected infection is discovered.[2,6,12,30] Infection should be strongly suspected in patients with postoperative wound drainage that has subsided spontaneously who subsequently develop hip pain. Surin[18] reported that patients with early superficial wound drainage have a threefold greater chance of developing a deep wound infection than do patients without drainage. The risk is doubled if the patient has had prior hip surgery.[18]

Most reported cases of hematogenously acquired infection are late in onset, often years after implantation.[15,32–35] Hematogenous infection occurs infrequently in patients with THA (0.29 percent in patients who had been followed for 2 to 8 years by Ahlberg and associates[34]); however, this accounts for 17 to 32 percent of all infections in prosthetic joints.[7,15,22,30] The clinical presentation of an infection of hematogenous origin differs from that of the subacute late infection. The patient is usually asymptomatic after surgery until there is an abrupt onset of pain, often accompanied by fever, chills, and signs of inflammation of the hip.[15,33,34] Reported sources of bacteremia include pneumonia,[33,36] pharyngitis,[22,32,37] teeth or gums,[22,32,33,37,38] skin lesions,[22,32–34] urinary tract infections,[22,37] and the gastrointestinal tract.[33] Occasionally the origin of the bacteremia may be suspected only retrospectively on the basis of the patient's history. However, Stinchfield and associates[33] convincingly documented the etiology of nine consecutive hematogenous infections of total hip and knee arthroplasties, in all of which the infecting organism was isolated from blood (seven cases), an infected distant focus (four cases), or both (two cases).

Laboratory Findings

The erythrocyte sedimentation rate (ESR) is elevated in 67 to 94 percent of patients with prosthetic joint infection.[15,30,39] Following an uncomplicated THA the ESR usually will return to normal within 6 months of surgery. If it remains elevated in a patient with a painful prosthesis, infection must be suspected. A patient found to have an elevated ESR without other obvious cause prior to THA should be evaluated further to exclude infection before implanting a prosthetic joint.[15] The leukocyte count is usually normal in patients with an infected THA.[15,30]

Radiologic Evaluation

Plain films, radionuclide scans, and arthography have each been used alone or in combination in evaluation of painful prosthetic joints. With each of these techniques there are findings that *suggest* infection but none that *prove* its presence. Loosening of the prosthesis occurs ultimately in all patients, and occasionally it is the only clue to the presence of infection. Unfortunately, aseptic loosening may closely resemble that due to infection.

Infection is likely if extensive, irregular, endosteal bony reabsorption or periosteal new bone is seen on plain film, but the sensitivity of each of these findings is 50 percent or less.[40,41] Plain radiographs are more sensitive in detecting loosening of the femoral component of a painful prosthetic hip (76 to 98 percent)[40,41] but are less reliable in identifying acetabular loosening.[40,41] Radiographic features indicating loosening of the prosthesis include: (1) a change in position of one of the prosthetic components[40,42]; (2) a lucent zone ≥ 2 mm between cement and bone or progressive widening on serial films[40,42]; (3) any lucency between cement and prosthesis[40]; (4) fracture of either acetabulum or femur[40]; and (5) extensive cystic defects in the cement.[40]

A radiographic scan with ^{99}Tc identifies areas of bone with increased blood supply or osteogenesis and is therefore quite sensitive. However it is nonspecific; a ^{99}Tc scan may be positive for months in an asymptomatic, uninfected patient following THA.[42] However, the pattern of uptake may help to distinguish infection from other abnormalities. According to Williamson and his associates, increased uptake in a diffuse pattern over both the femoral and acetabular components is suggestive of infection.[43] In contrast, locally increased uptake is characteristic of a fracture, heterotopic bone formation, or an area of increased stress.[43] Using Williamson's criteria, Tehranzadeh and his coworkers[41] correctly identified all nine cases of infected THA in their series of patients with bone scans. Because of the sensitivity of ^{99}Tc scans, some believe that a negative scan should mitigate against surgical intervention in a patient with a painful prosthesis.[43,44]

Gallium, like ^{99}Tc, becomes localized at areas of increased blood flow, although binding to leukocytes seems to be a more important determinant of abnormal uptake on delayed films. Some authors have found gallium scans to be more specific than ^{99}Tc scans for infection[40,44] although they are perhaps less sensitive.[40] A positive gallium scan in a patient with a painful total joint arthroplasty (TJA) and a positive ^{99}Tc scan accurately predicted the presence of positive intraoperative cultures in 19 of 20 infected patients in Reing's series. There were no falsely positive gallium scans among the 58 patients in this series who did not have infection.[44]

An arthrogram in conjunction with aspiration of the hip has the potential for providing an accurate, sensitive evaluation of the anatomy of the joint and confirming the diagnosis of infection suggested by other findings. If radiopaque cement has been implanted, subtraction angiography is necessary for accurate visualization of the interface between cement and prosthesis. Cultures of aspirated intracapsular fluid are positive in 66 to 90 percent of cases in which infection is documented at surgery.[40,42] Arthrographic findings suggested by Lyons and her co-workers to be associated with infection are irregularity of the pseudocapsule, and the presence of a sinus tract, fistula, or extracapsular cavity.[40]

Arthographic criteria for loosening are defined differently by different investigators based upon the observation of radiographic contrast in the bone-cement interface. Using criteria for loosening based on the size of the pseudocapsule surrounding the joint, Lyons and her co-workers[40] found subtraction angiography to be 96 percent accurate in diagnosing femoral and acetabular loosening. In contrast, Tehranzadeh and his associates[41] found almost 25 percent false negatives in 38 patients. Murray and Rodrigo[45] evaluated 12 patients with painful THA by arthrography and found only 58 percent correspondence to the operative findings. Murray and Rodrigo also performed arthrograms on 53 patients who were asymptomatic after THA and found evidence of acetabular loosening in 12 (23 percent). Differences in technique and in definition of loosening may account in part for the disparate results.

Microbiology

Staphylococcus aureus (25 to 61 percent)[7,15,18,22,39] and *Staphylococcus epidermidis* (5 to 26 percent)[7,15,18,22,39] are the most common bacteria isolated from infected THAs in most series. Streptococci, aerobic gram-negative rods, and anaerobes[7,15,18,22,39,46] also cause infection in some patients and seem to be more frequent isolates in patients who have received preoperative antibiotic prophylaxis.[18,22] Some investigators have obtained intraoperative cultures at the time of routine THA in an attempt to predict eventual infection. The incidence of positive cultures reported varies widely, and the significance of finding bacterial growth in the hip at the time of THA is not clear. Surin and his group[18] found no deep infections in any of 18 patients (11 percent of total) who had positive intraoperative cultures and who were followed for at least 3 years. Tietjen[47] reported that 2.3 percent of 1,187 patients with primary hip arthroplasty had positive intraoperative cultures, but none developed infection. In Murray's series[12] a striking 31 percent of 740 capsular cultures were positive. In an attempt to account for the high proportion of positive cultures Murray autoclaved half of each specimen obtained from subsequent patients and found that even the sterilized fragments of tissue were reported as having bacterial growth 8 percent of the time.

Murray[12] found that the incidence of positive cultures at the time of THA was the same in patients having primary and secondary hip arthroplasty. However, others report a higher incidence of positive intraoperative cultures in patients with prior hip surgery (6.4 versus 2.3 percent[47] and 38 versus 25 percent[48]). It is not clear how much importance should be attached to a positive intraoperative culture. Fitzgerald and his associates[48] identified subsequent infection in 4.8 percent of hips with prior surgery which had positive intraoperative cultures. However, Murray[12] found no correlation between a positive culture and risk of subsequent infection. Furthermore, infection, when encountered, was often due to different bacteria than those isolated from intraoperative cultures.[47,48] Tietjen[47] suggested that perioperative antibiotics may have altered the bacterial flora and resulted in the growth of different bacteria. Some investigators[14,47,48] recommend a prolonged course of antibiotics when positive cultures are obtained at time of THA in patients with prior hip surgery. Unfortunately, the value of this approach has not been assessed in rigorously designed prospective studies.

Prevention

Contamination of the surgical wound may be either endogenous (from organisms on the patient's skin or from a distant source) or exogenous (from direct contact with a member of the surgical team or from airborne particles containing bacteria). Preventative measures have been aimed at limiting access of bacteria to the wound at the time of surgery, eradicating bacteria present in the wound perioperatively, and preventing hematogenous seeding of the prosthetic joint. The number of bacteria gaining access to the wound may be decreased by thoroughly cleansing the operative field, by using a separate pair of gloves for draping the patient,[49] and by wearing impermeable gowns. Although very few airborne bacteria are measurable in an empty operating room, bacterial counts rise when the room is occupied.[50,51] Charnley contended that "the living body of personnel in an operating room is by far the most important source of pathogenic organisms."[29] In support of his contention, it has been found that decreasing traffic in the surgical suite, eliminating unnecessary conversation,[50] and wearing masks that are covered on three sides by the hood[50] all minimize the number of airborne bacteria.

Much attention has been directed toward the ventilation systems in operating rooms used for joint replacements since Charnley demonstrated a decrease in deep infection rate from 8.9 to 1.3 percent with the introduction of the "clean" operating room.[52] Conventional ventilation systems provide approximately 12 air exchanges per hour. Patients operated on in this environment without perioperative antibiotic prophylaxis have incurrred infection at rates ranging from 3.7 to 11 percent.[3,16,52] The more sophisticated laminar flow systems championed by Charnley and others provide 130 to 480 air exchanges per hour. Filtration of the recirculated air in most laminar flow systems is accomplished by HEPA (high-efficiency particulate air) filters which remove 99.9 percent of particles 0.3 μm or larger. Infection rates in patients operated on in laminar flow rooms without preoperative antibiotic prophylaxis range from 0.7 to 3.3 percent.[16,17,52]

In order to further decrease the emission of bacteria from the operative team, Charnley introduced body exhaust systems for the operating team in 1970; other surgeons have used personnel isolator systems. Infection rates with these systems in the absence of perioperative antibiotics range from 0 to 1.0 percent.[16,24,53] However, the installation of laminar flow systems costs from $20,000 for a horizontal system to $40,000 for a vertical system, while a helmet-aspirator personnel isolator system for four people costs $1,000.[54] These costs have prevented the use of laminar flow systems in many hospitals.

Another, less expensive method for eliminating airborne bacteria is ultraviolet (UV) lighting. UV light of 2650 Å in a dry environment rapidly decreases bacterial counts in operating room air.[55] The use of UV lighting has been associated with a decrease in the deep infection rate following THA from 3.06 to 0.74 percent at Harvard Medical Center.[55] Installation of this system at the Duke University Medical Center has been followed by a deep infection rate of 0.96 percent in hip arthroplasties.[51]

Prevention of infection in TJA may also be accomplished by use of prophylactic systemic antibiotics perioperatively. Ericson[56] and his associates found a drop in the early infection rate following THA from 17 to 0 percent when patients operated on in a conventional room were given 14 days of cloxacillin beginning 1 hour before surgery. Carlsson and his co-workers[57] then followed Ericson's patients for 5 to $6\frac{1}{2}$ years postoperatively. They found a deep infection rate of 3.3 percent in those who had received cloxacillin in comparison with 24 percent in patients who had received no perioperative antibiotic. Pollard[58] found that prophylaxis with three doses of cephaloridine perioperatively was as effective as 14 days of flucloxacillin. Most investigators now prefer relatively brief courses of antibiotics for prophylaxis. Others operating in a conventional operating room have had similar results using antibiotic prophylaxis, with infection rates ranging from 0 to 2.0 percent.[7,13–15,24,59]

There is no question that in the setting of a conventionally ventilated operating room perioperative antibiotic administration significantly decreases the deep infection rate following THA. However, the benefit of antibiotic prophylaxis to a patient operated on in a "clean" operating room has not been demonstrated. The infection rates reported are 0.7 to 3.3 percent[16,17,52] without and 0 to 1.2 percent[16,17,59] with antibiotics in a clean room. A review by Nelson[16] of 15,520 cases in the literature comparing these two groups of patients found comparable rates of infection: 0.7 percent without and 0.6 percent with antibiotics. No studies have compared the use of ultraviolet light with and without antibiotic prophylaxis.

If a systemic antibiotic is to be given perioperatively, which drug should be chosen? To be effective as prophylaxis, an antibiotic theoretically must achieve a concentration in bone that exceeds the minimum inhibitory concentration (MIC) for the bacteria of concern. Cephalosporins have been widely used because the in vitro spectrum of activity of these drugs includes most of the bacteria that commonly cause infection in TJA. The penetration into bone of these antibiotics varies. Williams[60] and Cunha[61] found higher bone concentrations with cefazolin,[60,61] ceforanide,[60] and cephradine[61] than with cefamandole,[60] cefoxitin,[60] and cephalothin,[60,61] and attributed the differences to the longer half-lives[60] and higher peak serum concentrations[60,61] of the former drugs. However, these observations may not extrapolate directly to the clinical situation. First, both free (active) and protein-bound (inactive) antibiotics are measured by assays currently in use for bone specimens. Second, the assay for cephalothin in bone may give falsely low levels because of the drug's instability in the laboratory. Finally, long-term studies have not compared the clinical outcome of patients based on the concentration of antibiotic in bone at the time of THA. Williams and his group[60] have recommended selection of cefazolin for systemic prophylaxis because of its proven efficacy and relative cost effectiveness. Because peak levels of antibiotic in bone were found within 60 minutes of antibiotic administration,[60] proper timing in the administration of the preoperative dose is necessary to maximize activity at the operative site.

In an attempt to direct antibiotic prophylaxis locally, precluding the necessity for systemic antibiotics, some investigators have used cement mixed with antibiotic for implanting THAs. The addition of up to 4.5 g antibiotic in powdered form to 40 g cement does not significantly decrease the compressive or tensile strength of the mixture.[62–64] Most surgeons who use antibiotic-loaded acrylic cement (ALAC) mix 0.5 to 1.0 g of antibiotic with 40 g Palacos brand cement because more antibiotic is released from Palacos than from other brands.[63,65,66] Many antibiotics have been added to cement, including aminoglycosides, erythromycin, and colistin, but the pharmacokinetics of the aminoglycosides have been studied the most extensively. Peak serum concentrations of tobramycin were less than 1.5 μg/ml in all 10 patients studied by Soto-Hall and co-workers.[67] In contrast, wound and urine concentrations reached peaks of 20 and 15 μg/ml respectively and were in the therapeutic range for hours after surgery. Tobramycin was excreted in the urine for up to 14 days. Torhulm and co-workers[68] detected gentamicin in the urine of one patient 2 years after a hip implant with ALAC. Wahlig and Dingeldein[65] found therapeutic concentrations of gentamicin in periprosthetic soft tissues for up to $5\frac{1}{2}$ years after THA with ALAC.

Few large clinical studies have evaluated the efficacy of ALAC in humans in preventing deep wound infection, and none have conclusively proven ALAC more useful than systemic antibiotic prophylaxis. Buchholz and his group have been using ALAC without systemic antibiotic prophylaxis since 1970. They reported a deep infection rate of less than 1.0 percent in their first patients after short-term follow-up.[64] However, in a later series of 1,655 patients with at least 3 years follow-up at the same institution, the infection rate was 1.6 percent.[64] This result was comparable with the infection rate found following systemic antibiotic prophylaxis. Murray at the University of California San Francisco has also employed ALAC cement. The infection rate in 1,112 patients at that institution was 1.0 percent after addition of erythromycin to Palacos cement.[62] When colistin was also routinely added, the infection rate fell to 0.4 percent.[62] However, other changes were made at the same time: ultraviolet lights were added in the operating room and systemic antibiotic prophylaxis was given. Thus the true impact of ALAC on the infection rate is difficult to ascertain. Josefsson and his co-investigators[69] in a multicenter collaborative trial compared the efficacy of systemic perioperative antibiotics and genta-micin-loaded Palacos cement in preventing infections of THA performed in a conventional operating room. Unfortunately, there were variations in methodology between centers, including the systemic antibiotic chosen, the duration of its administration, and the interval of preoperative dosing. A significant difference in infection rate was found early in the study: 1.6 percent in the systemic antibiotic group versus 0.4 percent for the group with gentamicin-impregnated cement. However, patients were followed for only 1 to 2 years. Another potentially confounding factor was identified: one of the eight centers participating in the study contributed fewer than 20 percent of the patients but accounted for half of the infected patients in the systemic antibiotic group. If that center's patients are excluded, the infection rate for the systemic antibiotic group falls to 1.0 percent. At present, it appears prudent to consider use of ALAC investigational. Rigorous, prospective studies are necessary to evaluate efficacy and quantify risks of hypersensitivity reactions and development of antibiotic resistance.

Prevention of hematogenous infection in a TJA should be an ongoing concern of primary care physicians as well as orthopedic surgeons. During the preoperative period it behooves the surgeon to evaluate the patient with regard to potential sources of hematogenous infection, for example, urinary tract, teeth, or skin lesions. If active infection is found, it should be treated prior to surgery.[22,33] Foci that may cause bacteremia later, such as extensively diseased teeth, should be removed before surgery if possible. Some advocate systemic antibiotic prophylaxis for patients with prosthetic joints prior to procedures known to cause bacteremia, such as dental work and genitourinary surgery, which is analogous to the prophylaxis given to patients with prosthetic heart valves.[33,37,38,70] However, Norden[71] has recommended against this approach following his cost-benefit analysis of antibiotic prophylaxis for dental work in patients who have THA. He suggests that a nationwide registry of infections following dental, gastrointestinal, and genitourinary procedures be established to document and quantitate the risks of subsequent infection of prosthetic joints. Clearly, if a patient with a TJA develops an acute infection at a distant site, appropriate cultures should be obtained and systemic antibiotic therapy started promptly in order to minimize the risk of hematogenous infection.

Therapy

There are three alternatives for therapy of an infected THA: (1) debridement and antibiotics, with or without irrigation; (2) revision arthroplasty, done either at the time of excision of the infected prosthesis or later; or (3) complete excision of the hip, with formation of a pseudarthrosis.

The use of debridement and antibiotics has been reported to be successful occasionally when symptoms occur abruptly.[22,72,73] In such cases there is less likely to be involvement of the cement-bone interface and of the bone itself, which makes a conservative approach feasible. Radical debridement of deep soft tissue with extensive intraoperative irrigation and irrigation-suction after surgery, together with prolonged systemic antibiotic therapy, is usually employed. The presence of irrigation-suction tubes has been associated with colonization of the wound with more resistant organisms.[74] Although clinical failure has not been documented as a result, the possibility of superinfection exists if irrigation tubes are left in place for prolonged periods. Debridement combined with antibiotics has also been tried in patients with a more indolent onset of symptoms; the results have been disappointing, with success rates of only 4 to 20 percent.[72,74,75]

Since 1970 Buchholz and his group have championed the primary exchange arthroplasty as the treatment of choice for infected THA. They add as much as 6.0 g of antibiotic to Palacos cement, depending on the infecting organism, and give no systemic antibiotics routinely. With this protocol they report a 77 percent success rate for first exchange procedures and 90 percent success for subsequent exchanges.[76] Their success rate was best in cases in which no organism was cultured (89 percent) or anaerobic *Corynebacterium* spp (84 percent), *Peptococcus* (76 percent), or *S. aureus* (72 percent) was isolated. Their success rate was lower with aerobic gram-negative bacilli (50 percent) and group D streptococci (53 percent). Overall mortality was 2.78 percent. Similar results have been reported by Carlsson[77] and Lindberg,[78] who judged 88 percent of 59 primary exchange and 83 percent of 18 delayed exchange procedures healed after 3 to 4 years of follow-up. However, only six of these infections involved gram-negative organisms, and systemic antibiotics were administered for 6 months postoperatively. Miley and his co-investigators,[79] using antibiotic-laden cement combined with prolonged (mean 13.2 month) administration of multiple systemic antibiotics also had excellent results, 87 percent success of 47 infected THA so treated. However, their criteria for selection of patients for a primary exchange procedure were quite strict: infection with a single gram-positive organism sensitive to multiple antibiotics, the presence of healthy deep tissues, with enough healthy bone to support cement fixation (as determined at the time of surgery), and the absence of a draining sinus.

The results following a one-step revision have not been universally excellent. Hunter and Dandy[39] reported a success rate of only 33 percent in their review of 30 Canadian cases treated with primary revison arthroplasty although neither ALAC nor long-term systemic antibiotics were used in these cases. Hunter[80] later reported a series of his own patients in whom the rate of success of this approach was equally low (25 percent). Using both ALAC and systemic antibiotics, Murray[75] also had poor results in a small series of patients. Available data indicate that infection with gram-negative organisms[75,76,79] and extensive bony or soft tissue involvement[78,79] are predictive of an unfavorable outcome for a one-step revision arthroplasty. This procedure appears better suited to patients with smoldering, low-grade infection (such as that caused by *S. epidermidis*) with minimal soft tissue inflammation.

Surgeons at the Mayo Clinic have used a two-step revision arthroplasty, with prolonged systemic antimicrobial therapy after excision, for some years. They found that 88 percent of their 131 patients were free of infection after 2 to 9 years of follow-up. The chances for recurrent infection were increased if any cement was left in place at the time of excision and if the prosthesis was reinserted less than 429 days after excision. There was a trend toward failure in patients with infection caused by gram-negative bacteria although the difference was not statistically significant.[81] Excision of the prosthesis and formation of a pseudarthrosis is the least desirable treatment option for infected THA. Gait instability,[82,83] persistent pain,[83] and wound drainage[82,83] are reasons for poor clinical results with this procedure.

KNEES

The analysis of factors that may increase the risk of infection after total knee arthroplasty (TKA) has not been as complete as has that for THA. The type of prosthesis does seem to influence risk of infection, which ranges from 4.8 to 10.9 percent in hinged, fully constrained prostheses in which both components are metal[22,84,85] and from 0.57 to 6.0 percent for minimally or partially constrained prostheses in which the articulation occurs between a metal and a plastic surface.[19,85–92] Although many patients with infected TKA have received intra-articular steroid injections prior to arthroplasty,[92] there is no evidence that this increases the risk of infection. Neither is there evidence that prior surgery on the knee increases the risk of infection.[91] An observed increase in infection rate of TKAs was ascribed to the change in position of the surgical team upwind from the wound during part of the procedure, which did not occur in conventional operating rooms or when hip arthroplasties were inserted.[59]

Infections in TKA tend to present earlier than infections in THA,[30,91] perhaps because of the proximity of the joint to the examiner.[85] Hematogenous infections, as with hips, may occur at any time. Presenting symptoms of deep infection in one series of 23 patients included drainage in 10, swelling in 13, and fever in 8.[92]

The principles of radiographic analysis of the prosthetic knee are the same as for the prosthetic hip. The major difference between the findings in the two joints is that the radionuclide bone scan may remain positive, with mild to moderately increased uptake, in asymptomatic individuals for years after knee replacement. Therefore, a scan that is minimally positive in a symptomatic patient is not evidence of infection by itself.[93]

The treatment options for an infected TKA are essentially the same as for an infected THA. Salvage of the prosthesis by debridement and antibiotics is likely to succeed only if the infection is mild and detected early, before the prosthesis loosens, and if the causative organism is sensitive to oral antibiotics.[86,91,94] For cases in which these conditions are not met, removal of the prosthesis and fusion of the joint, while not entirely satisfactory, is an option.[95] Delayed implantation of the prosthesis is a more attractive choice, and has been successful when preceded by extensive debridement and prolonged parenteral antibiotics prior to reimplantation.[86,95] The total number of cases reported in which any of these methods of treatment have been used is relatively small. More data are clearly needed. Encouragingly, attempts at salvage of prosthetic knees appear to be successful more often than with hips, perhaps because of earlier identification of infection.

CONCLUSION

Knowledge of infections of prosthetic joints has increased exponentially over the past 15 years. At present, infection rates of less than 1 percent appear to be realistic goals wherever prosthetic joint surgery is performed. Despite the progress made, a number of important questions remain unanswered. They are: (1) Is ALAC as safe and effective as systemic antimicrobial prophylaxis? (2) Is the combination of UV light and antimicrobial prophylaxis more effective than either alone? (3) Is the concentration of drug in bone at the time of surgery a critical determinant for success in prophylaxis? (4) Are intraoperative cultures of predictive value following first implantation and if so, will specific antimicrobial treatment reduce the rate of subsequent infection? (5) Is antibiotic prophylaxis indicated in patients with TJA before dental, gastrointestinal, or genitourinary procedures? The great progress made to date should provide momentum for performance of the studies to answer these remaining questions.

REFERENCES

1. Melton LJ III, Stauffer RN, Chao EYS, et al: Rates of total hip arthroplasty. A population based study. N Engl J Med 307:1242, 1982
2. Patterson FP, Brown CS: The McKee-Farrar total hip replacement. Preliminary results and complications of 368 operations performed in five general hospitals. J Bone Joint Surg [Am] 54A:257, 1972
3. Wilson PD Jr, Amstutz HC, Czerniecki A, et al: Total hip replacement with fixation by acrylic cement. A preliminary study of 100 consecutive McKee-Farrar prosthetic replacements. J Bone Joint Surg [Am] 54A:207, 1972

4. Todd RC, Lightowler CDR, Harris J: Total hip replacement in osteoarthrosis using the Charnley prosthesis. Br Med J 2:752, 1972

5. Harris J, Lightowler CDR, Todd RC: Total hip replacement in inflammatory hip disease using the Charnley prosthesis. Br Med J 2:750, 1972

6. Charnley J, Cupic Z: The nine and ten year results of the low-friction arthroplasty of the hip. Clin Orthop 95:9, 1973

7. Andrews HJ, Arden GP, Hart GM, et al: Deep infection after total hip replacement. J Bone Joint Surg [Br] 63B:53, 1981

8. Smith RE, Turner RJ: Total hip replacement using methylmethacrylate cement. An analysis of data from 3,482 cases. Clin Orthop 95:231, 1973

9. Ring PA: Total replacement of the hip joint. Clin Orthop 95:34, 1973

10. Buchholz HW, Noack G: Results of the total hip prosthesis design "St. George." Clin Orthop 95:201, 1973

11. Nicholson OR: Total hip replacement. An evaluation of the results and techniques, 1967–1972. Clin Orthop 95:217, 1973

12. Murray WR: Results in patients with total hip replacement arthroplasty. Clin Orthop 95:80, 1973

13. Collis DK, Steinhaus K: Total hip replacement without deep infection in a standard operating room. J Bone Joint Surg [Am] 58A:446, 1976

14. Eftekhar NS, Kiernan HA Jr, Stinchfield FE: Systemic and local complications following low-friction arthroplasty of the hip joint. A study of 800 consecutive operations. Arch Surg 111:150, 1976

15. Fitzgerald RH, Jr, Nolan DR, Ilstrup DM, et al: Deep wound sepsis following total hip arthroplasty. J Bone Joint Surg [Am] 59A:847, 1977

16. Nelson JP, Glassburn AR Jr, Talbott RD, et al: The effect of previous surgery, operating room environment, and preventive antibiotics on post-operative infection following total hip arthroplasty. Clin Orthop 147:167, 1980

17. Ha'eri GB, Wiley AM: Total hip replacement in a laminar flow environment with special reference to deep infections. Clin Orthop 148:163, 1980

18. Surin VV, Sundholm K, Bäckman L: Infection after total hip replacement. With special reference to a discharge from the wound. J Bone Joint Surg [Br] 65B:412, 1983

19. Engh CA: Hip arthroplasty with a Moore prothesis with porous coating. A five-year study. Clin Orthop 176:52, 1983

20. Lord G, Bancel P: The madreporic cementless total hip arthroplasty. New experimental data and a seven-year clinical follow-up study. Clin Orthop 176:67, 1983

21. Morscher EW, Dick W: Cementless fixation of "isoelastic" hip endoprostheses manufactured from plastic materials. Clin Orthop 176:77, 1983

22. Poss R, Thornhill TS, Ewald FC, et al: Factors influencing the incidence and outcome of infection following total joint arthroplasty. Clin Orthop 182:117, 1984

23. Rhinelander FW, Nelson CL, Stewart RD, et al: Experimental reaming of the proximal femur and acrylic cement implantation. Vascular and histologic effects. Clin Orthop 141:74, 1979

24. Fitzgerald RH Jr, Bechtol CO, Eftekhar N, et al: Reduction of deep sepsis after total hip arthroplasty. Arch Surg 114:803, 1979

25. Petty W: The effect of methylmethacrylate on chemotaxis of polymorphonuclear leukocytes. J Bone Joint Surg [Am] 60A:492, 1978

26. Leake ES, Wright MJ, Gristina AG: Comparative study of the adherence of alveolar and peritoneal macrophages, and of blood monocytes to methylmethacrylate, polyethylene, stainless steel, and vitallium. J Reticuloendothel Soc 30:403, 1981

27. Costerton JW, Geesey GG, Cheng K-J: How bacteria stick. Sci Am 238:86, 1978
28. Gristina AG, Costerton JW: Bacterial adherence to biomaterials and tissue. The significance of its role in clinical sepsis. J Bone Joint Surg [Am] 67A:264, 1985
29. Charnley J: Postoperative infection after total hip replacement with special reference to air contamination in the operating room. Clin Orthop 87:167, 1972
30. Inman RD, Gallegos KV, Brause BD, et al: Clinical and microbial features of prosthetic joint infection. Am J Med 77:47, 1984
31. Gristina AG, Kolkin, J: Total joint replacement and sepsis. J Bone Joint Surg [Am] 65A:128, 1983
32. Downes EM: Late infection after total hip replacement. J Bone Joint Surg [Br] 59B:42, 1977
33. Stinchfield FE, Bigliani LU, Neu HC, et al: Late hematogenous infection of total joint replacement. J Bone Joint Surg [Am] 62A:1345, 1980
34. Ahlberg A, Carlsson AS, Lindberg L: Hematogenous infection in total joint replacement. Clin Orthop 137:69, 1978
35. D'Ambrosia RD, Shoji H, Heater R: Secondarily infected total joint replacements by hematogenous spread. J Bone Joint Surg [Am] 58A:450, 1976
36. Mallory TH: Sepsis in total hip replacement following pneumococcal pneumonia. A case report. J Bone Joint Surg [Am] 55A:1753, 1973
37. Cruess RL, Bickel WS, von Kessler KLC: Infections in total hips secondary to a primary source elsewhere. Clin Orthop 106:99, 1975
38. Rubin R, Salvati EA, Lewis R: Infected total hip replacement after dental procedures. Oral Surg 41:18, 1976
39. Hunter G, Dandy D: The natural history of the patient with an infected total hip replacement. J Bone Joint Surg [Br] 59B:293, 1977
40. Lyons CW, Berquist TH, Lyons JC, et al: Evaluation of radiographic findings in painful hip arthroplasties. Clin Orthop 195:239, 1985
41. Tehranzadeh J, Schneider R, Freiberger RH: Radiological evaluation of painful total hip replacement. Radiology 141:355, 1981
42. Schneider R, Freiberger RH, Ghelman B, et al: Radiologic evaluation of painful joint prostheses. Clin Orthop 170:156, 1982
43. Williamson BRJ, McLaughlin RE, Wang GJ, et al: Radionuclide bone imaging as a means of differentiating loosening and infection in patients with a painful total hip prosthesis. Radiology 133:723, 1979
44. Reing CM, Richin PF, Kenmore PI: Differential bone-scanning in the evaluation of a painful total joint replacement. J Bone Joint Surg [Am] 61A:933, 1979
45. Murray WR, Rodrigo JJ: Arthrography for the assessment of pain after total hip replacement. J Bone Joint Surg [Am] 57A:1060, 1975
46. Kamme C, Lidgren L, Lindberg L, et al: Anaerobic bacteria in late infections after total hip arthroplasty. Scand J Infect Dis 6:161, 1974
47. Tietjen R, Stinchfield FE, Michelsen CB: The significance of intracapsular cultures in total hip operations. Surg Gynecol Obstet 144:699, 1977
48. Fitzgerald RH Jr, Peterson LFA, Washington JA II, et al: Bacterial colonization of wounds and sepsis in total hip arthroplasty. J Bone Joint Surg [Am] 55A:1242, 1973
49. McCue SF, Berg EW, Saunders EA: Efficacy of double-gloving as a barrier to microbial contamination during total joint arthroplasty. J Bone Joint Surg [Am] 63A:811, 1981
50. Letts RM, Doermer E: Conversation in the operating theater as a cause of airborne bacterial contamination. J Bone Joint Surg [Am] 65A:357, 1983

51. Moggio M, Goldner JL, McCollum DE, et al: Wound infections in patients undergoing total hip arthroplasty. Ultraviolet light for the control of airborne bacteria. Arch Surg 114:815, 1979
52. Charnley J, Eftekhar N: Postoperative infection in total prosthetic replacement arthroplasty of the hip-joint. With special reference to the bacterial content of the air of the operating room. Br J Surg 56:641, 1969
53. Brady LP, Enneking WF, Franco JA: The effect of operating-room environment on the infection rate after Charnley low-friction total hip replacement. J Bone Joint Surg [Am] 57A:80, 1975
54. Nelson JP: Prevention of postoperative infection by airborne bacteria. Orthop Rev 8:77, 1979
55. Lowell JD: The ultraviolet environment. Orthop Rev 8:111, 1979
56. Ericson C, Lidgren L, Lindberg L: Cloxacillin in the prophylaxis of postoperative infections of the hip. J Bone Joint Surg [Am] 55A:808, 1973
57. Carlsson AS, Lidgren L, Lindberg L: Prophylactic antibiotics against early and late deep infections after total hip replacements. Acta Orthop Scand 48:405, 1977
58. Pollard JP, Hughes SPF, Scott JE, et al: Antibiotic prophylaxis in total hip replacement. Br Med J 1:707, 1979
59. Salvati EA, Robinson RP, Zeno SM, et al: Infection rates after 3,175 total hip and total knee replacements performed with and without a horizontal unidirectional filtered air-flow system. J Bone Joint Surg [Am] 64A:525, 1982
60. Williams DN, Gustilo RB, Beverly RG, et al: Bone and serum concentrations of five cephalosporin drugs. Relevance to prophylaxis and treatment in orthopedic surgery. Clin Orthop 179:253, 1983
61. Cunha BA, Gossling HR, Pasternak HS, et al: The penetration characteristics of cefazolin, cephalothin, and cephradine into bone in patients undergoing total hip replacement. J Bone Joint Surg [Am] 59A:856, 1977
62. Murray WR: Use of antibiotic-containing bone cement. Clin Orthop 190:89, 1984
63. Marks KE, Nelson CL, Lautenschlager EP: Antibiotic-impregnated acrylic bone cement. J Bone Joint Surg [Am] 58A:358, 1976
64. Buchholz HW, Elson RA, Heinert K: Antibiotic-loaded acrylic cement: current concepts. Clin Orthop 190:96, 1984
65. Wahlig H, Dingeldein E: Antibiotics and bone cements. Experimental and clinical long-term observations. Acta Orthop Scand 51:49, 1980
66. Elson RA, Jephcott AE, McGechie DB et al: Antibiotic-loaded acrylic cement. J Bone Joint Surg [Br] 59B:200, 1977
67. Soto-Hall R, Saenz L, Tavernetti R, et al: Tobramycin in bone cement. An in-depth analysis of wound, serum, and urine concentrations in patients undergoing total hip revision arthroplasty. Clin Orthop 175:60, 1983
68. Törholm C, Lidgren L, Lindberg L, et al: Total hip joint arthroplasty with gentamicin-impregnated cement. A clinical study of gentamicin excretion kinetics. Clin Orthop 181:99, 1983
69. Josefsson G, Lindberg L, Wiklander B: Systemic antibiotics and gentamicin-containing bone cement in the prophylaxis of postoperative infections in total hip arthroplasty. Clin Orthop 159:194, 1981
70. Lattimer GL, Keblish PA, Dickson TB, Jr, et al: Hematogenous infection in total joint replacement. Recommendations for prophylactic antibiotics. JAMA 242:2213, 1979
71. Norden CW: Prevention of bone and joint infections. Am J Med 78:suppl. 6B, 229, 1985

72. Coventry MB: Treatment of infections occurring in total hip surgery. Orthop Clin North Am 6:991, 1975
73. Burton DS, Schurman DJ: Salvage of infected total joint replacements. Arch Surg 112:574, 1977
74. Canner GC, Steinberg ME, Heppenstall RB, et al: The infected hip after total hip arthroplasty. J Bone Joint Surg [Am] 66A:1393, 1984
75. Murray WR: Treatment of the established deep wound infection after total hip arthroplasty: A report of 65 cases. p. 382. In Leach RE, Hoaglund FT, Riseborough EJ (eds): Controversies in Orthopaedic Surgery. W. B. Saunders, Philadelphia, 1982
76. Buchholz HW, Elson RA, Engelbrecht E, et al: Management of deep infection of total hip replacement. J Bone Joint Surg [Br] 63B:342, 1981
77. Carlsson AS, Josefsson G, Lindberg L: Revision with gentamicin-impregnated cement for deep infections in total hip arthroplasties. J Bone Joint Surg [Am] 60A:1059, 1978
78. Lindberg L: Treatment of septic total hip arthroplasty by immediate exchange with antibiotic-containing cement. p. 399. In Leach RE, Hoaglund FT, Riseborough EJ (eds): Controversies in Orthopaedic Surgery. W. B. Saunders, Philadelphia, 1982
79. Miley GB, Scheller AD Jr, Turner RH: Medical and surgical treatment of the septic hip with one-stage revision arthroplasty. Clin Orthop 170:76, 1982
80. Hunter GA: The results of reinsertion of a total hip prosthesis after sepsis. J Bone Joint Surg [Br] 61B:422, 1979
81. Fitzgerald RH Jr, Jones DR: Hip implant infection. Treatment with resection arthroplasty and late total hip arthroplasty. Am J Med 78:suppl. 6B, 225, 1985
82. Clegg J: The results of the pseudarthrosis after removal of an infected total hip prosthesis. J Bone Joint Surg [Br] 59B:298, 1977
83. Bittar ES, Petty W: Girdlestone arthroplasty for infected total hip arthroplasty. Clin Orthop 170:83, 1982
84. Deburge A, Aubriot JH, Genet JP, et al: Current status of hinge prosthesis (Guepar). Clin Orthop 145:91, 1979
85. Insall JN, Ranawat CS, Aglietti P, et al: A comparison of four models of total knee-replacement prostheses. J Bone Joint Surg [Am] 58A:754, 1976
86. Walker RH, Schurman DJ: Management of infected total knee arthroplasties. Clin Orthop 186:81, 1984
87. Lewallen DG, Bryan RS, Peterson LFA: Polycentric total knee arthoplasty. A ten-year follow-up study J Bone Joint Surg [Am] 66A:1211, 1984
88. Kaufer H, Matthews LS: Spherocentric arthroplasty of the knee. Clinical experience with an average four-year follow-up. J Bone Joint Surg [Am] 63A:545, 1981
89. Insall J, Scott WN, Ranawat CS: The total condylar knee prosthesis. A report of two hundred and twenty cases. J Bone Joint Surg [Am] 61A:173, 1979
90. Skolnick MD, Coventry MB, Ilstrup DM: Geometric total knee arthroplasty. A two-year follow-up study. J Bone Joint Surg [Am] 58A:749, 1976
91. Skolnick MD, Bryan RS, Peterson LFA, et al: Polycentric total knee arthroplasty. A two-year follow-up study. J Bone Joint Surg [Am] 58A:743, 1976
92. Petty W, Bryan RS, Coventry MB, et al: Infection after total knee arthroplasty. Orthop Clin North Am 6:1005, 1975
93. Schneider R, Hood RW, Ranawat CS: Radiologic evaluation of knee arthroplasty. Orthop Clin North Am 13:225, 1982
94. Brause BD: Infected total knee replacement. Diagnostic, therapeutic, and prophylactic considerations. Orthop Clin North Am 13:245, 1982
95. Insall JN, Thompson FM, Brause BD: Two-stage reimplantation for the salvage of infected total knee arthroplasty. J Bone Joint Surg [Am] 65A:1087, 1983

17 | Opportunistic Infections in Burn Patients: Diagnosis and Treatment*

Basil A. Pruitt, Jr

Infection is the most frequent cause of morbidity and mortality following burns and other injuries.[1] The risk of infection is proportional to the severity of injury, which can be quantified in the burn patient as the extent of body surface burned. Both host and microbial factors are important in the pathogenesis of infection, and disturbance of the normal balance between host resistance and microbial invasiveness determines whether an injured patient will develop an infection. The local and systemic effects of injury not only predispose the severely injured patient to infection but, by confounding the diagnosis of infection, may also delay the institution of therapy. An understanding of the host-microbial interactions which influence the occurrence of infection and a knowledge of the whole-body and organ-system responses to both injury and infection will facilitate the timely diagnosis of infection and the early institution of therapy, which are necessary to enhance patient salvage.

---

* The opinions or assertions contained herein are the private views of the author and are not to be construed as official or as reflecting the views of the Department of the Army or the Department of Defense.

BURN WOUND INFECTIONS

In burn patients the incidence of wound infections is influenced by extent of burn, patient age, and depth of injury. Life-threatening burn wound infections are uncommon in patients with burns over less than 30 percent of the body surface; they increase with frequency as burn size increases above that level.[2] The importance of the extent of burn injury has been emphasized by recent studies by Yurt et al., who showed that a partial-thickness burn resistant to bacterial inoculation became susceptible to invasive infection after an additional burn injury was inflicted.[3] Yurt has also reported a lesser wound neutrophil density in animals subjected to a 60 percent burn than in animals subjected to a 30 percent burn.[4] Invasive burn wound infections due to gram-negative opportunists are most common in pediatric age burn patients, least common in the young adult age group (15 to 40 years), and of intermediate frequency in burn patients above 40 years old.[5]

The local blood supply is the most important host factor in resistance to wound infection. In recognition of that fact, early surgical debridement is carried out in mechanical trauma patients to remove all nonviable tissue susceptible to infection and ensure the viability of the remaining tissue. Burn wound infections are uncommon in partial-thickness burns, in which the local blood supply is only transiently impaired, but characteristically occur in areas of full-thickness injury, in which local tissue damage results in ischemia. The avascularity of tissue coagulated by thermal injury not only makes the protein-rich eschar an ideal site for microbial proliferation but also prevents delivery of systemically administered antibiotics and of the host's immune cells to the site of microbial proliferation within the eschar.[6] The importance of the local blood supply is further indicated by the occurrence of invasive infection in partial-thickness burns and even at split-thickness skin graft donor sites in which local ischemia due to systemic shock has compromised tissue viability.

Additional host factors which influence the occurrence of infection include: (1) wound pH (invasive fungal infections are more common in acidotic patients[7]; (2) wound temperature (coolness not only decreases local blood flow but impairs phagocytic cell matabolism); (3) maceration, which promotes suppuration and may even cause further tissue damage[8]; and (4) the presence of foreign bodies. Although the interval between injury and treatment appears to be most important in mechanical trauma wounds, topical antimicrobial therapy is most effective in preventing the proliferation of wound microorganisms when applied early postburn and is significantly less effective once the burn wound microbial density has exceeded the critical level.

A number of microbial characteristics and properties determine not only the clinical characteristics of a wound infection but the likelihood of invasion and systemic spread. The microbial flora of a burn wound changes across time in a pattern which recapitulates the history of prevalence of life-threatening infections in burn patients. In the immediate postburn period the microbial population of a burn wound is sparse, is localized to the surface, and consists principally of gram-positive cocci. Early postinjury burn wound infection commonly takes the form of cellulitis, most frequently caused by group A beta-hemolytic streptococci, which respond promptly to penicillin therapy.

Although staphylococci may persist on the wound throughout the postburn course, gram-negative organisms become the predominant flora of the burn wound, and by the end of the first postburn week *Pseudomonas* organisms are recoverable from over 60 percent of burn wounds.[9] In burn wounds that are not treated with topical antimicrobial agents, such bacteria proliferate and migrate along hair follicles and other skin appendages, progressively penetrating the eschar to reach the nonviable-viable tissue interface (the subeschar space). Here further proliferation occurs and causes the lysis of denatured collagen, which permits the eschar to slough. If microbial proliferation results in a density which exceeds host defense capacity, invasion of unburned tissue will occur. The critical bacterial density appears to be 10^5 organisms per gram of tissue; invasive infection is rare if the density is below that level even in the immunocompromised burn patient.[10]

Other microbial factors which influence the occurrence of invasion, local tissue destruction, and systemic spread include products of microbial metabolism (e.g., endotoxins, exotoxins, vascular permeability factor, and enzymes)[11] and bacterial motility. Using a murine model McManus et al. found that the seeding of a burn wound with a motile control strain derived from a motile parent strain resulted in the same mortality as occurred with the parent strain, while mortality was significantly reduced when the burn was seeded with a nonmotile mutant of the parent strain.[12] Either intrinsic or therapy-induced microbial resistance to antibiotics not only makes treatment of an existing infection more difficult but may permit development of resistant secondary infections in remote locations. Prior to the development of topical burn wound chemotherapy the uncontrolled proliferation of gram-negative opportunistic bacteria, most often *Pseudomonas* organisms, within the eschar, followed by invasion of viable tissue and systemic spread, was a common occurrence and was the principal cause of death in 60 percent of those burn patients who died.[13]

TOPICAL CHEMOTHERAPY

The studies which defined the pathogenesis of invasive burn wound infection led directly to the development of topical chemotherapeutic agents, which control the proliferation of bacteria in the nonviable eschar and have reduced the incidence of invasive burn wound infection.[14] Three widely used topical agents—mafenide acetate burn cream, 0.5 percent silver nitrate soaks, and silver sulfadiazine burn cream—are of verified effectiveness.[2] All these agents appear to be equally effective when applied to burn wounds before microbial proliferation has generated a significant bacterial density within the eschar. Mafenide acetate burn cream, from which the bacteriostatic agent can freely diffuse into the eschar, is specifically indicated for use in patients in whom delayed institution of topical therapy has permitted growth of a signif-

Table 17-1. Effective Topical Chemotherapeutic Agents for Burn Wound Care

	Mafenide Acetate Burn Cream	Silver Sulfadiazine Burn Cream	Silver Nitrate Soaks
Active component concentration	11.1%	1.0%	0.5%
In vitro spectrum of antibacterial activity	Gram-negative—good Gram-positive—fair Yeast—minimal	Gram-negative— selectively good Gram-positive—good Yeast—good	Gram-negative—good Gram-positive—good Yeast—good
Method of wound care	Exposure	Exposure or light dressing	Occlusive dressings
Advantages	Penetrates eschar Wound appearance readily monitored Easily applied Joint motion unrestricted No gram-negative resistance	Painless Wound appearance readily monitored when exposure method used Easily applied Joint motion unrestricted when exposure method used Greater effectiveness against yeasts	Painless No hypersensitivity reactions No gram-negative resistance Dressings reduce evaporative heat loss Greater effectiveness against yeasts
Disadvantages	Painful on partial-thickness burns Acidosis due to inhibition of carbonic anhydrase Hypersensitivity reactions in 7% of patients	Possible neutropenia (batch-related) Hypersensitivity (infrequent) Limited eschar penetration Resistance of certain gram-negative bacteria Selection of plasmid-mediated multiple antibiotic resistance	Deficits of sodium, potassium, and calcium No eschar penetration Limitation of joint motion by dressings Methemoglobimemia (rare) Argyria (rare) Staining of environment and equipment

icant microbial population within the eschar. Other advantages and limitations of each of the commonly used topical chemotherapeutic agents are listed in Table 17-1. If significant side effects develop while one of the agents is being used, application of that agent should be stopped and topical therapy should be continued with one of the other agents. A knowledge of the characteristics of each topical agent will enable the physician to employ topical therapy with the flexibility necessary to meet the wound care needs of the individual patient. At the present time I utilize alternate application of two of the topical agents (mafenide acetate following the daily morning cleansing and silver sulfadiazine burn cream 12 hours later) to achieve optimum antimicrobial coverage and reduce the incidence of the side effects of both agents.

During two decades of use, year-to-year fluctuation of the sensitivity of burn wound flora to mafenide acetate has been observed but no true resistance has appeared. Although the recently described plasmid-mediated sulfonamide resistance appears to be of little consequence with regard to wound care, such plasmids may also confer resistance to the aminoglycosides, the penicillins, the tetracyclines, chloramphenicol, and even mercurials and may thus severely complicate the treatment of other infections such as pneumonia, which frequently develop in severely burned patients.[15]

The use of topical burn wound chemotherapy has significantly reduced the incidence of invasive burn wound infection and decreased the mortality of patients with burns of up to 60 percent of the total body surface.[13] However, none of the topical antimicrobial agents sterilize the burn wound, and the burn wound flora of individual patients, commonly those with burns of more than 50 percent of the total body surface, may escape from control with resulting invasive burn wound infection.

MONITORING THE BURN WOUND

The incomplete protection provided by topical antimicrobial agents requires that the wounds of every patient be examined on at least a daily basis to identify signs of wound infection. This examination is best carried out when all topical agent has been removed from the wound surface by the daily wound cleansing. Color change of the wound is the most frequent sign of burn wound infection[16] (Fig. 17-1). The initial focal or multifocal dark brown, black, or violaceous discolorations, if untreated, spread to become generalized. Local wound trauma and even the maturation of uninfected eschar can produce tinctorial changes in the wound which mimic those of infection. The most reliable clinical sign of burn wound infection is the conversion of an area of partial-thickness burn to full-thickness necrosis, but severe focal trauma and pressure necrosis may cause similar changes.[17] The other clinical signs of burn wound infection are listed in Table 17-2. As noted, infection may cause unexpectedly rapid eschar separation, but fat liquefaction caused by deep thermal injury may also produce early slough of the eschar. In addition to the previously noted wound changes that may be confused with wound infection, the presence of the eschar per se, edema in the wound, and destruction of the local nerve supply by the burn injury conspire to make the diagnosis of burn wound infection on the basis of clinical signs alone unreliable. This uncertainty necessitates the use of other techniques to differentiate between microbial colonization of the burned tissue and invasion of the viable tissue underlying the burn.

Qualitative surface cultures provide information about the microbial population on the surface of the burn wound but do not provide a reliable assessment of the bacterial density at the nonviable-viable tissue interface.[18] A wound biopsy is the most reliable means by which to differentiate microbial colonization of the eschar from microbial invasion of viable tissue. By use of a scalpel a 500-mg lenticular sample of eschar and underlying and/or adjacent unburned tissue should be obtained from that area of the wound in which the changes indicative of wound infection are the most prominent (Fig. 17-1).

The biopsy specimen should be bisected, with one portion sent to the microbiology laboratory for quantitative culture and the other portion sent to

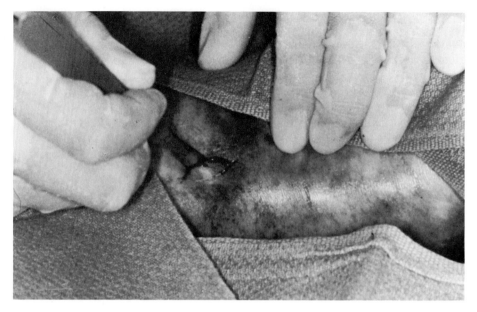

Fig. 17-1   The focal areas of dark discoloration of the burns on the arm of this patient appeared on the fifth postburn day and prompted the biopsy shown here. Note that the biopsy must include unburned viable tissue, as confirmed by the bleeding from the biopsy incision.

the pathology laboratory for histologic examintion. Before bisection the biopsy specimen should be inspected for areas of hemorrhage or saponification in unburned subcutaneous tissue, which occur in association with invasive *Pseudomonas* and phycomycotic infections, respectively. A quantitative culture report of 10^5 organisms per gram of tissue is consistent with but not diagnostic of burn wound infection because of the variability of such culture techniques.[19]

Table 17-2. Clinical Signs of Burn Wound Infection

Focal discoloration of wound (dark red, dark brown, violaceous, or black)
Erythema and edema of unburned skin at wound margin
Conversion of partial-thickness burn to full-thickness necrosis
Hemorrhagic discoloration of subeschar tissue
Presence of green pigment (pyocyanin) in subcutaneous fat[a]
Erythematous nodules in unburned skin (ecthyma gangrenosum)[a]
Unexpectedly rapid separation of eschar
Rapidly spreading subcutaneous edema with central ischemic necrosis[b]
Vesicular lesions in healing or healed partial-thickness burn[c]
Crusted serration of margins of partial-thickness burns[c]

[a] Characteristic of *Pseudomonas* infections
[b] Characteristic of fungal infections
[c] Characteristic of viral infections

Table 17-3. Histologic Signs of Invasive Burn Wound Infection

Microorganisms present in viable tissue:
    Microorganisms in unburned subcutaneous tissue
    Perivascular, perilymphatic, and perineural clustering of
      bacteria
    Microorganisms present within vessels
Dense microbial growth within eschar and in subeschar space
Heightened inflammatory response in unburned tissue
Hemorrhage present in uninjured subcutaneous tissue
Small-vessel thrombosis and ischemic necrosis of unburned tissue
Intracellular viral inclusions

The other half of the specimen is processed for histologic examination by a newly described frozen section technique requiring 30 minutes,[20] with subsequent preparation of permanent sections to provide confirmation of the rapid section diagnosis. The prepared sections are examined to identify the histologic signs of invasive burn wound infection listed in Table 17-3. In order to make a diagnosis of invasive burn wound infection, microorganisms must be identified in unburned tissue—the other histologic findings are only confirmatory or indicative of burn wound infection[21] (Fig. 17-2). The pathlogist should examine the microvasculature of the biopsy specimen with particular care since

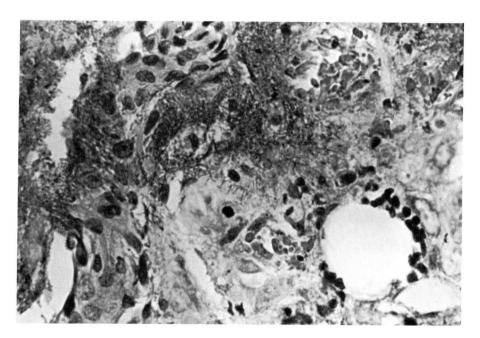

Fig. 17-2 Photomicrograph of biopsy specimen, showing eschar to left and dark staining mass of bacillary organisms in unburned tissue in upper half of field (biopsy stage IIB). Note the "cuffing" of organisms around the vessel at 1 o'clock, characteristic of *Pseudomonas* infections.

Table 17-4. Grading Schema of Burn Wound Biopsies

Microbial Status of Wound	Histologic Characteristics	Biopsy Stage
Colonization	Microorganisms confined to nonviable eschar	I
Invasion	Microorganisms present in and spreading through viable unburned tissue	II
Microinvasion	Microorganisms show limited focal spread	II A
Generalized invasion	Microorganisms widely invading and proliferating	II B
Microvascular invasion	Microorganisms present within capillaries and lymphatics	II C

lymphangitic or vasculitic involvement indicates the possibility of local and even systemic dissemination of the infection.

The microbial status of the burn wound can be graded according to microbial density and depth of penetration. The most important differentiation to be made is that between colonization and invasion. In those biopsies in which only colonization is evident further stratification can be made, ranging from sparse surface colonization to full eschar penetration and proliferation of bacteria in the subeschar space. In those biopsies showing invasive infection further stratification can also be made, ranging from the earliest microinvasion to generalized invasion and microvascular involvement[17] (Table 17-4).

Inappropriate sampling and improper processing can result in either falsely positive or falsely negative biopsy results. The patient's general condition must always be considered when interpreting burn wound biopsy findings. In a patient with systemic signs of sepsis, a negative biopsy report should prompt a repeat biopsy as well as a thorough search for another source of infection. The microbial status of wounds showing any of the clinical changes characteristic of infection should be monitored by serial burn wound biopsies. An increase in microbial density or depth of penetration on sequential biopsies, even in the absence of invasion, indicates a need for alteration of wound care to arrest microbial proliferation.

TREATMENT OF BURN WOUND INFECTION

Changes in both local and systemic treatment are necessary if a diagnosis of invasive burn wound infection is made. If a nondiffusible topical agent is being used, it should be discontinued and application of mafenide acetate burn cream begun, since the bacteriostatic agent in that cream can diffuse into and through the eschar to arrest bacterial proliferation. As guided by the culture and sensitivity results of the institution's microbial surveillance program, systemic antibiotic therapy should be initiated and later adjusted according to the sensitivity testing results of the organisms recovered from the patient in question. General supportive measures to correct hypovolemia, anemia, pulmonary dysfunction, hypothermia, and nutritional deficits should be instituted.

The extent and depth of microbial invasion are the principal determinants of the local treatment required for burn wound infection. The type of infecting organism also influences wound care requirements. Staphylococcal infections, which typically begin as microabscesses that may expand with time, commonly remain localized and seldom extend beyond the subcutaneous tissue. Removal of the burned tissue overlying a staphylococcal abscess is usually sufficient treatment, but it may be necessary to excise extensive areas of overlying eschar to provide adequate drainage of multiple abscesses. Although certain strains of *Proteus* may cause rapidly invasive wound infections, gram-negative burn wound infections are most often caused by *Pseudomonas aeruginosa* and should be treated as such until culture results indicate differently.[22] Other gram-negative opportunists may gain entry to the general circulation through other portals but show little tendency to invade through a surface wound.

Focal or even multifocal invasive *Pseudomonas* burn wound infections involving less than 2 percent of the body surface have been controlled by the subeschar infusion of an antibiotic-containing solution. A solution of normal saline containing a semisynthetic penicillin (10 g of antibiotic and 150 ml of saline) should be injected into the infected tissue twice daily until the focal septic process is arrested, as indicated by desiccation of the necrotic tissue. Extension of the focal infection during such treatment indicates the need for prompt excision of the infected tissue. In patients with more extensive burn wound infections, such subeschar injections should be carried out 6 hours before and again immediately prior to debridement of the infected tissue in order to reduce the risk of systemic dissemination of viable bacteria during the debridement procedure. The high sodium content of the semisynthetic penicillins may necessitate adjustment of fluid therapy to prevent the development of hypernatremia.

As a general rule, all areas of infected burn wound should be surgically debrided. In the majority of instances the investing fascia defines the lower limit of the excision but if invasion of the fascia and underlying muscle has occurred, that tissue should be debrided, and if extensive subfascial extension has occurred (most commonly owing to invasive fungal infection), amputation may be necessary. The excised wounds should be protected from desiccation by application of a biologic dressing or skin substitute or, if one is uncertain as to the adequacy of the excision, application of antimicrobial containing soaks.[23] The patient is returned to the operating room 24 to 48 hours later to assess the adequacy of excision and carry out further debridement as necessary. The wound is closed by skin grafting only when the wound infection has been definitively controlled.

No matter what treatment is employed, the mortality of patients with generalized burn wound infection is almost universal. Clearing of the infection and salvage of patients with focal burn wound infection has been achieved by the use of subeschar antibiotic infusion followed by surgical excision of the infected tissue. The importance of early diagnosis and prompt treatment of burn wound infection is emphasized by the fact that in the survivors reported by McManus et al. the wound infection was diagnosed in the absence of positive blood cultures, i.e., before hematogenous dissemination had occurred.[24]

NONBACTERIAL WOUND INFECTIONS

Effective topical antimicrobial burn wound therapy has reduced the occurrence of bacterial burn wound infection, but nonbacterial burn wound infections have increased in frequency, accounting for approximately 8 percent of burn admissions in recent years. *Candida* species are the most common nonbacterial colonizers of the burn wound but they seldom cause invasive infection.[25] *Aspergillus* and *Fusarium* species are the true fungi that most often colonize burn wounds.[2] These organisms also appear to be of limited invasiveness, causing infections which are typically localized and seldom traverse fascial planes. The Phycomycetes are much more aggressive fungi, characteristically spread rapidly along and across fascial planes, and may even disseminate hematogenously to remote tissues.[26] The propensity of the Phycomycetes to invade vessels and cause thrombosis is responsible for the sudden appearance and rapid centrifugal spread of ischemic necrosis of the wound and for the rapidly expanding peripheral margin of subcutaneous edema characteristic of infections caused by those fungi (Fig. 17-3).

The treatment of fungal burn wound infections is similar to that of bacterial burn wound infections. Wide local excision is carried out for infections involving only the subcutaneous tissue. Subfascial fungal infection of an extremity may require amputation for control.[27] Following initial excision, the wound must be examined daily to determine the adequacy of excision, with further debridement performed as necessary until all foci of infection have been ablated. Extensive subfascial extension of the infection or evidence of systemic spread are indications for systemic administration of antifungal agents. Amphotericin B is the primary agent for the systemic treatment of fungal infections. Although most invasive infections caused by true fungi have shown little response to 5-fluorocytosine alone,[28] a combination of 5-fluorocytosine and amphotericin B has been used, with the dosage of the latter lowered to reduce its toxicity.

Herpes simplex is the virus most frequently causing burn wound infections.[29] Histologic examination of a wound biopsy or lesion scrapings is the most reliable means of diagnosing viral burn wound infections. Burn wound infections due to herpes simplex virus occur most commonly in healing or recently healed partial-thickness burns in the nasolabial area, are commonly self-limited, and require no specific treatment. Fatal systemic herpetic infections, with involvement of liver, spleen, bone marrow, and adrenals, have occurred in a few patients. Unexplained systemic signs of infection in a burn patient who shows extension of cutaneous herpetic lesions should prompt the institution of systemic antiviral therapy. Adenine arabinoside is widely recommended for such use, but its effectiveness remains unconfirmed.

A variable incidence of cytomegalovirus infections has also been reported

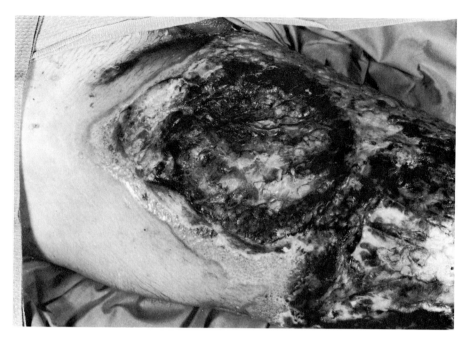

Fig. 17-3 Surgical removal of the burned tissue from the leg of this patient with phycomycotic burn wound infection revealed the extensive involvement of subcutaneous tissue shown here. The intense black discoloration and peripheral edema denote the extent of subcutaneous spread of the infection. Note the typical saponified character of the indurated fatty tissue exposed in the central portion of the lesion on the upper thigh.

in burn patients.[30] The clinical signs of such infections are nonspecific, and diagnosis depends upon a documentation of significant increase in viral antibodies. The clinical importance of cytomegalovirus infections in burn patients is undefined, but recognition of such an infection will prevent the unwarranted administration of antibiotics.

OTHER INFECTIONS

The refractory mortality of patients with burns of more than 60 percent of the body surface and the persistence of infection as the most frequent cause of death in burn patients (even though topical burn wound chemotherapy has significantly reduced the occurrence of invasive burn wound infections) are manifestations of the immunosuppressive effects of thermal injury.[31] Studies by numerous investigators have identified impaired function of all limbs of the immune system following burn injury with the severity of dysfunction proportional to burn size. Burn injury not only destroys the mechanical barrier of the skin but alters the circulating levels of immunoglobulins and various com-

Table 17-5. Characteristics of Pneumonia in Burn Patients

	Hematogenous Pneumonia	Bronchopneumonia
Initial lesion	Capillaritis	Bronchiolitis
Distribution	Random: scattered nodules in all lobes	Nonrandom: dependent areas
Average time of occurrence	Third postburn week	Second postburn week
Radiographic findings		
Early	Solitary nodular infiltrate	Diffuse or multifocal irregular infiltrate
Late	Multiple solitary or coalescent infiltrates	Dense lobular or lobar infiltrate
Mortality	Greater than 80% but infrequently a primary cause of death	Less than 50% but often a primary cause of death

ponents of the complement system, as well as the number and function of all the cellular elements of the immune system. As a consequence of these changes and the microbial colonization of the burn wound, infection has maintained its prominence as a cause of morbidity and mortality in the burn patient.

The effectiveness of topical chemotherapy in reducing the occurrence of invasive burn wound sepsis has not only made pneumonia the most frequent septic complication of burn patients but has brought about a change in the predominant form of pneumonia.[32] Hematogenous pneumonia arising from a site of pulmonary capillaritis caused by the lodgement of bloodborne bacteria was the most common form of pneumonia prior to the use of topical burn wound chemotherapy. This form of pneumonia commonly presents relatively late in the postburn course as a solitary nodular infiltrate evident on chest roentgenogram. If the primary source of infection is unidentified and untreated, subsequent chest roentgenograms may show randomly distributed multiple infiltrates, which may coalesce and become virtually indistinguishable from the infiltrates of bronchopneumonia.

Airborne pneumonia, or bronchopneumonia, has replaced hematogenous pneumonia as the predominant form of pulmonary infection occurring in burn patients. Bronchopneumonia begins as a bronchiolitis, spreads to adjacent alveoli, and if uncontrolled involves a progressively greater volume of lung tissue. This form of pneumonia, commonly diagnosed early in the second postburn week, occurs earlier following injury than does hematogenous pneumonia. As a reflection of its primary pulmonary origin, bronchopneumonia is more commonly a principal cause of death than is hematogenous pneumonia even though the mortality associated with bronchopneumonia is lower than that associated with hematogenous pneumonia (Table 17-5).

The secretions of the bronchial tree of any patient with pneumonia should be sampled for both microscopic and culture examination. The bronchial origin of the sample, i.e., the characteristic presence of a significant number of polymorphonuclear leukocytes and paucity of squamous epithelial cells, should be verified by methylene blue staining. Gram staining should also be carried out to determine the predominant organism, and cultures should be obtained to identify the causative bacteria and antibiotic sensitivities. Inasmuch as the organisms causing pulmonary infections in burn patients are those which predominate on the burn wound and the predominant flora of the burn wound change across time and are institute-specific, the initial choice of antibiotic therapy should be based on the culture and sensitivity results of the microbial surveillance program of the individual burn unit.

The appearance of a nodular infiltrate of apparent hematogenous origin on the chest roentgenogram of a burn patient necessitates a search to identify the primary septic focus.[33] Common sources of such metastatic infection include an infected burn wound, a site of suppurative thrombophlebitis, an inapparent soft tissue abscess, and intraperitoneal infection due to an occult visceral perforation. Treatment of this form of pneumonia includes control and elimination of any identified primary site of infection, systemic administration of specific antibiotics, and, as in the case of bronchopneumonia, ventilatory support as necessary.

Suppurative thrombophlebitis is another septic complication which occurs with relatively high frequency in burn patients. This septic complication, which occurred in 4.2 percent of 4,636 burn patients treated at the U.S. Army Institute of Surgical Research during a 19-year period, can serve as the source of hematogenous pneumonia and acute bacterial endocarditis.[34] The incidence of suppuration in individual veins reflects the frequency of cannulation, and an increase in central vein suppurative thrombophlebitis has paralleled an increase in the use of central vein cannulas in recent years. The causative organisms are the predominant members of the burn wound flora. Recovery of a positive blood culture in a clinically septic patient is the most frequent clinical presentation, and local signs of infection are present in less than half of patients with suppurative thrombophlebitis. In patients with a positive blood culture but no identifiable focus of infection and in patients with roentgenographic signs of hematogenous pneumonia, all currently and previously cannulated veins should be examined and, if indicated, explored for the presence of intraluminal suppuration. If an area of suppurative thrombophlebitis is identified, the entire extent of vein involved in the septic process must be excised following institution of appropriate systemic antibiotic therapy.

SYSTEMIC SEPSIS

The systemic response to injury, seen in its most exaggerated form in patients with extensive burns, is characterized by many of the systemic changes which are produced by infection[35] (Table 17-6). The hyperthermia, tachycardia, and hyperventilation associated with postinjury hypermetabolism and injury-related peripheral neuropathy and disorientation may serve to obscure the systemic response to sepsis or, conversely, may be interpreted as manifestations of a nonexistent infection. Similarly, changes in white blood cell populations and function related to either injury or therapy may be confused with those due to sepsis. Resuscitation-related pulmonary edema may be mistakenly in-

Table 17-6. Systemic and Organ Responses to Injury Mimicking Responses to Sepsis

I. Hypermetabolism
  A. Fever
  B. Tachycardia
  C. Hyperventilation
II. Impaired CNS function
  A. Mentation
  B. Hypothalamic dysfunction
III. Immunosuppression
  A. Depression of humoral factors
  B. Change in number and function of cell populations
IV. Organ dysfunction
  A. Oliguria and variable uremia
  B. Ileus and gastrointestinal mucosal injury
  C. Hematologic changes
    1. Decreased red cell mass
    2. Chemical coagulopathy

terpreted as a response to infection. A familiarity with the whole body and organ system response to injury and careful monitoring of the patient's clinical trajectory by serial examination will minimize the overdiagnosis of infection.

Although fever is an unreliable indicator of infection in injured patients, hypermetabolism per se seldom increases body temperature to levels of 103°F or above, and hypothermia or normothermia in a previously hyperthermic patient is a frequent accompaniment of gram-negative sepsis. The sudden appearance of hyperglycemia and diffuse roentgenographic infiltrates in the absence of carbohydrate loading and fluid loading, respectively, are frequent manifestations of systemic infection and should alert the clinician to that possibility. In the absence of positive cultures, one should use caution in making the diagnosis of systemic sepsis. Conversely, the interpretation of blood culture results in severely injured patients may be difficult; not to be discounted are blood cultures showing growth of multiple organisms or sequential blood cultures showing growth of different organisms in patients with systemic signs of sepsis with or without an identifiable focus of infection. Such results reflect the immunologic impairment of the patient, not a technical error, and mandate systemic administration of multiple antibiotics to provide coverage of all the recovered organisms.

CONTROVERSIES AND FUTURE DIRECTIONS

Excision of the burn wound soon after injury is being performed with increasing frequency to reduce the risk of invasive burn wound infection by removing the nonviable eschar and to reduce the incidence of other infections by achieving early wound closure, thereby limiting the duration of systemic stress and organ dysfunction. A beneficial effect of burn wound excision on burn patient mortality remains unconfirmed. The use of historic controls and failure to randomize patients have flawed those studies claiming that excision improves survival. Recent studies have shown a reduction in hospital stay in patients with burns of less than 20 percent of the total body surface, but no improvement in mortality has been observed in patients with more extensive burns.[36,37]

One of the most severe limitations of excision therapy is the paucity of available donor sites for wound closure in patients with extensive burns. A variety of biologic dressings, skin substitutes, and, most recently, tissue culture–derived epidermal sheets have been utilized for the closure of excised wounds, but the limitations of such membranes restrict their usefulness. Technological modification of skin substitutes and immunologic modification of tissue culture–derived membranes may overcome the current limitations of those materials and enhance their effectiveness.[38]

The importance of early diagnosis and prompt treatment of infection and the time constraints and other limitations of available methods of diagnosing infection in severely injured patients serve to focus attention on the development of more sensitive methods of diagnosis. The identification of humoral indicators of infection and the observation that decreased neutrophil membrane–associated oxidase activity is prognostic of a fatal outcome, as well as those studies which have related outcome to circulating protease levels as assessed by a chromogenic assay, may ultimately lead to the development of more sensitive and rapid means of diagnosing infection (R. C. Allen, unpublished data, Powanda et al.,[39] and Smith-Erichson et al.[40]).

The susceptibility of the badly injured patient to infection by virtually any microorganism, the persistence of infection as the most frequent cause of morbidity and mortality in severely injured patients, and the identification of the global immunosuppression due to severe injury has focused attention on means to enhance the immune capabilities of the compromised host. Vaccines against whole organisms, specific components of organisms, and toxins have been studied, as have a large variety of immunomodulators and serologic agents. The protection afforded by many of the agents appears to be species-specific,[41] and the inadequacy of many of the reported trials makes interpretation of the results difficult.

The wide spectrum of antibody content of an IgG preparation which can be given systemically has prompted clinical trials of that material, which are now underway.[42] In summary, the protection afforded by all present-day adjunctive infection therapy is imperfect, but it may well be that administration of multiple immunomodulators will improve host defense capacity and reduce the mortality due to infection in injured patients.

REFERENCES

1. Pruitt BA Jr: The universal trauma model. Scudder Oration, Bull American College of Surgeons, in press
2. Pruitt BA Jr: The burn patient. II. Later care and complications of thermal injury. Curr Prob Surg 16(5):6, 1979

3. Yurt RW, McManus AT, Mason AD Jr, et al: Increased susceptibility to infection related to extent of burn injury. Arch Surg 119:183, 1984

4. Yurt RW, Pruitt BA Jr: Decreased wound neutrophils and indiscrete margination in the pathogenesis of wound infection. Surgery 98:191, 1985

5. Pruitt BA Jr, Curreri PW: The burn wound and its care. Arch Surg 103:461, 1971

6. Order SE, Moncrief JA: Vascular destruction and revascularization in severe thermal injuries. Surg Forum 15:37, 1964

7. Espinosa CG, Halkias DG: Pulmonary mucormycosis as a complication of chronic salicylate poisoning. Am J Clin Pathol 80:508, 1983

8. Wallace AB: Treatment of burns. A return to basic principles. Br J Plastic Surg 1:232, 1948–49

9. Pruitt BA Jr, Lindberg RB: *Pseudomonas aeruginosa* infections in burn patients. p. 339. In Doggett RG (ed): *Pseudomonas aeruginosa*. Academic Press, New York, 1979

10. Moncrief JA, Lindberg RB, Switzer WE, et al: Use of topical antibacterial therapy in the treatment of the burn wound. Arch Surg 92:558, 1966

11. Pruitt BA Jr: Infections of burn and other wounds caused by *Pseudomonas aeruginosa*. p. 55. In Sabath LD (ed): *Pseudomonas aeruginosa*: The Organism, Diseases It Causes, and Their Treatment. Hans Huber, Bern, Switzerland, 1980

12. McManus AT, Moody EE, Mason AD: Bacterial motility: a component in experimental *Pseudomonas aeruginosa* burn wound sepsis. Burns 6:236, 1980

13. Pruitt BA Jr, O'Neill JA Jr, Moncrief JA, et al: Successful control of burn wound sepsis. JAMA 203:1054, 1968

14. Lindberg RB, Brame RE, Moncrief JA, et al: Prevention of invasive *Pseudomonas aeruginosa* infection in seeded burned rats by use of a topical sulfamylon cream. Fed Proc 23:388, 1964

15. McManus AT, Denton CL, Mason AD Jr: Machanisms of in vitro sensitivity to sulfadiazine silver. Arch Surg 118:161, 1983

16. Pruitt BA Jr, Lindberg RB, McManus WF, et al: Current approach to prevention and treatment of *Pseudomonas aeruginosa* infections in burn patients. Rev Infect Dis 5:Suppl. 5, S889, 1983

17. Pruitt BA Jr: Burns in soft tissues. p. 113. In Polk HC (ed): Infection in the Surgical Patient. Churchill Livingstone, London, 1982

18. Pruitt BA Jr, McManus AT: Opportunistic infections in severely burned patients. Am J Med 76(3A):146, 1984

19. Woolfrey BF, Fox JM, Quall CO: An evaluation of burn wound quantitative microbiology. I. Quantitative eschar cultures. Am J Clin Pathol 75:532, 1981

20. Kim SH, Hubbard GB, McManus WF, et al: Frozen section technique to evaluate early burn wound biopsy: a comparison with the rapid section technique. J Trauma, in press

21. Pruitt BA Jr, Foley FD: The use of biopsies in burn patient care. Surgery 73:887, 1973

22. McManus AT, McCloud CG Jr, Mason AD Jr: Experimental *Proteus mirabilis* burn surface infection. Arch Surg 117:187, 1982

23. Curreri PW, Shuck JM, Flemma RJ, et al: Treatment of burn wounds with 5 percent aqueous sulfamylon and occlusive dressings. Surg Forum 20:506, 1969

24. McManus WF, Goodwin CW Jr, Pruitt BA Jr: Subeschar treatment of burn wound infection. Arch Surg 111:291, 1983

25. Bruck HM, Nash G, Stein JM, et al: Studies on the occurrence and significance of yeast and fungi in the burn wound. Ann Surg 146:108, 1972

26. Bruck HM, Nash G, Foley FD, et al: Opportunistic fungal infection of the burn wound with *Phycomycetes* and *Aspergillus*. Arch Surg 102:476, 1971

27. Pruitt BA Jr: Phycomycotic infections. p. 664. In Alexander JW (ed): Problems in General Surgery. J. B. Lippincott, Philadelphia, 1984

28. Wheeler MS, McGinnis MR, Shell WA, et al: *Fusarium* infection in burn patients. Am J Clin Pathol 75:304, 1981

29. Foley FD, Greenawald KA, Nash G, et al: Herpesvirus infection in burned patients. N Engl J Med 282:652, 1970

30. Pruitt BA Jr: The diagnosis and treatment of infection in the burn patient. AB Wallace Memorial Lecture, British Burn Association Meeting. Burns 11(2):79, 1984

31. Pruitt BA Jr: Opportunistic infections in the severely injured patient. Proc of the Second International Symposium on the Pathophysiology of Combined Injury and Trauma, Wintergreen, Va. (in press)

32. Pruitt BA Jr, Flemma RJ, DiVincenti FC, et al: Pulmonary complications in burn patients: A comparative study of 697 patients. J Thorac Cardiovasc Surg 59:7, 1970

33. Pruitt BA Jr, DiVincenti FC, Mason AD Jr, et al: The occurrence and significance of pneumonia and other pulmonary complications in burn patients: Comparison of conventional and topical treatments. J Trauma 10:519, 1970

34. Pruitt BA Jr, McManus WF, Kim SH, et al: Diagnosis and treatment of cannula related intravenous sepsis in burn patients. Ann Surg 191:546, 1980

35. Pruitt BA Jr, Goodwin CW Jr: Nutritional management of the seriously ill burn patient. p. 63. In Winters RW, Green HL (eds): Nutritional Support of the Seriously Ill Patient. Academic Press, New York, 1983

36. Engrav LH, Heimbach DM, Reus JL, et al: Early excision and grafting vs. non-operative treatment of burns of indeterminant depth: A randomized prospective study. J Trauma 23:1001, 1983

37. Gray DT, Pine RW, Harnar TJ, et al: Early surgical excision versus conventional therapy in patients with 20 to 40 percent burns: A comparative study. Am J Surg 144:76, 1982

38. Pruitt BA Jr, Levine NS: Characteristics and uses of biologic dressings and skin substitutes. Arch Surg 119:312, 1984

39. Powanda MC, Dubois J, Villareal Y, et al: Detection of potential biochemical indicators of infection in the burned rat. J Lab Clin Med 97:672, 1981

40. Smith-Erichson N, Aasen AO, Amundsen E: Treatment of sepsis in the surgical patient evaluated by means of chromogenic peptide substrate assays. Acta Chir Scand [Suppl] 509:33, 1982

41. Waymack JP, Miskell P, Gonce SJ, et al: Immunomodulators in the treatment of peritonitis in burned and malnourished animals. Surgery 96:308, 1984

42. Shirani KZ, Vaughan GM, McManus AT, et al: Replacement therapy with modified immunoglobulin G in burn patients: Preliminary kinetic studies. Am J Med 76(3A):175, 1984

18 Antibiotics: Future Directions by Understanding Structure–Function Relationships

J. Davis Allan, Jr.
George M. Eliopoulos
Robert C. Moellering, Jr.

Following the introduction of penicillin in the 1940s the focus of antibiotic development was primarily concerned with the discovery and isolation of new, naturally occurring antibacterial compounds. While obviously tedious work, such research led to the discovery of all the major classes of clinically useful antibiotics, including cephalosporins, tetracyclines, macrolides, aminoglycosidic aminocyclitols, chloramphenicol, polypeptide antibiotics such as vancomycin, the polymyxins, and bacitracin. However, over the past 10 to 15 years the major emphasis in antibiotic research has shifted toward understanding structure-function relationships and using such knowledge to modify the basic structure of the already known antibiotics to produce agents with improved characteristics.

While there has been some development of chloramphenicol analogs, macrolides, tetracyclines, and antifolates, the vast majority of important advances in recent years have involved the β-lactams, aminoglycosidic aminocyclitols, and more recently the quinolones. For this reason this chapter focuses on recent developments in our understanding of structure and function of these three classes of antibacterial compounds.

However, there have been several noteworthy discoveries of novel agents. Two are technically β-lactams but are significantly different in structure from the penicillins (penams) and cephalosporins (cephems). These two new subclasses of β-lactams are the monobactams and thienamycins (carbapenems). A third new class of antibacterial agents, the lipopeptides, will also be discussed. Though related to polypeptide antibiotics, the lipopeptides have a novel structure and appear to have a novel mechanism for action.

NEWER AGENTS WITH NOVEL STRUCTURES

Monobactams

Although monobactams are members of the large β-lactam family of compounds (Fig. 18-1), their monocyclic nuclear structure differs markedly from the bicyclic nuclei of penicillins or cephalosporins. The first monocyclic β-lactams discovered were the nocardiocins, which are extremely poor antibacterial compounds.[1] The naturally occurring monobactams, discovered in 1979, have a β-lactam ring that is activated relative to the nocardiocins by the presence of a sulfonic acid group at the 1 position of the ring.[1-3] Although the naturally occurring monobactams exhibit relatively weak antibacterial activity, a large series of monobactam structures have been produced, some with potent antibacterial activity.[1-3] The various modifications of the monobactam nucleus and their effects on in vitro activity and β-lactamase activity will be discussed

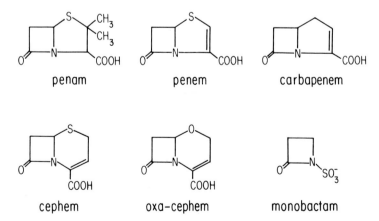

Fig. 18-1 Nuclear structure of the major classes of β-lactam antibiotics. (Reproduced with permission from Allan JD, Eliopoulos GM, Moellering RC Jr: Expanding spectrum of beta-lactam antibiotics. Adv Intern Med 31:119, 1986.)

in subsequent sections of this chapter. However, monobactams appear to have the same mechanism of action as the penicillins and cephalosporins and have been shown to bind to and inactivate penicillin-binding proteins (PBPs) of both gram-negative and gram-positive bacteria[4-6] The monocyclic β-lactam nucleus has also been activated by placement of carboxyl or phosphate moieties at the 1 position, but at this time the other monobactams appear more promising.[3]

Thienamycins

Thienamycins are a newly discovered class of compounds that, like the monobactams, are in the family of β-lactams. Like the penicillins and cephalosporins, the thienamycins are bicyclic but are carbapenems rather than penams or cephems (Fig. 18-1). Carbapenems are similar to penams (penicillins) but differ in having a carbon atom substituted for the sulfur atom and in having an unsaturated 2,3 carbon-carbon bond. Thienamycin is a naturally occurring product of *Streptomyces cattleya* and exhibits remarkable in vitro potency against a very broad spectrum of bacteria.[7,8] However, thienamycin is chemically unstable in concentrated solution or in solid form.[8] For this reason a semisynthetic derivative of thienamycin, N-formimidoyl thienamycin, or imipenem (Figs. 18-2, 18-3) was produced, which is stable and allowed further development leading to a pharmaceutical preparation.[8]

Imipenem exhibits extreme in vitro potency against a remarkably broad range of both gram-positive and gram-negative cocci and bacilli, including anaerobes, *Pseudomonas aeruginosa*, and enterococci.[9-12] Only *Pseudomonas maltophilia* is usually resistant to imipenem by virtue of being able to produce an unusual β-lactamase capable of hydrolyzing it.[13] With the exception of this enzyme and a recently reported, apparently rare enzyme in *Bacteroides fragilis*, imipenem is resistant to hydrolysis by virtually all other β-lactamases produced by bacteria.[14,15] In fact, imipenem markedly inhibits many different types of β-lactamase produced by gram-negative bacteria, probably by functioning as a competitive substrate.[16,17] However, like cefoxitin, imipenem appears to be a potent inducer of the chromosomal β-lactamase (Richmond and Sykes's type 1) that is present in a large number of gram-negative bacilli.[18-21] Owing to imipenem's exceptional intrinsic and broad-spectrum activity, it is unlikely that it will be combined with a second β-lactam (which might be susceptible to hydrolysis by the induced β-lactamase). Therefore, there would seem to be little clinical potential for antagonism with imipenem. Unfortunately, imipenem is rapidly hydrolyzed by a renal dehydropeptidase and must be administered with an inhibitor (cilastatin) of this enzyme.[8]

Lipopeptide Antibiotics

A21978C$_1$ (Fig. 18-4) is a natural product of *Streptomyces vaseosporus*, which is representative of a new class of cyclic polypeptide antibiotics.[22-24] While generally similar to vancomycin or teichoplanin by virtue of being a

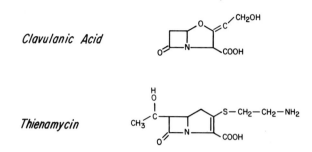

Clavulanic Acid

Thienamycin

Fig. 18-2 Structural formulas of clavulanic acid and thienamycin.

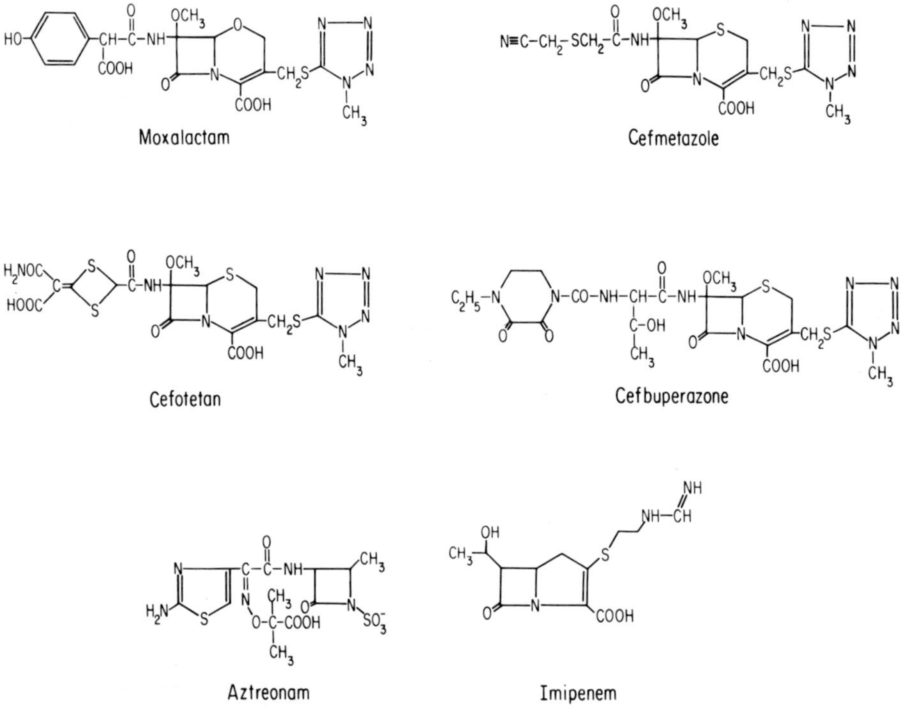

Moxalactam

Cefmetazole

Cefotetan

Cefbuperazone

Aztreonam

Imipenem

Fig. 18-3 Structural formulas of several new β-lactam antibiotics. (Modified from Allan JD, Eliopoulos GM, Moellering RC Jr: Expanding spectrum of beta-lactam antiobiotics. Adv Intern Med 31:119, 1986.)

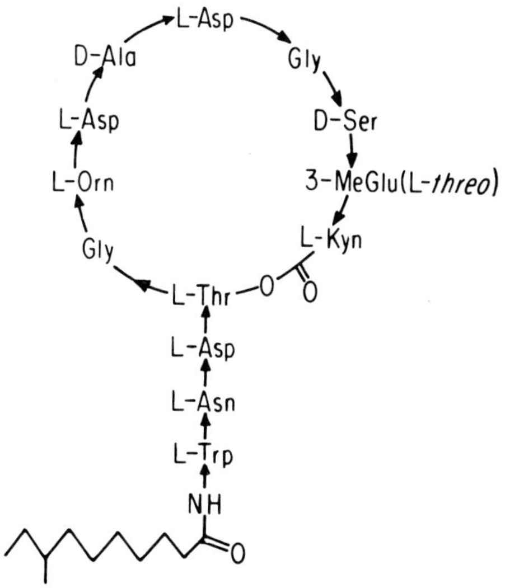

Fig. 18-4 Structural formula of A21978C$_1$. (Eliopoulos GM, Thauvin C, Gerson B, Moellering RC Jr: In vitro activity and mechanism of action of A 21978C$_1$. Antimicrob Agents Chemother 27:357, 1985.)

polypeptide, A21978C$_1$ differs from these compounds in that it has a much lower molecular weight and a large lipid side chain.[22-24] Derivatives of this compound have been produced by varying the lipid constituent (e.g., LY146032).[25] A21978C$_1$ also appears to differ from vancomycin and teichoplanin in its mechanism of action, which is not fully understood although its major target appears to be cell wall biosynthesis.[22,26] A21978C$_1$ exhibits in vitro activity that is comparable with or superior to that of vancomycin against a broad range of gram-positive bacteria, including enterococci, methicillin-resistant *Staphylococcus aureus* and *Staphylococcus epidermidis*, and penicillin-resistant pneumococci and viridans streptococci, but is less active than either vancomycin or teichoplanin against *Listeria monocytogenes*.[22-24] A potentially important difference between A21978C$_1$ and these other polypeptide antibiotics is that A21978C$_1$ exerts bactericidal activity against enterococci at concentrations close to the level at which it exerts bacteriostatic activity.[22]

RECENT MODIFICATIONS OF PREVIOUS STRUCTURES

Greater understanding of the chemistry and structure-function relationships involved in several of the classes of antibiotics, particularly the β-lactams, has enabled pharmaceutical chemists to produce a large number of compounds whose antibacterial or pharmacokinetic properties could in some degree be predicted in advance. The goals of such modifications of existing structures are to produce antibacterial agents with improved characteristics: increased or different intrinsic antibacterial activity, ability to circumvent mechanisms of bacterial antimicrobial resistance, improved pharmacokinetics, and improved absorption following oral administration. The greatest advances along these lines have occurred in the β-lactam class of antibiotics.

Modifications to Change Intrinsic Activity

β-Lactams

Alteration in the structure of the various β-lactam compounds may lead to improved intrinsic activity by altering the affinity of the β-lactam for target PBPs.[27,28] For gram-negative organisms in which the outer membrane represents a potential barrier that may prevent the β-lactam from reaching its target in the inner membrane, improved activity may also be produced by alterations that facilitate transit through the outer membrane.[29-31] Although the specific effect that a given side-chain substitution will exert is in large part a function of the entire β-lactam molecule, there is often enough similarity that knowledge derived from experience with a given substituent in one β-lactam structure can frequently be applied to the design of a new antibiotic belonging to a different class of β-lactams. However, application of knowledge gained with penam and cephem antibiotics has been less predictive of the effect of some substituents or side chains in monobactams.[3,32,33]

One of the earliest modifications of the penam nucleus was the addition of an amino group to the phenyl group that terminates the acyl side chain of penicillin. The resultant antibiotic, ampicillin (Fig. 18-5), exhibits significantly enhanced activity against many gram-negative bacteria, primarily owing to an improved ability to penetrate the outer membrane of these organisms.[29,30]

Significant antipseudomonal activity was obtained by substitution of a carboxylic acid group (instead of the amino group) at the same position in the acyl side chain of the penam nucleus. The resulting compounds, carbenicillin and ticarcillin, exhibit diminished activity against gram-positive organisms as compared with ampicillin or penicillin (Fig. 18-5).

It is clear that the acylamino side chain appears to be the major determinant of activity in the penam subclass. The new antipseudomonal penicillins, namely azlocillin, mezlocillin, piperacillin, and apalcillin, have all resulted from substitutions at the acylamino group of ampicillin (Fig. 18-6). As a rule these agents exhibit activity comparable with or superior to that of ticarcillin or carbenicillin against *P. aeruginosa*, have improved activity against many Enterobacteriaceae, and retain activity similar to that of ampicillin against most gram-positive organisms.[32-37]

Altered affinity for PBPs as a mechanism for altered intrinsic activity following structural modification of a β-lactam is perhaps best exemplified by amdinocillin. Amdinocillin differs structurally from penicillin by having an amidino group substituted at the 6 position of the penam nucleus (Fig. 18-6). As a result of this modification amdinocillin binds nearly exclusively to PBP2 of *Escherichia coli*.[27,28]

In many instances the exact mechanism by which a structural alteration

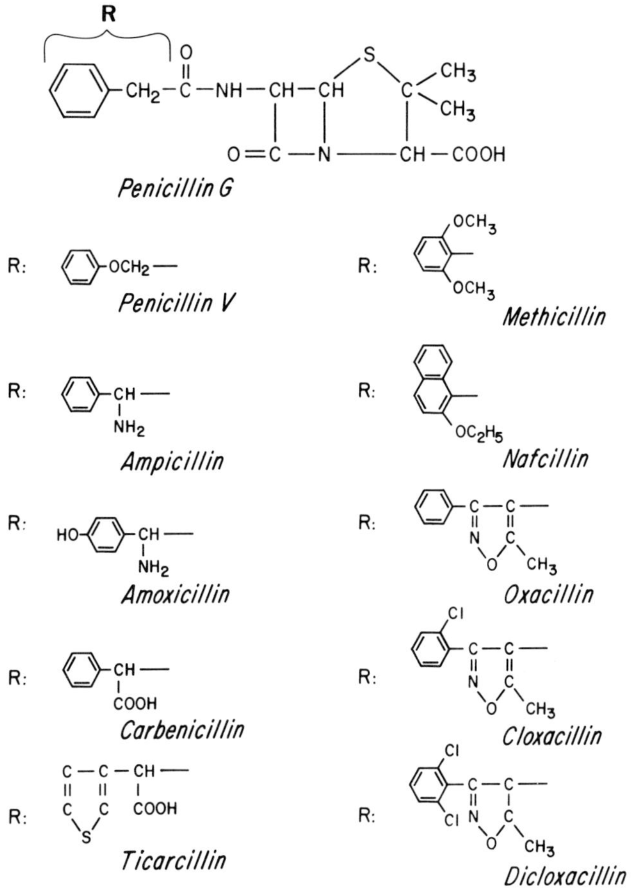

R

Penicillin G

R: Penicillin V

R: Ampicillin

R: Amoxicillin

R: Carbenicillin

R: Ticarcillin

R: Methicillin

R: Nafcillin

R: Oxacillin

R: Cloxacillin

R: Dicloxacillin

Fig. 18-5 Structural formulas of various penicillins.

produces the altered intrinsic activity of a β-lactam is not well understood since it is likely to be a result of a number of different effects.

The cephalosporin nucleus has been extremely amenable to a large number of modifications in an effort to produce compounds with greater intrinsic activity, as is evidenced by the rapidly expanding array of new cephalosporins. Substitutions of the cephem nucleus have primarily been made at positions 3 and 7 and on the acyl side chain (Figs. 18-7, 18-8). In general, substitutions of the acyl side chain have had the greatest effect on the intrinsic activity of the molecule although several substitutions at the 3 position have also had important effects on activity. For example, the methylthiotetrazole group at the 3 position of the cephem nucleus in cefamandole (Fig. 18-7) is associated with the significantly enhanced activity of this compound against gram-negative organisms, as compared with older cephalosporins lacking this structure.[32,33] Similar effects on activity have been demonstrated for several newer β-lactams

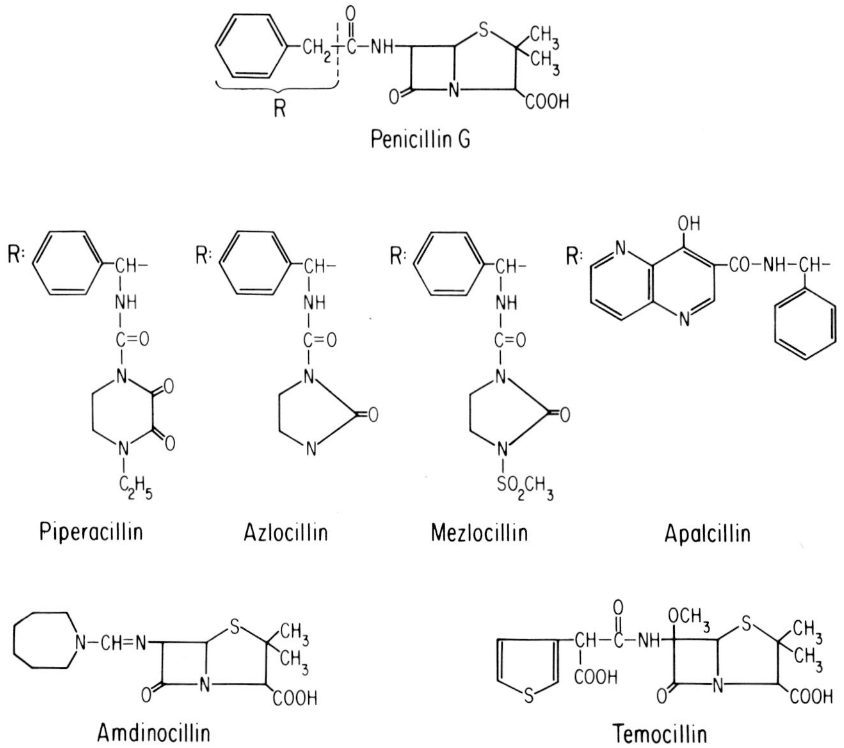

Fig. 18-6   Structural formulas of newer penicillins. (Allan JD, Eliopoulos GM, Moellering RC Jr: Expanding spectrum of beta-lactam antibiotics. Adv Intern Med 31:119, 1986.)

that also incorporate the methylthiotetrazole ring at the 3 position, including moxalactam, cefoperazone, cefmenoxime, cefmetazole, cefotetan, and cefbuperazone (Figs. 18-3, 18-8). However, this moiety also appears to be responsible for disulfuram-like reactions and prolongation of the prothrombin time.[33]

A very important structural modification of the cephalosporins has been the inclusion of an aminothiazolyl group in the acyl side chain of antibiotics such as cefotaxime (Fig. 18-8). This substitution greatly increases activity of the basic cephem nucleus against gram-negative bacilli and appears to affect the affinity for PBPs and perhaps the ability of the resulting β-lactam to penetrate the outer cell envelope of gram-negative bacilli.[32,33] The aminothiazolyl group has been a major part of the development of the third-generation cephalosporins and is present in many other cephalosporins in addition to cefotaxime, including ceftizoxime, ceftriaxone, cefmenoxime, ceftazidime, and cefpirome (HR810).

A major deficiency in the spectrum of most of the older cephalosporins is the lack of useful activity against *P. aeruginosa*. Several cephalosporins with significant antipseudomonal activity have been synthesized, including cefop-

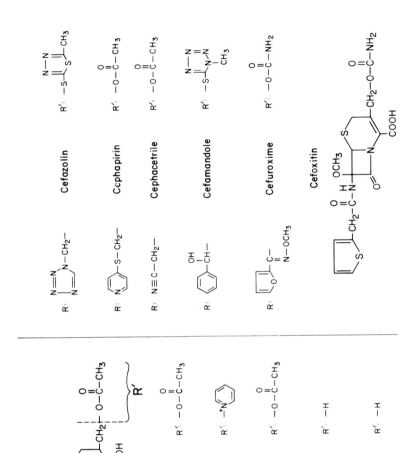

Fig. 18-7 Structural formulas of the older cephalosporins.

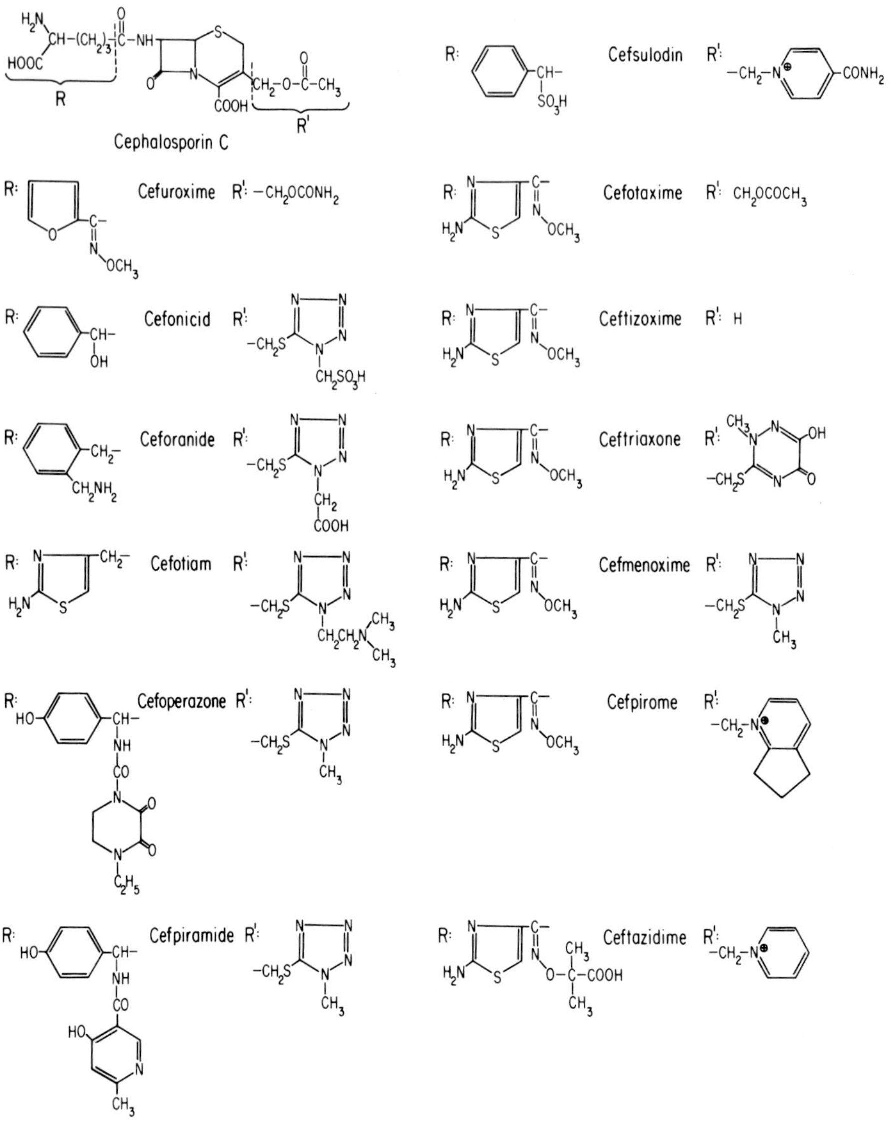

Fig. 18-8 Structural formulas of selected recently developed cephalosporins. (Allan JD, Eliopoulos GM, Moellering RC Jr: Expanding spectrum of beta-lactam antibiotics. Adv Intern Med 31:119, 1986.)

erazone, ceftazidime, cefsulodin and cefpiramide. The 2,3-dioxopiperazine moiety that contributes to the antipseudomonal activity of piperacillin was introduced onto the acyl side chain of the cephem nucleus, producing cefoperazone (Fig. 18-8), a cephalosporin that exhibits significant antipseudomonal activity.[32,33,38] A similar, though not identical, structure is present in cefpiramide and is probably responsible for the activity of this agent against *P. aeruginosa.*[36] Ceftazidime has a carboxypropyl group on the acyl side chain, which is reminiscent of the carboxyl group on carbenicillin and ticarcillin and is probably a major factor in this cephalosporin's antipseudomonal activity.[32,33] Similarly, the sulfonic acid group on the acyl side chain of cefsulodin (Fig. 18-8) is consistent with the observation in penicillins of the importance of an acidic function at this position in providing antipseudomonal activity.[32,33]

Another desirable goal in the further development of the cephalosporins is to produce structures that exhibit useful activity against the enterococcus. Cefathiamidine is a new cephalosporin, with a novel acyl side chain, that does exhibit significant antienterococcal activity.[39] The specific structural features of the acyl side chain that result in this improved activity against enterococci have not yet been elucidated.

Apart from manipulating side chains, it has been possible to alter activity characteristics of the cephems by altering components of the cephem nucleus itself. For example, the substitution of an oxygen atom for the sulfur atom in the cephem nucleus results in a new class of β-lactams, the 1-oxacephems, which includes moxalactam (Figs. 18-1, 18-3). This shift from sulfur to oxygen has several important consequences. It not only results in a structure with greatly enhanced activity against gram-negative bacteria but also in a structure that is more susceptible to hydrolysis by β-lactamase and has diminished activity against gram-positive bacteria.[32,33,40] It may be possible to develop a number of novel antibiotics based on the 1-oxacephem nucleus.

The development of the monobactams has benefited in many ways from the understanding of structure-function relationships elucidated in the development of the penicillins and especially the cephalosporins. As previously discussed, the naturally occurring monobactams exhibit weak antibacterial activity. It was therefore necessary to modify these agents in order to develop compounds with potential clinical usefulness. Literally thousands of such modifications have been made.[3] The compound that has undergone the most extensive testing and development is aztreonam (Fig. 18-3). Aztreonam was produced by α methylation at the 4 position as well as by incorporation of the aminothiazolyl and oxime moieties, so successfully used in the cephalosporins, resulting in an acyl side chain essentially identical to that found in ceftazidime.[3] Aztreonam exhibits marked activity against a broad spectrum of gram-negative bacteria, including *P. aeruginosa*, but exhibits little or no activity against anaerobes or gram-positive bacteria.[3,5,36] A number of newer monobactams have been produced by using different acyl side chains, some borrowed from those older penams and cephems, such as penicillin, piperacillin, and cephalothin, that exhibit significantly improved activity against gram-positive bacteria.[3]

Quinolones

Nalidixic acid was synthesized in 1962 and is the prototypical drug of a class of antimicrobial agents referred to as *quinolones* (Fig. 18-9). Nalidixic acid inhibits the enzyme DNA gyrase, which regulates supercoiling of DNA

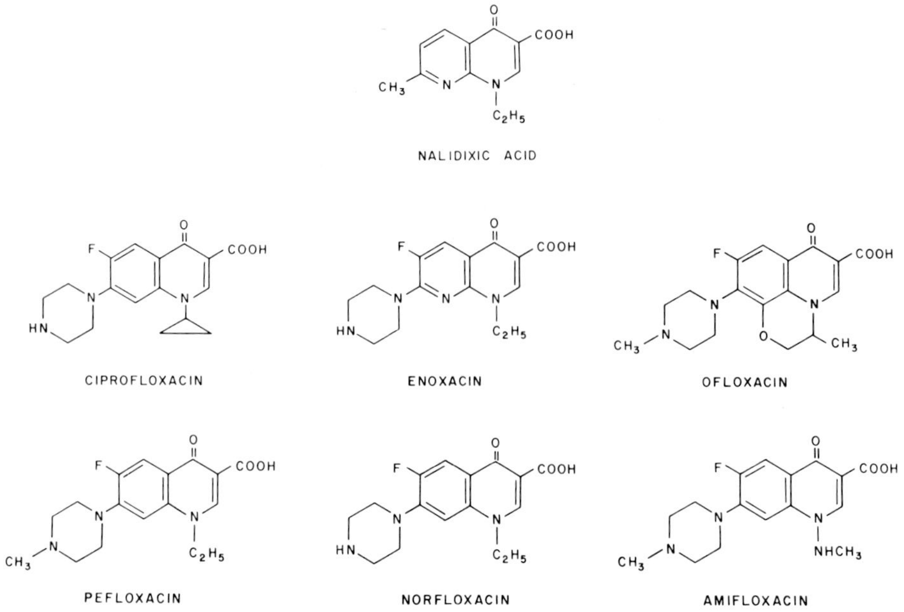

Fig. 18-9　Structural formulas of various quinolones and naphthyridines.

helices, and inhibition of this enzyme impairs DNA synthesis in bacteria.[41] Nalidixic acid is active in vitro against a wide range of gram-negative bacilli, with the notable exception of *P. aeruginosa*, but is inactive against gram-positive bacteria. Cinoxacin and oxolinic acid, which are older structural analogs of nalidixic acid, provided some advantages in terms of in vivo activity, but the spectrum of activity of these drugs is essentially identical to that of nalidixic acid. Recent advances in the understanding of structure-function relationships in this class of compounds have led to the synthesis of several new analogs with improved intrinsic antibacterial activity and with broad spectra of activity, including activity against *P. aeruginosa* and gram-positive organisms.

　Most of the newly developed quinolones contain a nucleus consisting of two fused six-membered rings (Fig. 18-9).[41] The quinolinecarboxylic acids contain one nitrogen atom at the 1 position of the bicyclic nucleus. Other analogs contain a second nitrogen atom in the nucleus and are known as 1,8-azaquinolines or naphthyridines. In general, the quinoline analogs are more potent in vitro than the corresponding naphthyridine compounds. The new and more potent compounds differ from the older drugs in having a fluorine atom at the 6 position and a piperazinyl constituent at the 7 position.[41] Both these substitutions result in enhanced activity against gram-negative bacteria, including *P. aeruginosa*, but also against staphylococci, enterococci, and other gram-positive bacteria.[42] Several new compounds are currently under development, including ciprofloxacin, enoxacin, norfloxacin, pefloxacin, and amifloxacin. All these drugs demonstrate greater potency against enteric gram-negative bacilli and gram-negative cocci than they do against gram-positive bacteria. Addition of a substituted pyrrolidine group for the piperazinyl moiety has led to the synthesis of a compound, designated CI-934, which shows enhanced activity against the gram-positive cocci.[43]

Modifications to Surmount Resistance

Perhaps the most important mechanism by which bacteria acquire resistance to antimicrobial agents is through the production of enzymes capable of inactivating antibiotics. Owing to the impressive ability of bacteria to produce different enzymes in response to new antibiotics, a major impetus for understanding structure-function relationships of antibiotics is provided by the need to produce compounds that preserve their intrinsic activity but are resistant to inactivation by these enzymes. In general, the two classes that have allowed the greatest success in attempts to produce compounds resistant to destruction by bacterial enzymes have been the β-lactams and the aminoglycosidic aminocyclitols.

β-Lactams

As a rule the penam structure has been more difficult than the cephem structure to protect from hydrolysis without causing an attendant loss of intrinsic activity.[32,44] However, one of the earliest modifications of the penam nucleus was the incorporation of a bulky moiety into the acyl side chain of penicillin, resulting in a compound, methicillin, that was resistant to hydrolysis by penicillinase-producing strains of *S. aureus* (Fig. 18-5). Nafcillin and all the isoxazolyl penicillins have similar modifications at this same position. Essentially only one other penicillin significantly resistant to hydrolysis by β-lactamase has been developed that retains useful antibacterial activity. This antibiotic, temocillin, which differs from ticarcillin because of the presence of a methoxy group in the 6 position (Fig. 18-6), will be discussed subsequently.[32]

One of the most important structural relationships to be identified in the cephems has been the effect of a methoxy group at the 7 position in increasing the resistance of the β-lactam ring to hydrolysis. The first β-lactam to be introduced for wide clinical use that incorporated this structural component was cefoxitin (Fig. 18-7).[32,33] Cefoxitin is extremely stable to most of the β-lactamases produced by gram-negative bacilli and therefore enjoys a significantly expanded spectrum of activity over the other cephems that do not incorporate this structural feature. However, in general the methoxy group in this position in cephems significantly reduces the activity of the β-lactam compound against gram-positive bacteria.[32,33,45,46] This structural feature is present in moxalactam, cefotetan, cefmetazole, and cefbuperazone, as well as cefoxitin (Figs. 18-3, 18-7, 18-8). All cephems that have the 7-methoxy group are considered cephamycins. As mentioned previously, the methoxy moiety has also been employed in one penam, temocillin. This penicillin is very stable to many of the gram-negative β-lactamases and predictably has an expanded spectrum of activity against most gram-negative bacilli, but it is relatively inactive against *P. aeruginosa* and is less active than most other penicillins against gram-positive bacteria.[33,44] A similar structural feature that has been widely utilized in cephalosporins is a methoxy group in the acyl side chain (methoxyimino cephalosporins). This feature also improves the resistance of the β-lactam ring to hydrolysis by β-lactamase and is present in a large number of cephalosporin antibiotics, including cefuroxime, cefotaxime, ceftizoxime, ceftriaxone, cefmenoxime, and cefpirome (HR810) (Fig. 18-8).[32,33,44]

In terms of stabilizing the monobactam nucleus, the lessons learned from development of the cephalosporins have been more difficult to apply. The naturally occurring monobactams are all highly resistant to hydrolysis by β-lactamase but have poor intrinsic activity.[1,3,44] Both characteristics are in part due to the presence of a methoxy group at the 3 position, which is analogous to the 6 position in penams and 7 position in cephems.[3,44] Therefore, the methoxy group used so effectively in the cephems unfortunately had to be discarded in order to produce a monobactam with useful antibacterial activity.[3] The semisynthetic monobactams are rendered resistant to hydrolysis by α methylation at the 4 position. This feature is incorporated into the structure of aztreonam, accounting for its β-lactamase stability (Fig. 18-3).[3]

A different approach to the problem of resistance to β-lactam activity due to β-lactamase production by bacteria is to develop compounds that are potent inhibitors of β-lactamase. A number of such compounds have been produced, but thus far only clavulanic acid (Fig. 18-2) and sulbactam have received extensive evaluation. Both compounds are β-lactams; clavulanic acid is a 1-oxapenam and sulbactam a penam sulfone.[17,18,44] Although poor antibacterial agents, these compounds are potent inhibitors of staphylococcal penicillinase and most of the plasmid-mediated β-lactamases produced by gram-negative bacilli (TEM, OXA, SHV, PSE).[17,18,44] However, they are generally poor inhibitors of the chromosomally mediated enzymes (Richmond and Sykes type 1) that are common in gram-negative bacilli such as *P. aeruginosa, Enterobacter* spp, *Proteus* spp, *Citrobacter* spp, and *Serratia marcescens*.[17,18,44] These compounds may be combined with another β-lactam to protect the latter from hydrolysis and allow it to exert an antibacterial effect.

Both sulbactam and clavulanic acid have been demonstrated to be effective in vitro and in vivo when combined with a number of different penicillins and cephalosporins. Thus far clavulanic acid has been combined with amoxicillin (Augmentin) or ticarcillin (Timentin), and sulbactam has been chemically linked to ampicillin (sultamicillin) for clinical use.

Aminoglycosidic Aminocyclitols

Bacteria may resist the activity of aminoglycosidic aminocyclitols by a number of mechanisms, including alterations in permeability, production of enzymes capable of inactivating the aminoglycoside, and alterations in the tar-

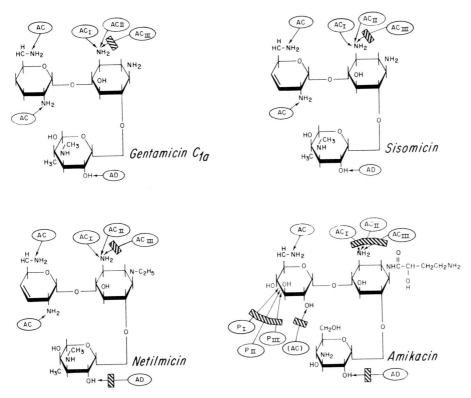

Fig. 18-10 Site of activity of various aminoglycoside-modifying enzymes. (Abbreviations: AC = acetyltransferase; P = phosphotransferase; AD = adenylyltransferase.)

get site. Of these mechanisms, resistance due to the production of plasmid-mediated aminoglycoside-modifying enzymes is the most common mechanism encountered in clinical isolate.[47]

There are three major modifications of the aminoglycoside molecule produced by bacterial enzymes that inactivate the antibiotic. These modifications are acetylation of an amino group, phosphorylation of a hydroxyl group, and adenylylation of a hydroxyl group (Fig. 18-10). Each type of enzyme—acetyltransferase (AAC), phosphotransferase (APH), and adenylyltransferase (ANT)—has a number of subtypes which differ in their substrate specificities.[47] The knowledge of the structural sites of modification and mechanisms of action of these aminoglycoside-modifying enzymes has allowed for the development of some semisynthetic derivatives of aminoglycosides that are resistant to attack by these enzymes. However, the current understanding of the structural features of aminoglycosides that are important for preserving intrinsic antibacterial activity is much less detailed, which often makes it difficult to produce agents resistant to enzymatic attack without the loss of significant antibacterial activity.

A number of agents have been produced by blocking or deleting known sites of enzymatic attack that retain antibacterial activity.[47-48] Kanamycin A is susceptible to modification by a number of enzymes of each of the three classes. Amikacin is produced by acylating the amino group of the C-1 position of the aminocyclitol ring of kanamycin A with a hydroxybutyric acid moiety. This resultant structure is resistant to most of the aminoglycoside-modifying enzymes capable of using kanamycin A as a substrate. Similarly, netilmicin is the semisynthetic C-1 *N*-ethyl derivative of sisomicin. The presence of an ethyl group at this position renders the molecule resistant to several enzymes that are capable of inactivating sisomicin and gentamicin, including ANT (2″), which is the most common enzyme found among gentamicin-resistant *E. coli* in the United States.[47]

Several other modifications of naturally occurring or older aminoglycosidic aminocyclitols have been made in an effort to produce new compounds resistant to enzyme inactivation. However, this has often resulted in significant loss of antibacterial activity. There are several recent reviews that discuss these agents.[47,48]

Modifications to Improve Pharmacokinetics

An area of increasing importance to pharmaceutical chemists centers on those structural characteristics of antibiotic compounds that primarily determine serum protein binding, distribution, metabolism, and excretion in order to develop compounds with improved pharmacokinetic properties. Other considerations being equal, a parenteral antibiotic with a prolonged half-life that can be administered on a once daily basis can significantly decrease administration costs and facilitate the ambulatory management of infections requiring parenteral antibiotics. In this area the β-lactam structure has proved very flexible for such manipulation. One of the early modifications in the cephalosporin class of agents that resulted in improved pharmacokinetics was the inclusion of a *para*-hydroxy group on the acyl side chain. Cefadroxil and cephalexin differ structurally from one another only in the presence of a *para*-hydroxy group in cefadroxil. Although their degree of serum protein binding is similar, cefadroxil has a serum half-life nearly twice as long as that of cephalexin.[49] Similarly, in the development of moxalactam, which contains the *para*-hydroxy group (Fig. 18-3), several analogs lacking this structure but otherwise identical to moxalactam were found to have a significantly shorter serum elimination half-life than moxalactam.[40]

An important observation in the development of the cephalosporins has been the recognition that the nature of the substitution of the cephem nucleus at the 3 position has an important influence on the pharmacokinetic properties of the compound.[33] This is perhaps well illustrated by the different pharmacokinetics exhibited by cefotaxime, ceftizoxime, and ceftriaxone. These cephems are all aminothiazolyl methoxyimino cephalosporins that differ only in the type of substitution at position 3 of the cephem nucleus. Ceftizoxime has only a hydrogen atom at the 3 position and is excreted unchanged in the urine, with an elimination half-life of 1.7 hours. Cefotaxime has an acetoxymethyl side chain at position 3, is metabolized in the liver by deacetylation, and exhibits an elimination half-life of approximately 1.0 hour. Ceftriaxone has a relatively complex side chain, triazinylthiol, and is highly protein-bound ($\geq$90 percent compared with about 30 percent for ceftizoxime and cefotaxime). Furthermore, ceftriaxone has a markedly prolonged elimination half-life of 8 hours and is excreted in both the urine and bile.[49] Alterations in structure that result in a β-lactam that is highly bound to serum proteins often result in prolongation of the elimination half-life, as in the case of ceftriaxone. Cefonicid is another recently released cephalosporin for which advantage was taken of this same approach. Cefonicid is structurally identical to cefamandole except that it has a sulfomethyl instead of a methyl group at the 1 position of the thiotetrazole ring that is attached to the 3 position of the cephem nucleus. As a consequence, cefonicid is bound more tightly to serum protein than is cefamandole (67 to 80 versus 98 percent) and has a half-life that is increased severalfold (0.5 to 0.9 versus 4.5 hours).[49–51]

Modifications to Improve Oral Absorption

A final important factor influencing the course of antibiotic development and chemical modification of previous structures has been the interest in improving the oral absorption of poorly or moderately absorbed compounds as well as in developing orally absorbable derivatives of nonabsorbable parent compounds.

In general, this goal has been easier to achieve with the penicillins than it has with the cephalosporins. In most cases, if a penicillin is acid-stable, it exhibits better absorption following oral administration than analogs which are not stable to gastric acid. Several modifications of penicillins have been shown to improve acid stability and result in improved oral absorption. For example, phenoxymethyl penicillin (penicillin V) (Fig. 18-5), which is more stable in acid than is benzyl penicillin (penicillin G), is better absorbed following oral administration. Similarly, the isoxazolyl penicillins (cloxacillin, dicloxacillin, oxacillin, and flucloxacillin) (Fig. 18-5) are generally more acid-stable than is methicillin and exhibit better oral absorption. However, the relative acid stability of cephalosporins as a group did not accurately predict their poor oral absorption.[52] All the currently available cephalosporins that exhibit significant oral absorption share a common phenylglycyl moiety in the acyl side chain. The cephalosporins with this structure are cephaloglycine, cephalexin, cephradine, cefadroxil, and cefaclor.[49,52] Similarly, in the penicillin class modifications may significantly improve oral absorption without having an acid-stabilizing effect, as is the case with the *para*-hydroxy group of amoxicillin (Fig. 18-5).[53]

The presence of a carboxyl group at position 3 of the penam nucleus (or position 4 of the cephem nucleus) is necessary for activation of the β-lactam ring (Fig. 18-1). However, the polarity of this moiety impairs absorption from the gastrointestinal tract. A very useful approach to improving the oral absorption of several penicillins has been the esterification of the penam nucleus at the 3 position. During or shortly after absorption the ester is hydrolyzed by nonspecific esterases in tissues and serum yielding the active parent compound.[53,54] Esters of ampicillin exhibiting significantly increased oral absorption include bacampicillin (1-ethoxycarboxyloxyethyl ester), pivampicillin (pivaloyloxymethyl ester), and talampicillin (phthalidyl ester).[53-55]

This approach has also been applied to β-lactams such as mecillinam and cefuroxime, which unlike ampicillin are not absorbed to any appreciable degree following oral administration. Mecillinam is available as a pivaloyloxymethyl ester (pivmecillinam) and cefuroxime as a 1-acetoxyethyl ester (cefuroxime axetil).[56-58] Esters of other extended-spectrum cephalosporins are under development.

A final interesting esterified molecule is sultamicillin. This compound is a double ester of both ampicillin and the β-lactamase inhibitor sulbactam. The esterification improves the absorption of both agents, and hydrolysis on absorption releases both active parent compounds to achieve higher serum levels than is obtainable from either agent alone.[59]

CONCLUSION

In this chapter we have outlined some of the insights achieved by pharmaceutical chemists into the relationship between chemical structure and the activity and pharmacokinetic properties of several antibacterial compounds, primarily penams and cephems. It is clear that over the last two decades the penam and cephem β-lactam nuclei have proved to be extremely flexible frameworks upon which to build new agents, and it is likely that further useful modifications will be developed. In addition, there is additional potential in the β-lactam family, as evidenced by the rapidly expanding numbers of monobactams and carbapenems (e.g., thienamycins). Modifications of the specific ring structures of the β-lactam antibiotics have been explored, but thus far, except for atomic substitutions at the 1 position of the cephem ring, none of these has resulted in compounds with clinically useful antimicrobial properties. This area clearly deserves further study, however, especially in view of the successes being achieved in synthesizing new monobactams with enhanced activity and stability to enzymatic inactivation.

Modifications of aminoglycosidic aminocyclitols have resulted in compounds with increased resistance to enzymatic inactivation, but often at a significant cost in terms of antimicrobial potency. Attempts to modify these agents to significantly decrease clinical toxicity seem unlikely to be successful on the basis of current knowledge.

It seems probable that modifications to alter pharmacokinetic properties will receive increased attention given the current economic pressures, since parenteral agents with prolonged half-lives that can be administered less frequently can result in significant reductions in cost. Similarly, the development of esters or other orally absorbable derivatives of some of the new, more potent cephalosporins might allow ambulatory therapy of some infections that now can only be treated with parenteral agents.

Significant improvements in absorption can also be achieved by exploring new methods of administration, such as slow-release capsules targeted at specific areas in the gastrointestinal tract, and by more judicious rectal administration of certain agents, especially in combination with adjuvants, to enhance per rectum absorption.[60]

Finally, the use of certain vehicles such as liposomes to reduce toxicity and enhance delivery of antibiotics to specific sites of infection is a most promising approach, which clearly deserves further investigation.[61–64]

REFERENCES

1. Sykes RB, Cimarusti CM, Bonner DP, et al: Monocyclic β-lactam antibiotics produced by bacteria. Nature 291:489, 1981
2. Imada A, Kitano K, Kintaka K: Sulfazecin and isosulfazecin, novel β-lactam antibiotics of bacterial origin. Nature 289:590, 1981
3. Bonner DP, Sykes RB: Structure-activity relationships among the monobactams. J Antimicrob Chemother 14:313, 1984
4. Georgopapadakou NH, Smith SA, Cimarusti CM: Interaction between monobactams and *Streptomyces* RG1 DD-carboxypeptidase. Eur J Biochem 124:507, 1982
5. Sykes RB, Bonner DP, Bush K, et al: Aztreonam (SQ 26.776), a synthetic monobactam specifically active against aerobic gram-negative bacteria. Antimicrob Agents Chemother 21:85, 1982
6. Bush K, Freudenberger JS, Sykes RB: Interaction of aztreonam and related monobactams with β-lactamases from gram-negative bacteria. Antimicrob Agents Chemother 22:414, 1982
7. Kahan JS, Kahan FM, Goegelman R, et al: Thienamycin, a new β-lactam antibiotic. I. Discovery, taxonomy, isolation and physical properties. J Antibiot 32:1, 1979
8. Kahan FM, Kropp H, Sundelof JG, Birnbaum J: Thienamycin: development of imipenem-cilastatin. J Antimicrob Chemother 12:suppl. D, 1, 1983
9. Kropp H, Sundelof JG, Kahan JS, et al: MK 0787 (*N*-formimidoyl thienamycin): Evaluation of in vitro and in vivo activities. Antimicrob Agents Chemother 17:993, 1980
10. Kesado T, Hashizume T, Asahi Y: Antibacterial activities of a new stabilized thienamycin, *N*-formimidoyl thienamycin, in comparison with other antibiotics. Antimicrob Agents Chemother 17:912, 1980
11. Kesado T, Watanabe K, Asahi Y, et al: Susceptibilities of anaerobic bacteria to *N*-formimidoyl thienamycin (MK 0787) and to other antibiotics. Antimicrob Agents Chemother 21:1016, 1982
12. Eliopoulos GM, Moellering RC: Susceptibility of enterococci and *Listeria monocytogenes* to N-formimidoyl thienamycin alone and in combination with an aminoglycoside. Antimicrob Agents Chemother 19:789, 1981
13. Saino Y, Kobayashi F, Matsuhisa I, Mitsuhashi S: Purification and properties of inducible penicillin β-lactamase isolated from *Pseudomonas maltophilia*. Antimicrob Agents Chemother 22:564, 1982

14. Yotsuji A, Minami S, Inoue M, Mitsuhashi S: Properties of a novel β-lactamase produced by *Bacteroides fragilis*. Antimicrob Agents Chemother 24:925, 1983
15. Neu HC, Labthavikul P: Comparative in vitro activity of *N*-formimidoyl thienamycin against gram-positive and gram-negative aerobic and anaerobic species and its β-lactamase stability. Antimicrob Agents Chemother 21:180, 1982
16. Toda M, Sato K, Nakazawa H, et al: Effect of *N*-formimidoyl thienamycin (MK 0787) on β-lactamases and activity against β-lactamase-producing strains. Antimicrob Agents Chemother 18:837, 1980
17. Bush K, Sykes RB: β-Lactamase inhibitors in perspective. J Antimicrob Chemother 11:97, 1983
18. Sykes RB: The classification and terminology of enzymes that hydrolyze β-lactam antibiotics. J Infect Dis 145:762, 1982
19. Sykes RB, Matthew M: The β-lactamases of gram-negative bacteria and their role in resistance to β-lactam antibiotics. J Antimicrob Chemother 2:115, 1976
20. Miller MA, Finan M, Yousaf M: In vitro antagonism by *N*-formimidoyl thienamycin and cefoxitin of second and third generation cephalosporins in *Aeromonas hydrophila* and *Serratia marcescens*. J Antimicrob Chemother 11:311, 1983
21. Tausk F, Evans ME, Patterson LS, et al: Imipenem-induced resistance to antipseudomonal β-lactams in *Pseudomonas aeruginosa*. Antimicrob Agents Chemother 28:41, 1985
22. Eliopoulos GM, Thauvin C, Gerson B, Moellering RC Jr: In vitro activity and mechanism of action of A-21978C$_1$, a novel cyclic lipopeptide antibiotic. Antimicrob Agents Chemother 27:357, 1985
23. Debono M, Barnhart M, Carrell CB, et al: A-21978C$_1$, a complex of new acidic peptide antibiotics: factor definition and preliminary chemical characterization. 20th Interscience Conf Antimicrob Agents Chemother, New Orleans, 1980. Abstract No. 68
24. Counter FT, Ensminger PW, Howard LC: A-21978C, a complex of new acidic peptide antibiotics: biological activity and toxicity. 20th Interscience Conf Antimicrob Agents Chemother, New Orleans, 1980. Abstract No. 69
25. Debono M, Abbott BJ, Krupinski VM, et al: Synthesis and structure-activity relationships of new analogs of the gram-positive lipopeptide antibiotic A-21978C. 24th Interscience Conf Antimicrob Agents Chemother, Washington, 1984. Abstract No. 1077
26. Allen N, Alborn W, Hobbs J, Percifield H: LY146032 inhibits the biosynthesis of cell wall peptidoglycan in gram-positive bacteria. 24th Interscience Conf Antimicrob Agents Chemother, Washington, 1984. Abstract No. 1081
27. Spratt BG: Penicillin-binding proteins and the future of β-lactam antibiotics. J Gen Microbiol 129:1247, 1983
28. Tomasz A: From penicillin-binding proteins to the lysis and death of bacteria: A 1979 view. Rev Infect Dis 1:434, 1979
29. Godfrey AJ, Bryan LE: Intrinsic resistance and whole cell factors contributing to antibiotic resistance. p. 113. In Bryan LE (ed): Antimicrobial Drug Resistance. Academic Press, New York, 1984
30. Nikaido H: Outer membrane permeability of bacteria: resistance and accessibility of targets. p. 249. In Sulton MRJ, Shockman GD (eds): β-Lactam Antibiotics. Academic Press, New York, 1981
31. Yoshimura F, Nikaido H: Diffusion of β-lactam antibiotics through the porin channels of *Escherichia coli* K-12. Antimicrob Agents Chemother 27:84, 1985
32. Christensen BG: Structure-activity relationships in β-lactam antibiotics. p. 101. In

Sulton MRJ, Shockman GD (eds): β-Lactam Antibiotics. Academic Press, New York, 1981

33. Neu HC: Structure-activity relations of new β-lactam compounds and in vitro activity against common bacteria. Rev Infect Dis 5:S319, 1983

34. Eliopoulos GM, Moellering RC Jr: Azlocillin, mezlocillin, and piperacillin: new broad spectrum penicillins. Ann Intern Med 97:755, 1982

35. Noguchi HY, Eda Y, Tobiki H, et al: PC904, a novel broad spectrum semisynthetic penicillin with marked antipseudomonal activity: microbiological evaluation. Antimicrob Agents Chemother 9:262, 1976

36. Allan JD, Eliopoulos GM, Ferraro MJ, Moellering RC Jr: Comparative in vitro activities of cefpiramide and apalcillin individually and in combination. Antimicrob Agents Chemother 27:782, 1985

37. Barry AL, Jones RN, Thornsberry C: Apalcillin (PC904): spectrum of activity and β-lactamase hydrolysis/inhibition. Diagn Microbiol Infect Dis 3:7, 1985

38. Saikawa I, Matsubara N, Minami S: Studies on new beta-lactam antibiotics having 2,3-dioxopiperazine group: piperacillin and cefoperazone. p. 353. In Sulton MRJ, Shockman GD (eds): β-Lactam Antibiotics. Academic Press, New York, 1981

39. Chen HY, Williams JD: The killing effects of cefthiamidine or ampicillin alone and in combination with gentamicin against enterococci. J Antimicrob Chemother 12:19, 1983

40. Yoshida T: Structure-activity relationships leading to the development of 1-oxa-cephem, 6059-S (moxalactam). p. 403. In Sulton MRJ, Shockman GD (eds), β-Lactam Antibiotics. Academic Press, New York, 1981

41. Wolfson JS, Hooper DC: The fluoroquinolones. Structure, mechanisms of action and resistance, and spectrum of activity in vitro. Antimicrob Agents Chemother 28:581, 1985

42. Matsumoto J, Miyamoto T, Minamida A, et al: Structure-activity relationships of 4-oxo-1,8-naphthyridine-3-carboxylic acids including AT-2266, a new oral antipseudomonal agent. p. 454. In Nelson JD, Grassi C (eds): Current Chemotherapy and Infectious Disease. American Society for Microbiology, Washington, 1980

43. Domagula JM, Nichols JB, Heifetz CL, Mich TF: The synthesis, activity, and preliminary structure-activity relationships of a new quinolone antibacterial agent. 24th Interscience Conference Antimicrob Agents Chemother, Washington, 1984. Abstract No. 80

44. Fisher J: β-Lactams resistant to hydrolysis by the β-lactamases. p. 33. In Bryan LE (ed) Antimicrobial Drug Resistance. Academic Press, New York, 1984

45. Stapley EO, Birnbaum J: Chemistry and microbiological properties of the cephamycins. p. 327. In Sulton MRJ, Shockman GD (eds): β-Lactam Antibiotics. Academic Press, New York, 1981

46. Sykes RB, Bush K: Interaction of new cephalosporins with β-lactamases and β-lactamase-producing gram-negative bacilli. Rev Infect Dis 5:S356, 1983.

47. Moellering, RC, Jr: In vitro antibacterial activity of the aminoglycoside antibiotics. Rev Infect Dis 5:S212, 1983

48. Bryan LE: Aminoglycoside resistance. p. 241. In Antimicrobial Drug Resistance. Academic Press, New York, 1984

49. Murray BE, Moellering RC Jr: Cephalosporins. Annu Rev Med 32:959, 1981

50. Actor P, Uri JV, Zajac I, et al: SK + F 75073, new parenteral broad-spectrum cephalosporin with high and prolonged serum levels. Antimicrob Agents Chemother 13:784, 1978

51. Barriere SL, Hatheway GJ, Gambertoglio JG, et al: Pharmacokinetics of cefonicid, a new broad-spectrum cephalosporin. Antimicrob Agents Chemother 21:935, 1982

52. Abraham EP: Discovery, chemistry and antibacterial properties of cephalosporins. p. 311. In Sulton MJR, Shockman GD (eds): β-Lactam Antibiotics. Academic Press, New York, 1981

53. Sjovall J, Magni L, Bergan J: Pharmacokinetics of bacampicillin compared with those of ampicillin, pivampicillin and amoxycillin. Antimicrob Agents Chemother 13:90, 1978

54. Neu HC: The pharmacokinetics of bacampicillin. Rev Infect Dis 3:110, 1981

55. Jones KH, Langley PF, Lees LJ: Bioavailability and metabolism of talampicillin. Chemotherapy 24:217, 1978

56. Kabir I, Rahaman MM, Ahmed SM, et al: Comparative efficacies of pivmecillinam and ampicillin in acute shigellosis. Antimicrob Agents Chemother 25:643, 1984

57. Sommers KD, Van Wyk M, Williams PEO, Harding SM: Pharmacokinetics and tolerance of cefuroxime axetil in volunteers during repeated dosing. Antimicrob Agents Chemother 25:344, 1984

58. Harding SH, Williams PEO, Ayrton J: Pharmacology of cefuroxime as the 1-acetoxyethyl esters in volunteers. Antimicrob Agents Chemother 25:78, 1984

59. Davies BI, Maesen FPV, van Noord JA: Clinical, bacteriological and pharmacokinetic results from an open trial of sultamicillin in patients with acute exacerbations of chronic bronchitis. J Antimicrob Chemother 13:161, 1984

60. Davis SS, Burnham WR, Wilson P, O'Brien J: Use of adjuvants for enhancement of rectal absorption of cefoxitin in humans. Antimicrob Agents Chemother 28:211, 1985

61. Bouventre PF, Gregoriadis G: Killing of intraphagocytic *Staphylococcus aureus* by dihydrostreptomycin entrapped within liposomes. Antimicrob Agents Chemother 13:1049, 1978

62. Desiderio JV, Campbell SG: Intraphagocytic killing of *Salmonella typhimorium* by liposome-encapsulated cephalothin. J Infect Dis 148:563, 1983

63. Nacucchio MC, Bellora MJG, Sordelli DO, D'Aquino M: Enhanced liposome-mediated activity of piperacillin against staphylococci. Antimicrob Agents Chemother 27:137, 1985

64. Grayhill JR, Craven PC, Taylor RL, et al: Treatment of murine cryptococcosis with liposome-associated amphotericin B. J Infect Dis 145:748, 1982

Index

Page numbers followed by *f* represent figures; those followed by *t* represent tables.

Abdomen, prevention of
    contamination
    from endogenous source, 168–169
    from exogenous source, 167–168
Abdominal abscess drainage
    catheter management and, 144–
        146
    catheter vs. surgical, 170–172
    diagnostic imaging and, 133–137
    guided-needle aspiration, 136f,
        137, 140, 142f
    percutaneous candidates, 137–142
    percutaneous, complications of,
        146–148
    percutaneous success rate, 148–
        149
    percutaneous technique, 143–144
    post-drainage radiologic
        evaluation, 144, 145f, 146f
Abdominal abscesses
    CT diagnosis, 169–170
    formation and prevention, 167–169
    multilocular, 140, 170
Abdominal injury, antibiotic
    prophylaxis, 180
Abscesses
    fluid, 37t, 41
    formation, 43t, 44
    intra-abdominal, 118
    pus formation factor in therapy,
        39t
    spontaneous drainage of, 43, 44
    tubo-ovarian in PID, 193, 194. *See
        also* individual types.
Abscess drainage, 43, 44
Abscesses, intra-abdominal
    CT diagnosis, 133, 134f, 136f, 137,
        140, 142f, 143
    radioisotope scans in, 133
Addict valve endocarditis, 152, 153t
Adnexal masses in PID, 195
AIDS (acquired immunodeficiency
    syndrome)

allograft contamination and, 98–99
    HIV and, 101
AIDS patients
    cerebral lesions in, 85, 86
    cerebral toxoplasmosis in, 84f
    CNS infections in, 87
    neurologic complications, 85–86
Alabama (University of) infectious
        endocarditis study
    clinical characteristics, 160t
    Gnann-Cobb point system and,
        159t
    therapy and outcome, 160, 161t
ALAC. *see* Antibiotic-loaded acrylic
    cement.
Allograft
    allograft-acquired infection, 97, 98
    donor suitability, 99
    rejection of, 95, 96. *See also*
        Organ transplantation.
Allograft recipient infection
        timetable, post-transplant,
        97t
    first month, 97, 98–100
    1 to 6 months, 97, 100–106
    6 months and later, 106
    differential diagnosis and, 98
    immunosuppression and, 96–97
Aminocyclitols, aminoglycosidic, 280
Aminoglycoside molecule
        modifications and
        hydrolysis resistance, 276–
        278
Aminoglycoside-modifying enzymes,
        277f
    hydrolysis resistance and, 276–278
Anastomatic leaks and abdominal
        abscesses, 171
Anoxia, 3
Antibacterial agents
    bacterial biofilms and, 17, 19
    classes of, 263–264
    structure-function relationships,
        263, 264

285